GENERAL DERMATOLOGY
An Atlas of Diagnosis and Management

GENERAL DERMATOLOGY
An Atlas of Diagnosis and Management

An Atlas of Diagnosis and Management

GENERAL DERMATOLOGY

John SC English, FRCP
Department of Dermatology
Queen's Medical Centre
Nottingham University Hospitals NHS Trust
Nottingham, UK

CLINICAL PUBLISHING
OXFORD

Clinical Publishing
An imprint of Atlas Medical Publishing Ltd
Oxford Centre for Innovation
Mill Street, Oxford OX2 0JX, UK

tel: +44 1865 811116
fax: +44 1865 251550
email: info@clinicalpublishing.co.uk
web: www.clinicalpublishing.co.uk

Distributed in USA and Canada by:
Clinical Publishing
30 Amberwood Parkway
Ashland OH 44805 USA

tel: 800-247-6553 (toll free within US and Canada)
fax: 419-281-6883
email: order@bookmasters.com

Distributed in UK and Rest of World by:
Marston Book Services Ltd
PO Box 269
Abingdon
Oxon OX14 4YN UK

tel: +44 1235 465500
fax: +44 1235 465555
email: trade.orders@marston.co.uk

© Atlas Medical Publishing Ltd 2007

First published 2007

All rights reserved. No part of this publication may be reproduced, stored in a retrieval system, or transmitted, in any form or by any means, without the prior permission in writing of Clinical Publishing or Atlas Medical Publishing Ltd.

Although every effort has been made to ensure that all owners of copyright material have been acknowledged in this publication, we would be glad to acknowledge in subsequent reprints or editions any omissions brought to our attention.

A catalogue record of this book is available from the British Library

ISBN-13 978 1 904392 76 7
ISBN-10 1 904392 76 8

The publisher makes no representation, express or implied, that the dosages in this book are correct. Readers must therefore always check the product information and clinical procedures with the most up-to-date published product information and data sheets provided by the manufacturers and the most recent codes of conduct and safety regulations. The authors and the publisher do not accept any liability for any errors in the text or for the misuse or misapplication of material in this work.

Printed by T G Hostench SA, Barcelona, Spain

Contents

Preface	vii
Acknowledgements	vii
Contributors	viii
Abbreviations	ix

1 *Introduction to diagnosing dermatological conditions (basic principles)*   1
G WHITLOCK, JOHN SC ENGLISH, AND IAIN H LEACH
- Essentials of cutaneous anatomy and physiology   1
- History taking   4
- Examination of the skin   5
- Investigations   10
- Further reading   11

2 *Paediatric dermatoses*   13
JANE C RAVENSCROFT
- Introduction   13
- Skin lesions   14
  - Birthmarks   14
  - Other childhood lesions   20
- Rashes   23
  - Neonatal and infantile rashes   23
  - Childhood rashes   28
- Further reading   32

3 *Widespread rashes*   33
GEORGINA E ELSTON AND GRAHAM A JOHNSTON
- Introduction   33
- Urticaria   33
- Erythroderma   35
- Atopic eczema   36
- Discoid eczema   38
- Psoriasis vulgaris   39
- Scabies   42
- Erythema multiforme   44
- Further reading   46

4 *Skin tumours*   47
VISHAL MADAN AND JOHN T LEAR
- Introduction   47
- Nonmelanoma skin cancers   47
  - Actinic (solar) keratosis   48
  - Intraepithelial carcinomas (IEC, Bowen's disease)   49
  - Cutaneous horn   50
  - Disseminated superficial actinic porokeratosis   50
  - Erythroplasia of Queyrat   51
  - Radiation-induced keratoses   51
  - Arsenical keratoses   52
  - Basal cell carcinoma   52
  - Squamous cell carcinoma   54
- Melanoma and melanoma precursors   56
  - Melanoma precursors   56
  - Malignant melanoma   59
- References   63

5 *Hand and foot dermatoses*   65
JOHN SC ENGLISH
- Introduction   65
- Hand and foot dermatitis   65
- Psoriasis   71
- Fungus infection   72
- Palmo-plantar pustulosis   74
- Miscellaneous conditions affecting the hands and feet   75
- Further reading   76

6 *Facial rashes*   77
PAUL FARRANT AND RUSSELL EMERSON
- Introduction   77
- History   77
- Acne   79
- Perioral dermatitis   80
- Rosacea   80
- Atopic eczema   82
- Contact dermatitis   82
- Seborrhoeic dermatitis   84
- Psoriasis   84

Melasma	86	
Lupus erythematosus	86	
Dermatomyositis	89	
Tuberous sclerosis	89	
Keratosis pilaris	90	
Further reading	90	

7 Genital and oral problems — 91
SHEELAGH M LITTLEWOOD

Introduction	91
Lichen sclerosus	91
Lichen planus	93
Zoon's balanitis	94
Zoon's vulvitis	95
Autoimmune bullous diseases	95
Malignant lesions	96
Eczematous conditions	97
Vulval ulceration	98
Further reading	98

8 Scalp and nail disorders — 99
STUART N COHEN

Introduction	99
Disorders of the scalp and hair	99
Alopecia areata	99
Trichotillomania	100
Tinea capitis	101
Folliculitis decalvans	102
Dissecting cellulitis of the scalp	102
Acne keloidalis nuchae	103
Lichen planopilaris	103
Discoid lupus erythematosus	104
Pseudopelade of Brocque	104
Naevus sebaceus	104
Diffuse hair loss	105
Traction alopecia	105
Disorders of nails	106
Onychomycosis	106
Psoriasis	107
Eczema	108
Lichen planus	109
Alopecia areata	110
Yellow nail syndrome	110
Onychogryphosis	110
Pincer nail	110
Median nail dystrophy	111
Tumours of the nail unit	111
Further reading	112

9 Skin infections and infestations — 113
NEILL C HEPBURN

Introduction	113
Bacterial infections	113
Impetigo	113
Cellulitis	114
Pitted keratolysis	115
Erythrasma	116
Atypical mycobacterium infection	116
Anthrax	118
Gonococcal septicaemia	118
Secondary syphilis	118
Viral infections	120
Herpes simplex	120
Herpes zoster	120
Molluscum contagiosum	120
Viral warts	122
Orf	122
Fungal and yeast infections	123
Pityriasis versicolor	124
Infestations	124
Cutaneous larva migrans	124
Tungiasis	125
Leishmaniasis	126
Cutaneous myiasis	127
Further reading	128

10 Leg ulcers and wound healing — 129
ANNA RICH AND JOHN SC ENGLISH

Introduction	129
Clinical presentation	129
Assessment and investigations	133
Differential diagnosis	133
Management	138
References	139

Index — 141

Preface

Dermatology is about diagnosis, as without the correct diagnosis the patient cannot be managed well. In medicine, treatments are often administered empirically, especially where there is uncertainty over the diagnosis. If one knows what the condition is then one can give the best treatment and an accurate prognosis. In this book we have tried to facilitate the process of making a diagnosis and formulating a differential diagnosis in dermatology patients. It is aimed primarily at dermatology naive practitioners and students, whether they be GPs, medical students, hospital doctors, specialist nurses or community pharmacists. Nevertheless, experienced practitioners will find much here to refresh their memory; for all health professionals, we hope this book will help them make the correct diagnosis and so be able to offer the best possible course of management.

John SC English

Acknowledgements

I thank Drs Andrew Affleck, Ruth Murphy, Kate Dalziel, and Roger Allen for providing illustrations where needed. My thanks also to all the chapter authors for their individual contributions.

Contributors

Stuart N Cohen, BMedSci, MRCP
Department of Dermatology
Queen's Medical Centre
Nottingham University Hospitals NHS Trust
Nottingham, UK

Georgina E Elston, MRCP
Department of Dermatology
Leicester Royal Infirmary
University Hospitals of Leicester NHS Trust
Leicester, UK

Russell Emerson, MD, MRCP
Department of Dermatology
Brighton General Hospital
Brighton, UK

John SC English, FRCP
Department of Dermatology
Queen's Medical Centre
Nottingham University Hospitals NHS Trust
Nottingham, UK

Paul Farrant, MRCP
Department of Dermatology
Brighton General Hospital
Brighton, UK

Neill C Hepburn, MD, FRCP
Dermatology Suite
Lincoln County Hospital
Lincoln, UK

Graham A Johnston, FRCP
Department of Dermatology
Leicester Royal Infirmary
University Hospitals of Leicester NHS Trust
Leicester, UK

Iain H Leach, MD, FRCPath
Department of Dermatology and Histopathology
Queen's Medical Centre
Nottingham University Hospitals NHS Trust
Nottingham, UK

John T Lear, MD, MRCP
Department of Dermatology
Manchester Royal Infirmary
Manchester, UK

Sheelagh M Littlewood, MBChB, FRCP
Department of Dermatology
Queen's Medical Centre
Nottingham University Hospitals NHS Trust
Nottingham, UK

Vishal Madan, MBBS, MD, MRCP
The Dermatology Centre
Hope Hospital
Manchester, UK

Jane C Ravenscroft, MRCP, MRCGP
Department of Dermatology
Queen's Medical Centre
Nottingham University Hospitals NHS Trust
Nottingham, UK

Anna Rich, RN (Dip BSc Hons)
Department of Dermatology
Queen's Medical Centre
Nottingham University Hospitals NHS Trust
Nottingham, UK

G Whitlock, PhD, MRCP
Department of Dermatology
Queen's Medical Centre
Nottingham University Hospitals NHS Trust
Nottingham, UK

Abbreviations

ABPI ankle brachial pressure index
ACD allergic contact dermatitis
ACE angiotensin-converting enzyme
ALA-based PDT 5-aminolaevulinic acid-based photodynamic therapy
BCC basal cell carcinoma
CIN cervical intraepithelial neoplasia
CMN congenital melanocytic naevus
CT computed tomography
CYP cytochrome P
DLE discoid lupus erythematosus
DLSO distal and lateral subungual onychomycosis
DSAP disseminated superficial actinic porokeratosis
DVT deep vein thrombosis
EM erythema multiforme
GST glutathione S-transferase
HPV human papilloma virus
HSP Henoch–Schönlein purpura
HSV herpes simplex virus
ICD irritant contact dermatitis
IEC intraepithelial carcinoma
JPD Juvenile plantar dermatosis
KID keratosis, ichthyosis, deafness
LE lupus erythematosus
LP lichen planus
LS lichen sclerosis
MRI magnetic resonance imaging
NMSC nonmelanoma skin cancers
PCR polymerase chain reaction
PIN penile intraepithelial neoplasia
PUVA ultraviolet A light with psoralen
PV pityriasis versicolor
SCC squamous cell carcinoma
SCLE subacute cutaneous lupus erythematosus
SLE systemic lupus erythematosus
SSSS staphylococcal scalded skin syndrome
UVB ultraviolet B
VIN vulval intraepithelial neoplasia

Chapter 1

Introduction to diagnosing dermatological conditions (basic principles)

G Whitlock PhD, MRCP, John SC English FRCP, and Iain H Leach MD, FRCPath

Essentials of cutaneous anatomy and physiology

The skin is a large and specialized organ, which covers the entire external surface of the body. It plays an important role in protecting the body against external traumas and injurious agents such as infection, trauma, UV radiation, and extremes of temperature as well as providing waterproofing. Additional functions include detection of sensory stimuli and thermoregulation.

The skin has two main layers, the superficial epidermis and the dermis, which lies between the epidermis and subcutaneous fat (**1.1**). The microanatomy of the skin is essentially similar throughout, but there is considerable regional variation. For example, the surface keratin layer is much thicker on the palms and soles (**1.2**) than elsewhere, whilst the dermis is much thicker on the back than on the eyelids. There is also considerable regional variation in the numbers and size of skin appendages such as hair follicles, sebaceous glands, and sweat glands.

The epidermis is the surface layer of the skin and is a keratinizing stratified squamous epithelium, the principle cell type being the keratinocyte. The basal layer of the epidermis contains small cuboidal cells that continually divide to replenish the cells lost from the skin surface. The bulk of the epidermis is composed of the stratum spinosum or 'prickle cell' layer, so called because the intercellular connections or desmosomes are visible on histological sections as prickles surrounding each cell. The cells in this layer are large with abundant cytoplasm containing keratin tonofilaments. With maturation towards the surface the cells

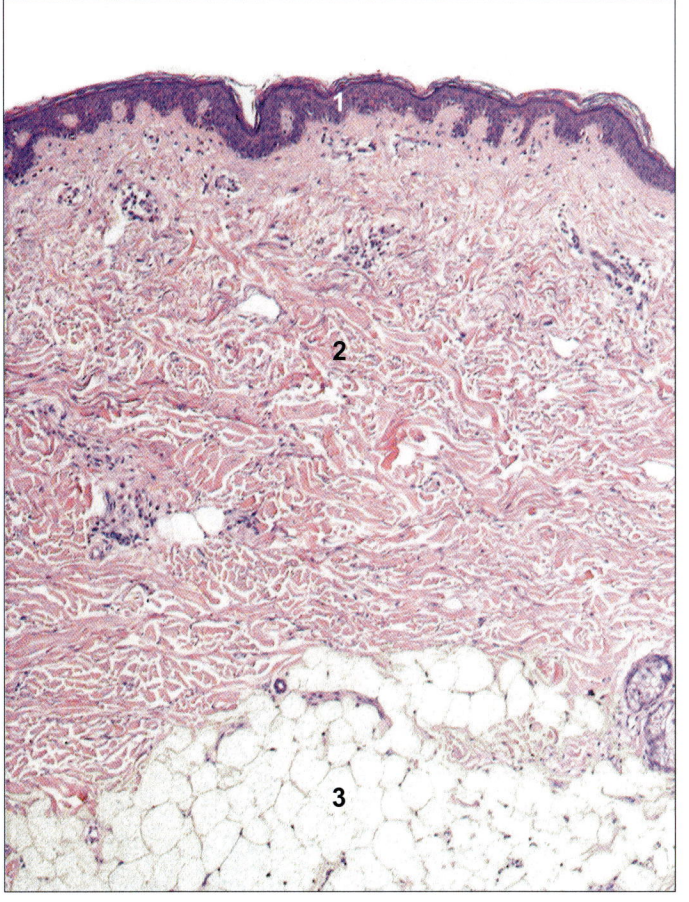

1.1 Normal skin: epidermis (1), dermis (2). and subcutis (fat) (3) (H&E x4).

become flatter and accumulate dark keratohyalin granules to form the granular layer. These cells then lose their nuclei and the keratohyalin granules, and keratin filaments

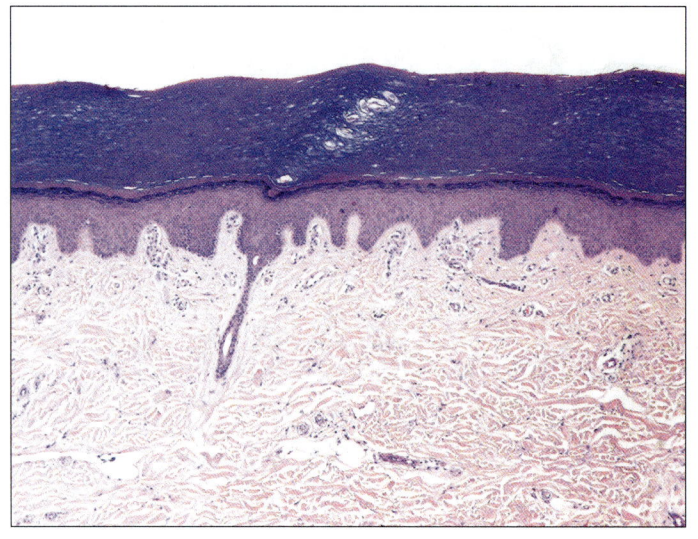

2 Introduction to diagnosing dermatological conditions (basic principles)

1.2 Acral skin (H&E x4).

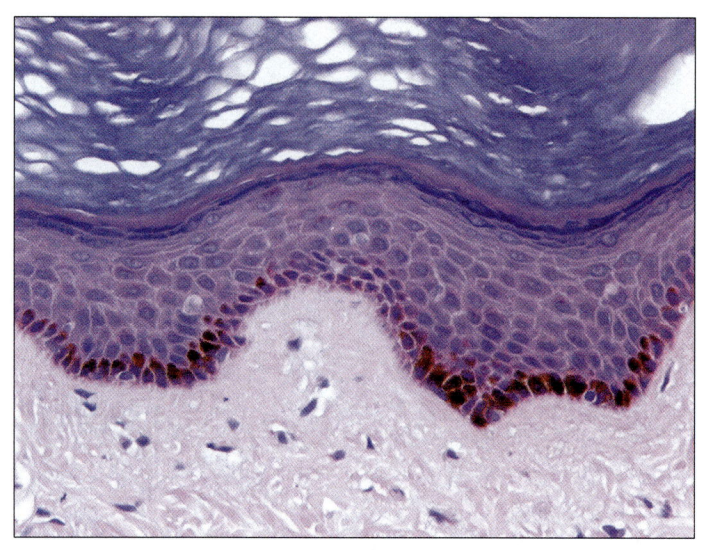

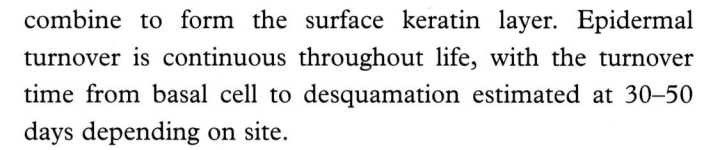

1.3 Racially pigmented skin (H&E x20).

combine to form the surface keratin layer. Epidermal turnover is continuous throughout life, with the turnover time from basal cell to desquamation estimated at 30–50 days depending on site.

The epidermis also contains small numbers of melanocytes, Langerhans cells, and Merkel cells. Melanocytes are present scattered along the basal epidermis. They have long dendritic cytoplasmic processes, which ramify between basal keratinocytes. Melanocytes synthesize melanin pigment that is passed to basal keratinocytes via the dendritic processes in the form of granules or melanosomes. Melanin pigment varies in colour from red/yellow to brown/black. It is responsible for skin pigmentation and has an important role in protecting the skin from the effects of UV radiation. There is some regional variation in the number of melanocytes, with more being present on sun-exposed sites though the number is fairly constant between individuals. Racial skin pigmentation is related to increased activity and increased amounts of pigment rather than increased numbers of melanocytes (**1.3**).

Langerhans cells are also dendritic cells and are located in the basal epidermis and stratum spinosum. They act as antigen presenting cells and are an important part of the immune system. Small numbers are present in normal skin, but numbers are increased in some inflammatory skin diseases, such as contact dermatitis. There are two types of allergic reaction in the skin: immediate reactions causing contact urticaria (hay fever is an immediate allergic reaction of the nasal mucosa), and delayed allergic reactions. This manifests as allergic contact dermatitis such as reactions from prolonged contact of nickel-containing metals with the skin. Merkel cells are difficult to visualize in routine histological sections but can be identified with special stains. Their precise function is not clear but they are thought to play a role in touch sensation. They can give rise to Merkel cell carcinoma, a rare aggressive malignant tumour most often seen in the elderly.

The dermis lies beneath the epidermis and is essentially fibrous connective tissue. The papillary dermis is a thin superficial layer containing fine collagen and elastic fibres, capillaries, and anchoring fibrils which help attach the epidermis to the dermis. The bulk of the dermis is formed by the reticular dermis which is mainly composed of thick collagen fibres and thinner elastic fibres. The collagen fibres provide much of the substance and tensile strength of the dermis, whilst elastic fibres provide the skin with elasticity. Small numbers of lymphocytes, macrophages, mast cells, and fibroblasts are present in the dermis together with blood vessels, lymphatic vessels, nerves, pressure receptors, and the skin appendages. The junction between the epidermis and dermis is not flat but has a complex three dimensional arrangement of downgrowths from the epidermis (rete ridges) and upgrowths from the papillary dermis (dermal papillae). This arrangement increases the surface area of the dermo-epidermal junction and enhances adhesion between the two layers.

The skin appendages comprise the hair follicles with their attached sebaceous glands, the eccrine sweat glands and the apocrine glands (**1.4–1.7**). Hair follicles are widely distributed but are not present on the palms and soles. They

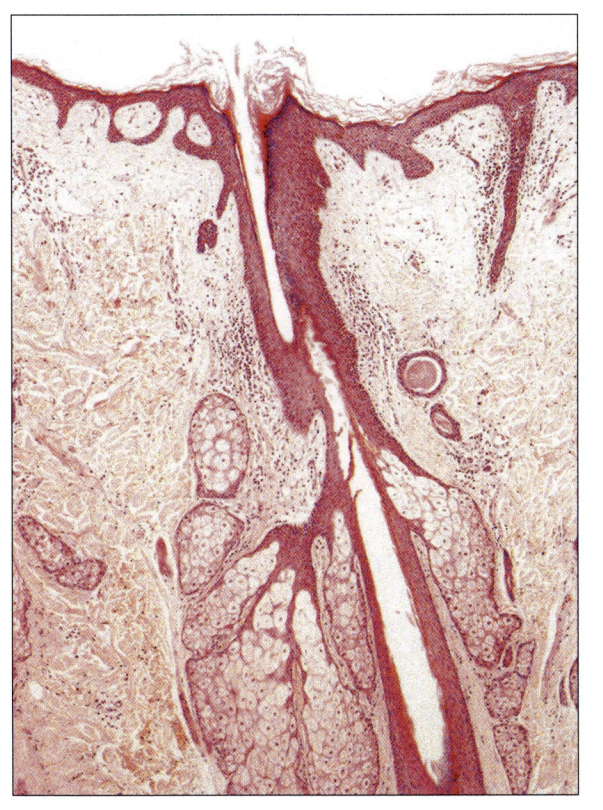

Introduction to diagnosing dermatological conditions (basic principles)

1.4 Pilo-sebaceous unit (H&E x4).

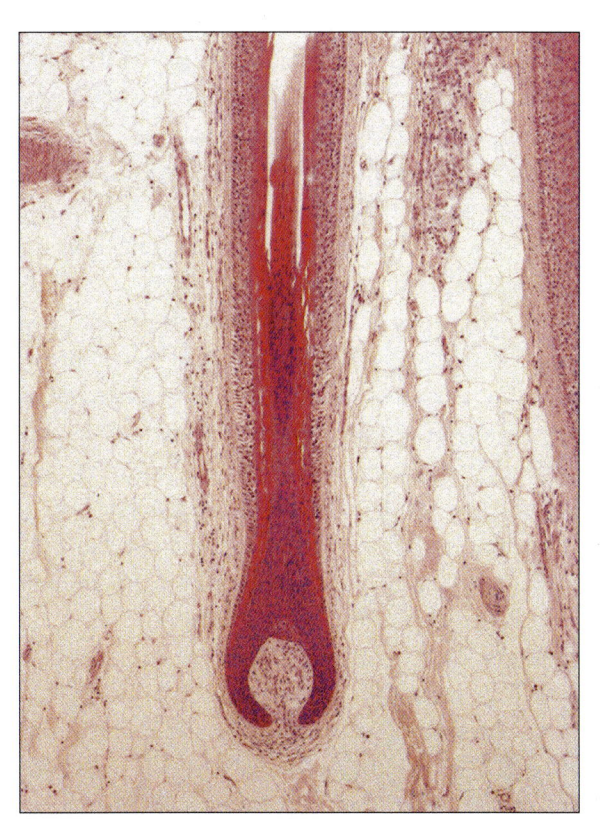

1.5 Hair bulb (H&E x4).

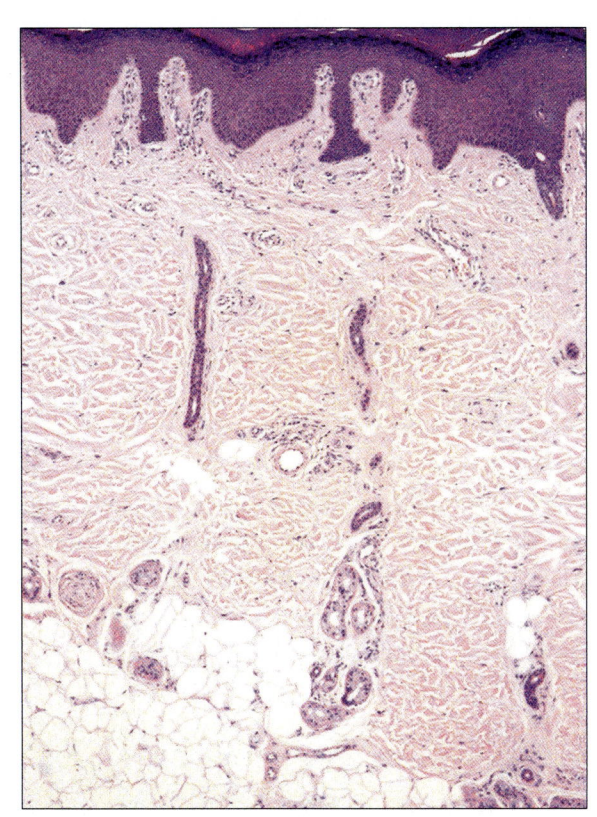

1.6 Eccrine glands (H&E x4).

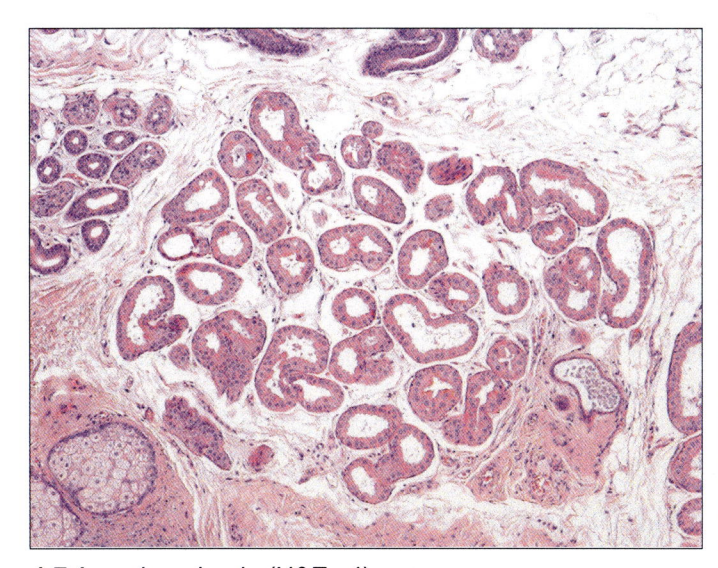

1.7 Apocrine glands (H&E x4).

vary considerably in size from the large follicles of the scalp and male beard area to the more widespread small vellus follicles, present on the female face for example. The hair follicle is a tubular epithelial structure, which opens onto the skin surface and is responsible for producing hairs. The deepest part of the follicle, the hair bulb, is situated in the dermis or subcutaneous fat. The germinal matrix of the bulb consists of actively dividing cells that give rise to the hair shaft and inner root sheath. Keratinization of the epithelial cells occurs without keratohyalin and with no granular layer; this produces 'hard' keratin as opposed to the 'soft' keratin of the epidermis, which is produced with keratohyalin. The outer root sheath of the follicle is derived from a downgrowth of the epidermis. Melanocytes in the hair bulb produce melanin pigment, which is incorporated into the hair shaft and is responsible for hair colouration.

Hair follicle growth is cyclical with an active growth phase (anagen phase), which is followed by an involutional phase (catagen), and a resting phase (telogen) during which time hairs are shed. The anagen phase (during which time hairs are growing) lasts for at least 3 years, catagen lasts for approximately 3 weeks, and telogen 3 months. At any one time the majority of hair follicles (>80%) are in anagen phase, 1–2% are in catagen, and the remainder are in telogen phase.

Sebaceous glands are normally associated with and attached to a hair follicle (**1.4**). They are widespread but are particularly large and numerous on the central face and are absent from the palms and soles. Sebaceous glands are largely inactive before puberty but subsequently enlarge and become secretory. The glands are composed of lobules of epithelial cells, the majority of which contain abundant lipid within the cytoplasm and appear clear on histological sections. The lipid-rich secretion, sebum, is formed through necrosis of the epithelial cells and is secreted into the upper portion of the hair follicle. The function of sebum may include waterproofing and protection of the hair shaft and epidermis as well as inhibition of infection. The other main component of the hair follicle is the arrector pili muscle. This is a small bundle of smooth muscle situated in the dermis but attached to the follicle. Contraction of the muscle makes the hair more perpendicular.

Eccrine sweat glands are responsible for the production of sweat and play an important role in temperature control. They are widely distributed and are particularly numerous on the palms and soles, the axillae, and the forehead. The secretory glandular component is situated in deep reticular dermis (**1.6**). The gland is composed of a tubular coil of secretory epithelial cells with an outer layer of contractile myoepithelial cells. Sweat is transported via a duct, which spirals upwards through the dermis to open onto the skin surface. Glandular secretion and sweating are controlled by the autonomic nervous system.

Apocrine glands are histologically similar to eccrine sweat glands but are slightly larger (**1.7**). They are much less widespread and are principally located in the axillae and ano-genital region. Their precise function in man is unclear, though in some other mammals they have an important role in scent production.

History taking

History taking is the first part of a skin consultation. This is no different to any other medical specialty: one seeks to know when the condition started, which part of the body is affected, and how the condition has progressed since presentation. Clues to the diagnosis may come from asking the patient's profession, if other family members or personal contacts are affected, and whether there has been exposure to allergens or irritants. Particular attention should be afforded to any treatments, both topical or systemic, that have been tried previously and if these have changed the character of the condition. In the past medical history, one considers whether the skin condition is a dermatological manifestation of a systemic disease, if there is a history of atopy (asthma, eczema, or hayfever), and also if the patient has suffered from previous skin complaints. Related to this, it is important to ask about family history of skin disease. Medications themselves can provoke skin eruptions and so a thorough drug history will include current and recent medications as well as any over-the-counter medicines or supplements. Often overlooked is the psychological impact of the skin condition. Changes in the patient's quality of life may be a major factor in the patient consulting the physician in the first place. Through questioning a patient about how the condition affects the patient's life, the physician will be able to assess what in particular is worrying the patient and explore the expectations for the consultation.

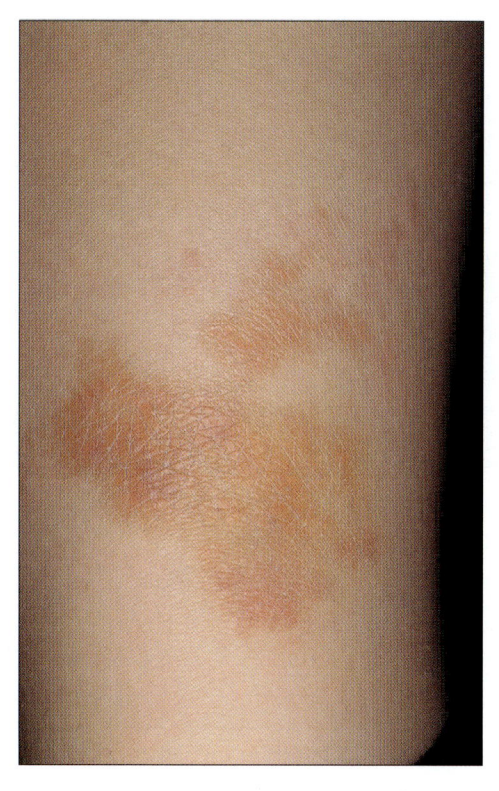

1.8 Macules and patches forming an area of lichen aureus on a child's leg. This is a harmless superficial capillaritis of the skin which leaks red cells leaving golden haemosiderin staining of the skin.

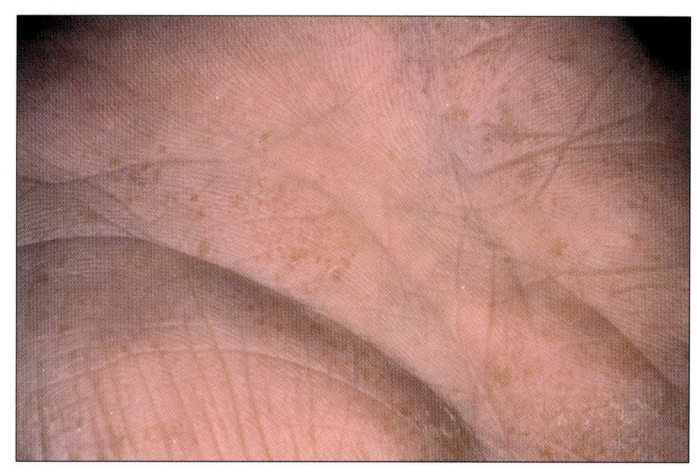

1.9 Vesicular hand eczema of the palms in a patient allergic to Compositae plants (see Chapter 5).

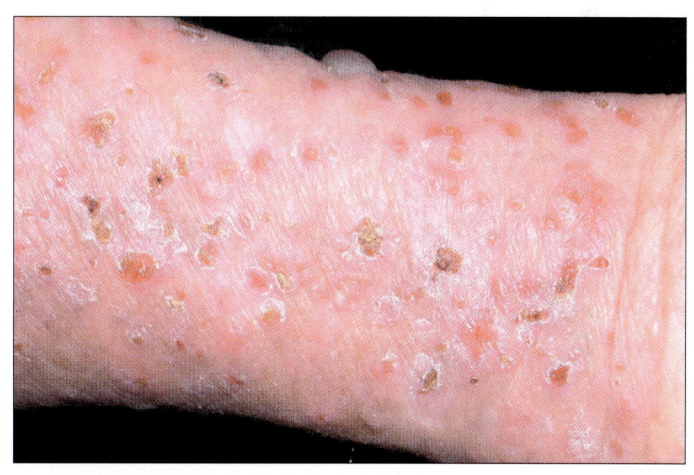

1.10 Vesicles and a bulla in a patient with bullous pemphigoid.

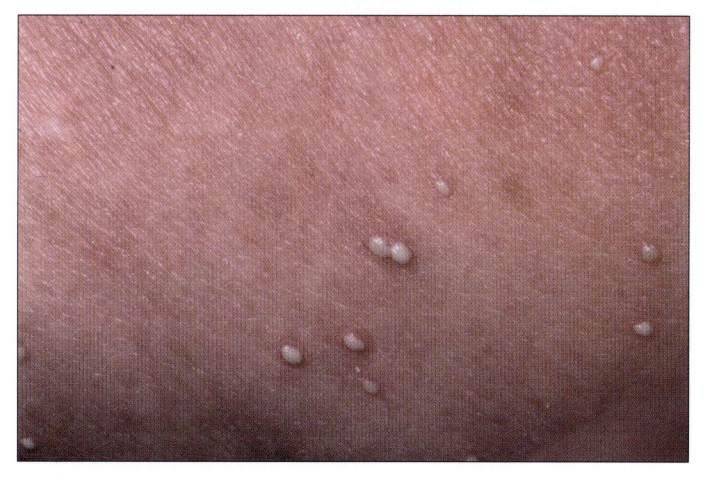

1.11 Pustular drug eruption.

Examination of the skin

Dermatology has its own vocabulary to describe skin lesions. Some of these terms (for example, nodule and plaque) are also used in nonmedical contexts, and special care must be given to their particular meaning in dermatology.

Flat lesions are discolourations of the skin and no change in texture is felt when passing a finger over the affected area. If the diameter of a flat lesion is smaller than 1–2 cm then it is called a macule. A larger flat lesion is known as a patch (**1.8**).

If the lesion is raised above the skin it may be a blister, a collection of free fluid beneath the skin. Again the terms used to refer to blisters depend on their diameter. A small blister is called a vesicle and large one, >0.5 cm in diameter, is a bulla (**1.9, 1.10**). If a lesion is raised above the skin and contains pus, then it is known as a pustule (**1.11**).

The description of a solid raised lesion, or what would commonly be called a 'lump', also depends on its diameter. A small lesion is referred to as a papule and a large lesion, >0.5 cm in diameter, as a nodule (**1.12–1.14**). However, some dermatologists distinguish between the two terms, with a nodule meaning a lesion that has a firmer consistency than a papule. Plaque is used for a raised lesion of large diameter (>2–3 cm) that is characteristically flat topped and often oval or disc shaped (**1.15**).

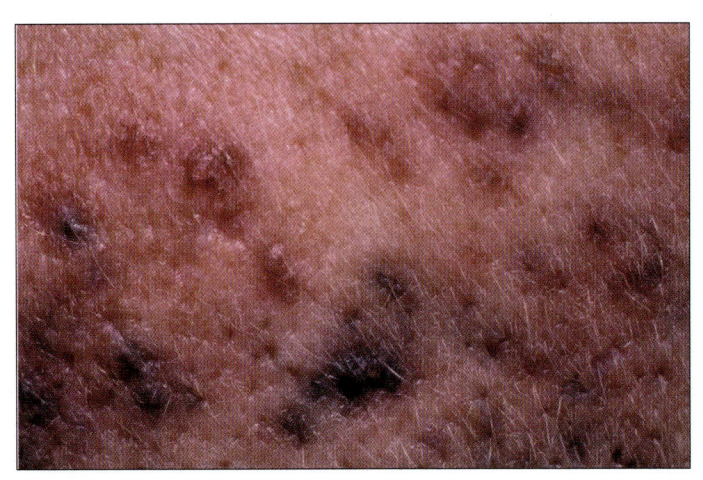

6   Introduction to diagnosing dermatological conditions (basic principles)

1.12 Papular acne lesions with inflammation and hyperpigmentation due to minocycline.

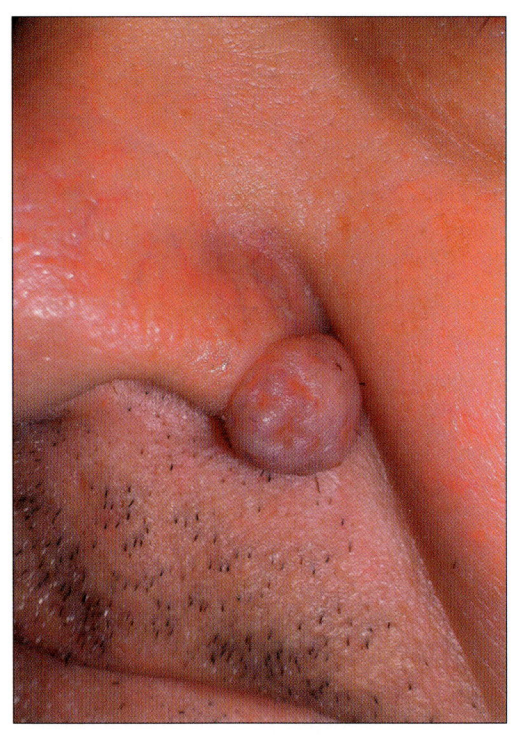

1.13 Nodular intradermal naevus on the side of the nose.

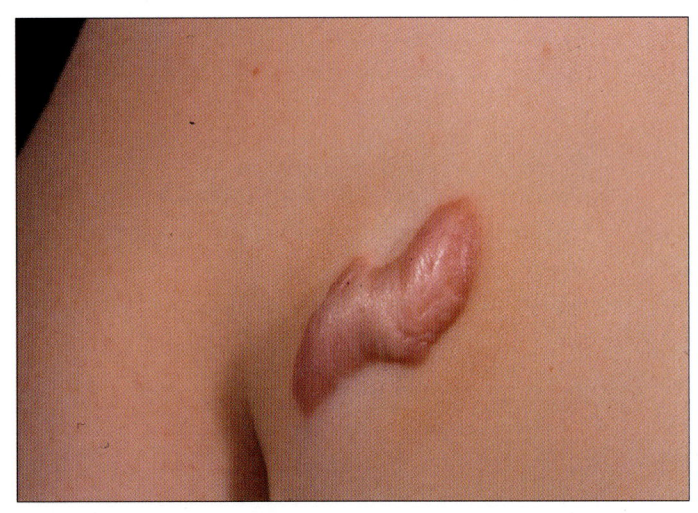

1.14 Keloid nodule on the back.

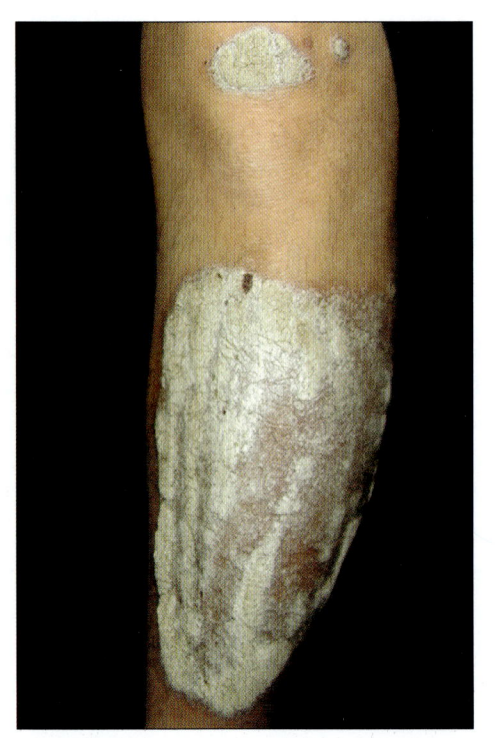

1.15 Hyperkeratotic plaques of psoriasis with obvious silvery scale.

Introduction to diagnosing dermatological conditions (basic principles)

Colour is also an important feature of a skin lesion. An area may be brown with pigment; it may be less pigmented than the surrounding skin or hypopigmented (**1.16**). In fact, it may have any colour. The physician should note if the area is uniformly coloured or not. Where a lesion is red, it is useful to compress the overlying skin to see if it blanches on pressure. Red macules that do not blanch on pressure are known as purpura (**1.17**). The redness is due to blood lying outside the blood vessels, which cannot be pushed away with compression. A small purpuric lesion is referred to as a petechia (plural: petechiae) and a large purpuric lesion as an ecchymosis (plural: ecchymoses), which is known to most people as a bruise (**1.18**). By contrast, erythema refers to skin reddening that does blanch on pressure.

There may be changes in the skin overlying the area of interest. The area may be scratched or excoriated, and with this there may be fresh or dried blood (**1.19**). Crust is dried serum that is typically golden in colour that can overlie a lesion; it suggests inflammation due to eczema or impetigo (**1.20, 1.21**). This must be differentiated from scale, which is the detached keratin of the top layer of skin. Depending on the skin condition, scale will be of differing adherence to

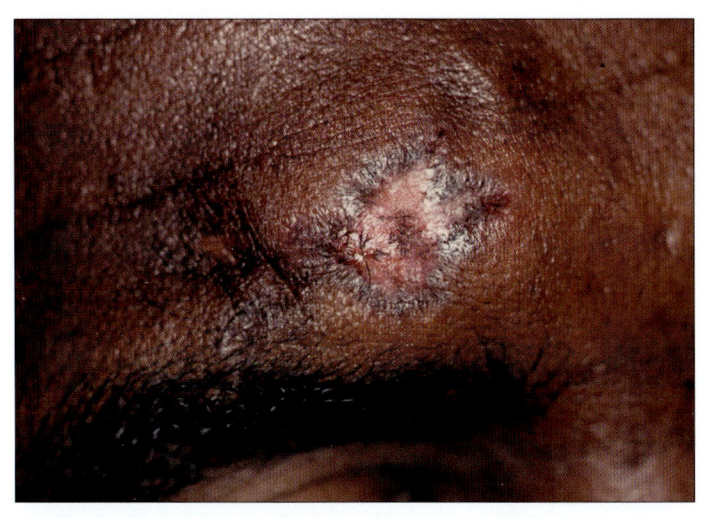

1.16 Hyper- and hypopigmentation in a small plaque of discoid lupus erythematosus on the forehead (see Chapter 6).

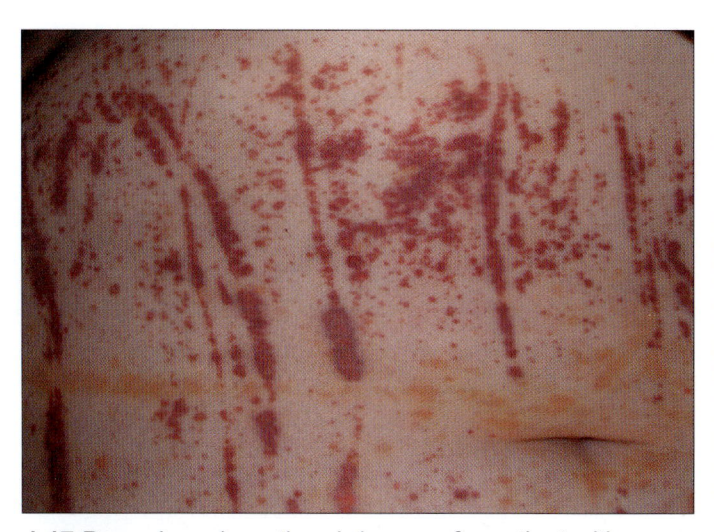

1.17 Purpuric rash on the abdomen of a patient with vasculitis. Not the Koebner phenomenon where she has scratched the skin and the yellow-brown pigmentation where the lesions have faded.

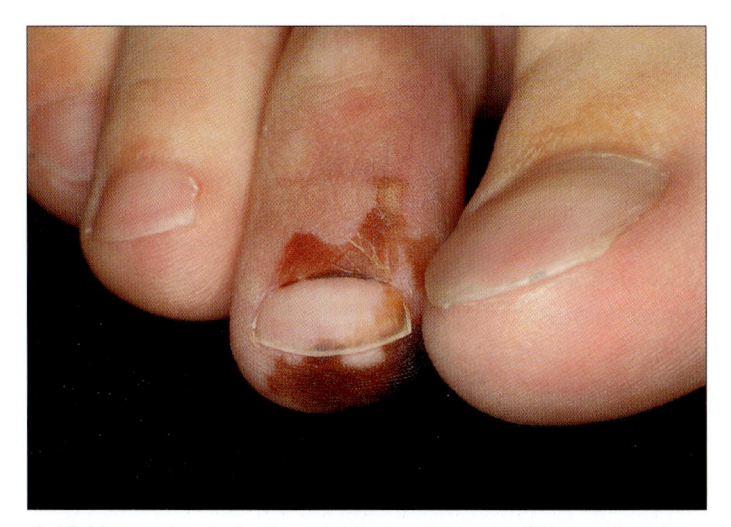

1.18 Haematoma in the stratum corneum of the second toe mimicking an acral lentiginous melanoma.

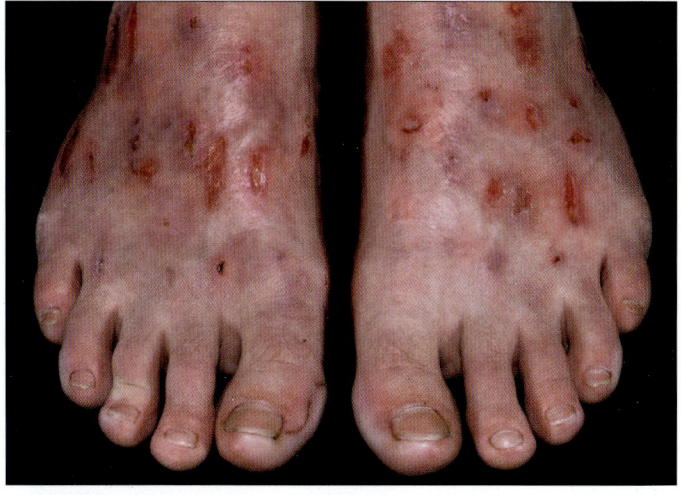

1.19 Excoriated lesions on the feet.

8 Introduction to diagnosing dermatological conditions (basic principles)

the lesion's surface. Often it is useful to remove overlying scale and crust in order to look at the underlying skin.

When examining in dermatology, good lighting must be used. The skin should be observed and then palpated. Rashes and isolated lesions should be approached in the same logical manner. The mnemonic DCM can be used to describe dermatological conditions: Distribution, Configuration, and Morphology.

- Distribution: which area or areas of the skin are affected; for instance does the rash tend to affect the flexor or extensor surfaces of the skin (**1.22**, **1.23**)?

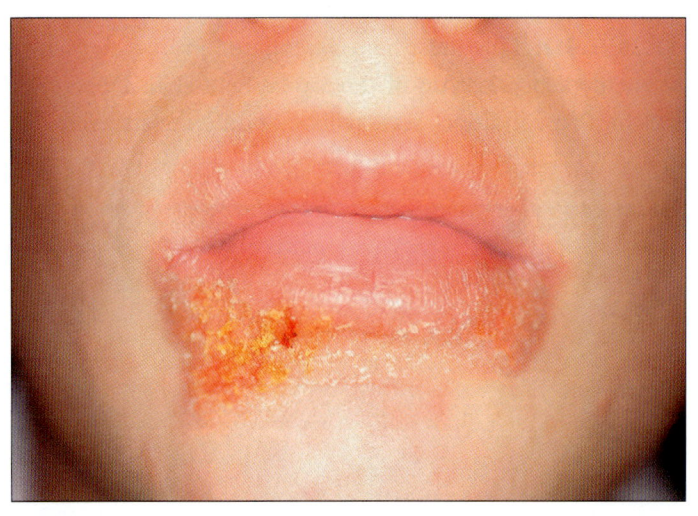

1.20 Impetiginized eczema of the lips and surrounding skin.

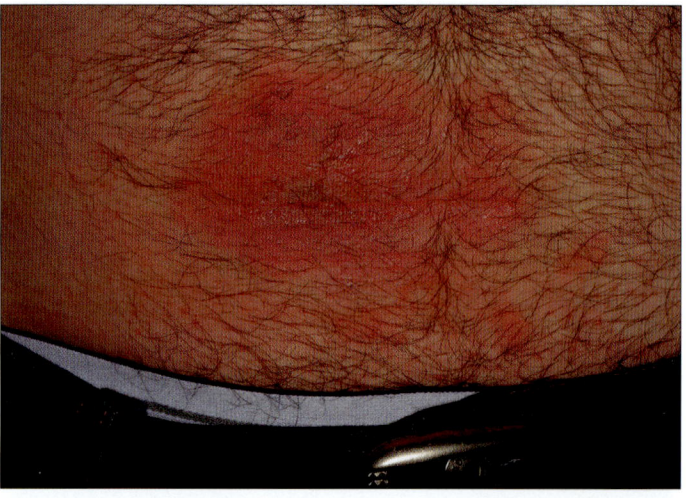

1.21 Weeping allergic dermatitis due to contact with nickel in the belt buckle.

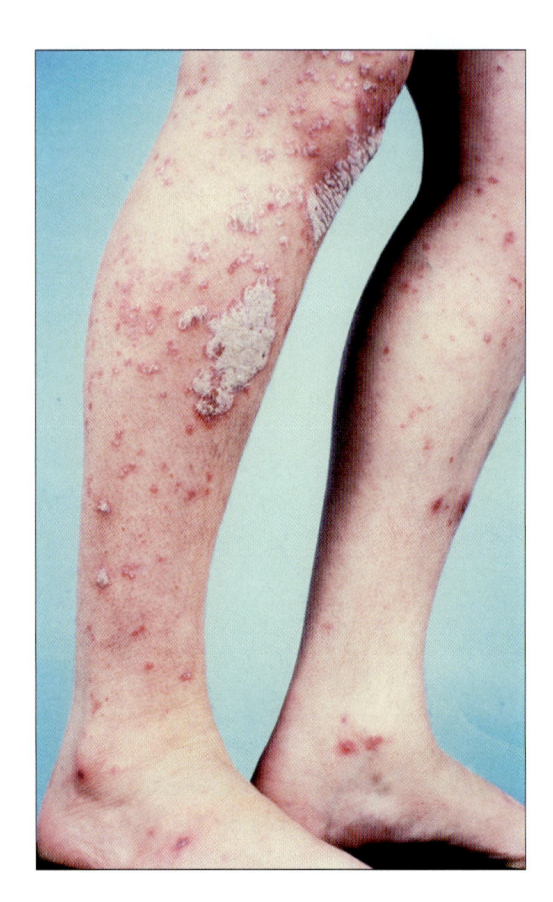

1.23 Dermatitis herpetiformis classically shows herpetiform lesions (vesicles grouped together like a cold sore) on elbows, knees, buttocks, and shoulders.

1.22 Plaques of psoriasis affecting the extensor surface of the lower leg.

Introduction to diagnosing dermatological conditions (basic principles)

- Configuration: first, does the condition affect the body symmetrically or not? Second, is there a pattern to the condition, such as linear, where lesions are in a line or annular, where they form a ring; are the lesions in groups or isolated (**1.24**, **1.25**)? When describing an isolated lesion, the physician should check if there are surrounding lesions and if so, do they form a pattern.
- Morphology: the form of the rash or lesion should be described, its size, colour, and any associated features. If the rash has different forms within it, each form should be described separately, using the terms described in the previous section. A general physical examination of the patient should not be overlooked, especially where the skin condition is a manifestation of systemic disease.

For a lesion that is changing, use of the **ABCDE** criteria can be a useful tool for suspecting malignancy (**1.26**, **1.27**). This rule has been validated in scientific studies in the prediction of malignant melanoma. Although it has not been validated for nonmelanoma skin lesions, it is a useful approach to all skin lesions that are reported as changing.

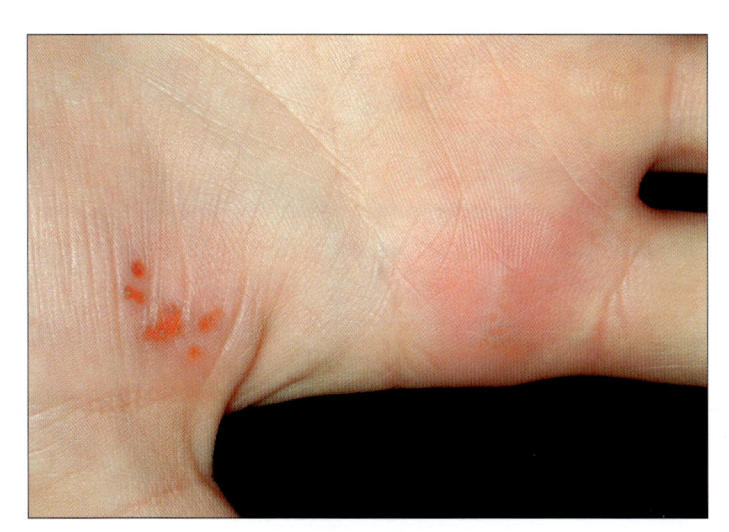

1.24 Herpes simplex infection of the palm.

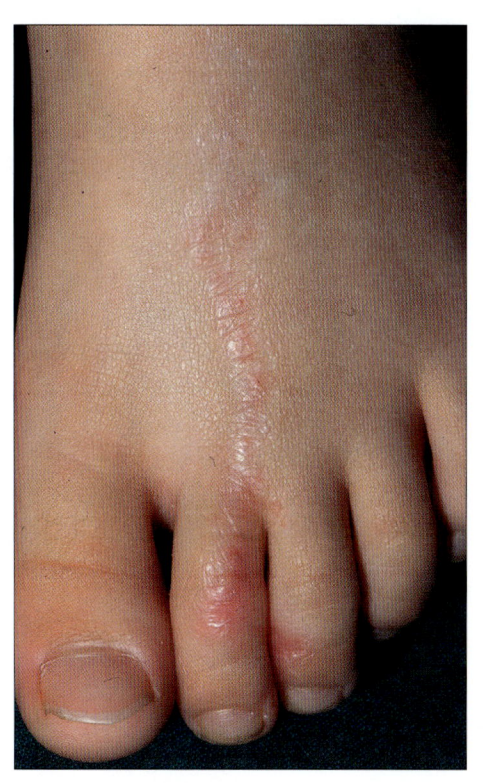

1.25 Lichen striatus.

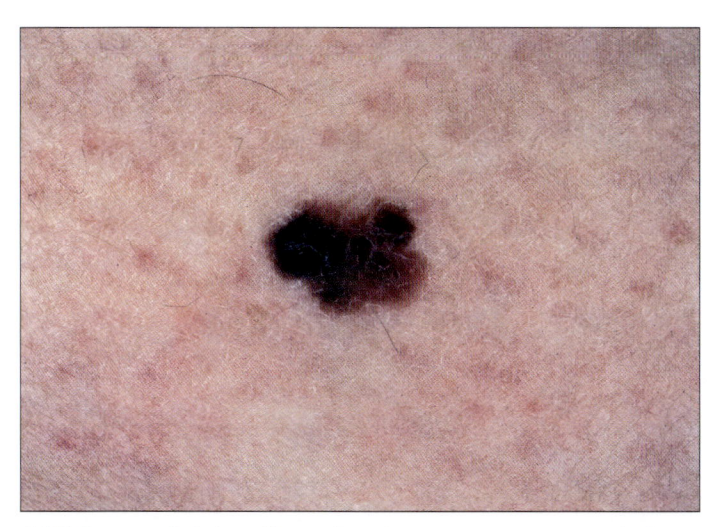

1.26 A superficial malignant melanoma on a woman's leg. It is **A**symmetrical, the **B**order is irregular, there is **C**olour variation, its **D**iameter is ≥6 mm, and it is **E**nlarging (**1.27**).

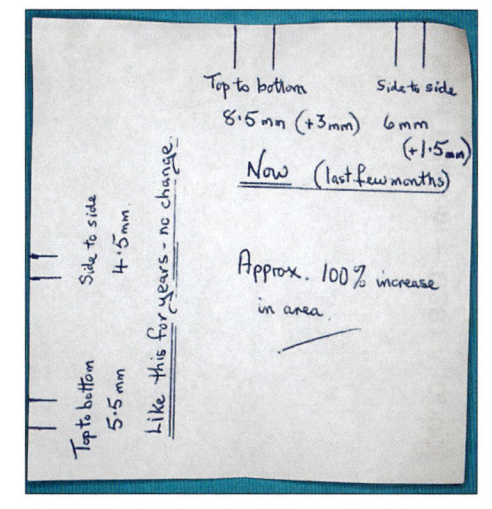

1.27 The husband of the patient in **1.26** regularly measured the lesion.

Introduction to diagnosing dermatological conditions (basic principles)

Malignancy should be suspected if one or more of the following criteria are fulfilled:
- Asymmetry: is the lesion asymmetrical in shape?
- Border: does the lesion have an irregular border?
- Colour: is the colour of the lesion irregular or changing?
- Diameter: is the diameter >6 mm?
- Enlargement: is the lesion growing, either vertically or horizontally along the skin surface?

Investigations

The skin can be viewed using a dermatoscope, a handheld device that magnifies the field of view ×10. This is especially useful when looking at pigmented lesions (see Chapter 4). Where a fungal infection is suspected, skin scrapings, collected using brisk strokes of a scalpel blade across the affected area, may be sent for analysis by microscopy and culture (**1.28**). Likewise, fluids within blisters or exuding from a lesion may be collected using a swab or syringe and analysed for the presence of bacteria or viruses.

An invasive investigation of skin disease is the removal of affected skin for analysis. Commonly, a core of skin measuring up to 6 mm in diameter is removed using a circular blade called a punch biopsy. Biopsies can be analysed in a number of ways including histology, culture, and immunofluorescence, which is a useful tool when considering the aetiology of immuno-bullous skin disease.

Patch testing is useful in suspected contact dermatitis (*Table 1.1*). Skin, usually on a patient's back, is exposed to different allergens; each is placed onto a separate disc and held in contact with the patient's skin using tape (**1.29**). These so-called patches are left in place for 2 days and then removed. The skin is inspected after a further 2 days for any reactions (**1.30**). Skill is required to discern irritant from allergic reaction. Various contact dermatitis groups set the number of standard chemicals used, although additional chemicals may be 'patched' if the history is relevant.

Skin prick tests are used to examine for atopy, latex allergy, and food allergy. A drop of allergen in solution is placed on the patient's forearm. The skin is pricked with a lancet through the drop and excess solution is then removed. Skin is inspected after 20 minutes (**1.31**). Skill is again required in interpretation of these tests. These tests are not commonly used because of the limited information afforded by them.

Table 1.1 Indications for patch testing

- Treatment-resistant eczema
- Chronic hand eczema
- Gravitational eczema
- Occupational contact dermatitis

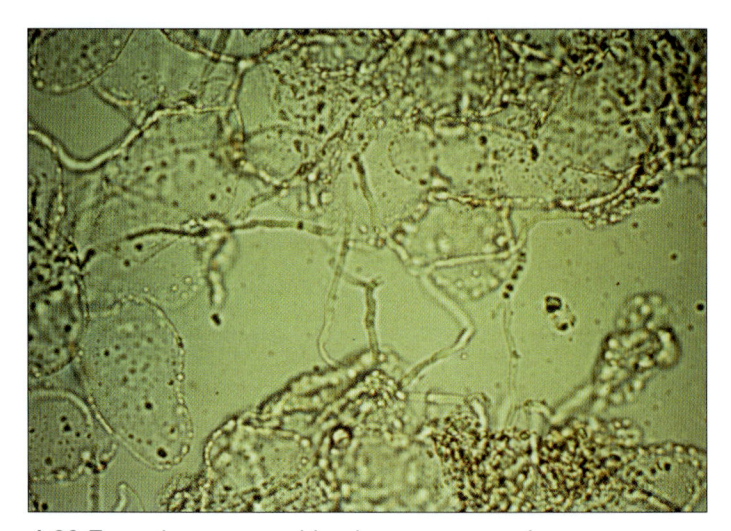

1.28 Fungal spores and hyphae seen on microscopy.

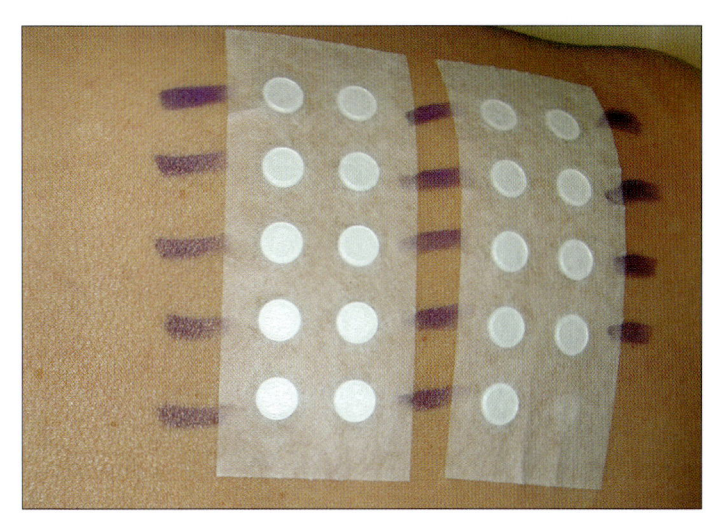

Introduction to diagnosing dermatological conditions (basic principles)

1.29 Patch tests in place.

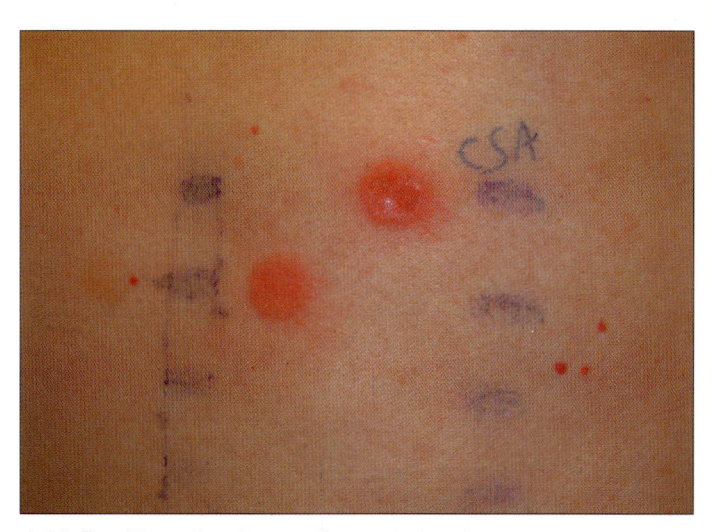

1.30 Positive allergic reactions at day 4.

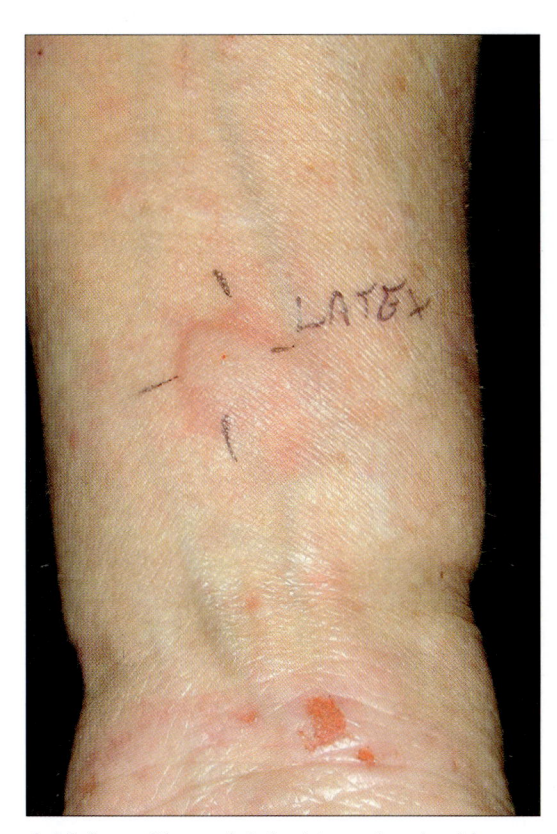

1.31 A positive prick test to natural rubber latex allergy.

Further reading

Burns T, Breathnach S, Cox N, Griffiths C (2004). *Rook's Textbook of Dermatology* (7th edn). Blackwell Science, Oxford.

McKee PH, Calonje E, Grauter SR (2005). *Pathology of the Skin* (3rd edn). Elsevier Mosby, Philadelphia.

Chapter 2

Paediatric dermatoses

Jane C Ravenscroft, MRCP, MRCGP

Introduction

Skin conditions are very common in children. Many are transient and of little importance; however, some may have important implications. Atopic eczema is very common, and because of this, any rash in a child is often diagnosed as atopic eczema. This chapter will illustrate some of the many different skin lesions (*Table 2.1*) and rashes (*Table 2.2*) which can affect children, and help in accurate diagnosis and management.

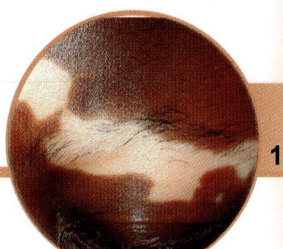

Table 2.1 Lesions presenting in children <10 years, by colour, or presence of blisters

Red/pink/blue
- Abscess/boil
- Infantile haemangioma
- Lymphangioma circumscriptum
- Naevus flammeus
- Pilomatricoma
- Port wine stain
- Pyogenic granuloma
- Ringworm
- Spider naevus
- Spitz naevus
- Vascular malformations

Skin coloured/yellow/orange
- Aplasia cutis
- Dermoid cyst
- Epidermal cyst
- Granuloma annulare
- Molluscum contagiosum
- Neurofibroma
- Sebaceous naevus
- Xanthogranuloma

Pigmented
- Acquired benign naevus
- *Café au lait* macule
- Congenital melanocytic naevus
- Dermatofibroma
- Epidermal naevus
- Mastocytoma
- Mongolian blue spot
- Naevus spilus

Hypopigmented
- Naevus depigmentosus
- Postinflammatory hypopigmentation
- Pityriasis alba
- Vitiligo

Blisters
- Bullous impetigo
- Chicken pox
- Chronic bullous disease of childhood
- Dermatitis herpetiformis
- Epidermolysis bullosa
- Herpes simplex
- Mastocytosis
- Miliaria
- Papular urticaria

14 Paediatric dermatoses

Table 2.2 Rashes in children <10 years

Neonatal and infantile rashes
• Atopic eczema
• Epidermolysis bullosa
• Erythema toxicum neonatorum
• Ichthyosis
• Infantile acne
• Miliaria crystallina
• Miliaria rubra
• Psoriasis
• Seborrhoeic dermatitis
 	
Rashes affecting the nappy area
• Atopic eczema
• Bullous impetigo
• *Candida* infection
• Irritant nappy rash
• Langerhans cell histiocytosis
• Perianal streptococcal disease
• Psoriasis
• Seborrhoeic dermatitis
 	
Acute childhood rashes
• Folliculitis
• Henoch–Schönlein purpura
• Infections:
  – Chicken pox
  – Erythema infectiosum
  – Hand, foot, and mouth disease
  – Herpes simplex
  – Kawasaki disease
  – Measles
  – Roseola
  – Rubella
  – Scabies
  – Scarlet fever
  – Staphylococcal scalded skin syndrome
• Pityriasis rosea
• Toxic erythema
• Urticaria
 	
Chronic childhood rashes
• Acne
• Atopic eczema
• Chronic bullous disease of childhood
• Dermatitis herpetiformis
• Ichthyosis
• Juvenile plantar dermatosis
• Keratosis pilaris
• Pityriasis versicolour
• Psoriasis
• Urticaria pigmentosum

SKIN LESIONS

Birthmarks

Infantile haemangioma (strawberry naevus)
Clinical presentation
Infantile haemangiomas are benign vascular tumours which affect 1–2% of infants, most commonly on the head and neck. They are not present, or just visible at birth, and grow rapidly in the first 6 months of life to become distinctive bright red nodules, sometimes with a deeper component (**2.1**). At around 12 months of age, they start to undergo spontaneous resolution (**2.2**). Fifty per cent of lesions will disappear by 5 years of age and 90% by 9 years. There may be residual flaccid skin and telangiectasia. Complications of ulceration (**2.3**), haemorrhage, and interference with function may occur during the phase of rapid proliferation. Rarely, multiple haemangiomas occur, which may be associated with internal haemangiomas. Very infrequently, large haemangiomas may be associated with structural brain and cardiac abnormalities, or consumptive coagulopathy.

Differential diagnosis
Differential diagnosis is from other vascular birthmarks. Vascular lesions which do not show characteristic proliferation after birth are not infantile haemangiomas and should be referred for accurate diagnosis.

Management
Due to the self-limiting nature of infantile haemangiomas, treatment is not required unless complications occur. Ulcerated lesions can be treated with topical steroid and antibiotics. Pulsed dye laser may be used for prolonged ulceration, and for residual telangiectasia after resolution. Interference with function may require intralesional or oral steroids.

Paediatric dermatoses

Naevus flammeus (salmon patch)
Clinical presentation
This is a pale pink vascular patch, present at birth, which commonly occurs on the nape of the neck, forehead, or eyelid (**2.4**).

Differential diagnosis
Naevus flammeus can be distinguished from port wine stain by its paler colour and typical site.

Management
Those on the forehead and eyelid tend to disappear during the first year of life, but those on the neck (stork marks) will persist. Treatment is not usually indicated, but they will respond to pulsed dye laser.

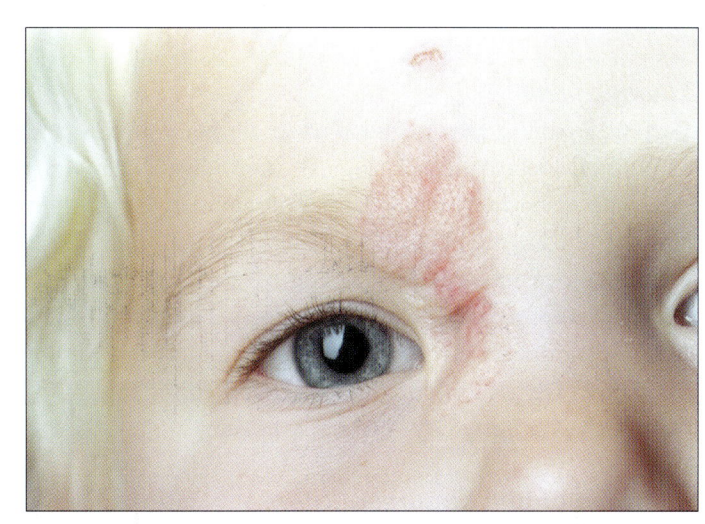

2.1 Infantile haemangioma at 5 months of age.

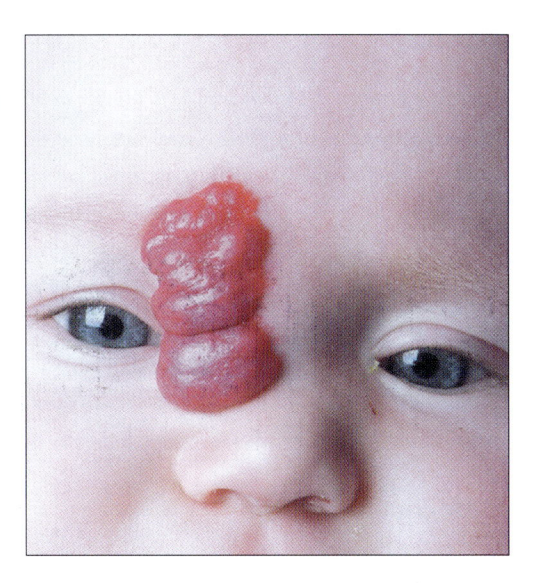

2.2 The same child as in **2.1** aged 3 years.

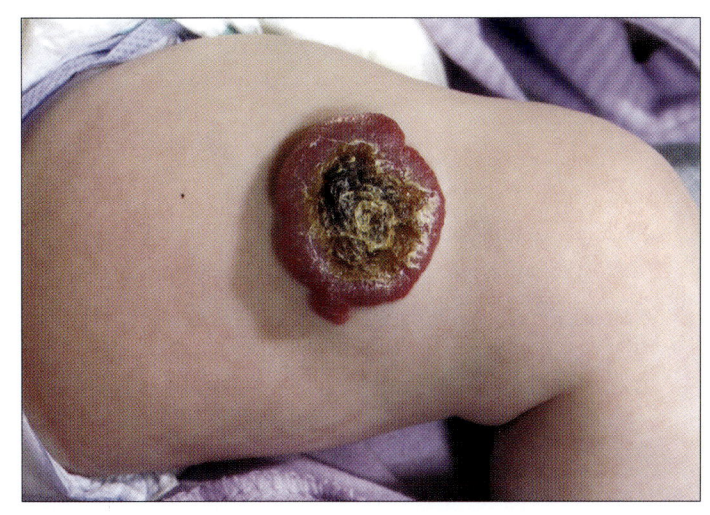

2.3 A proliferating infantile haemangioma, which is ulcerated.

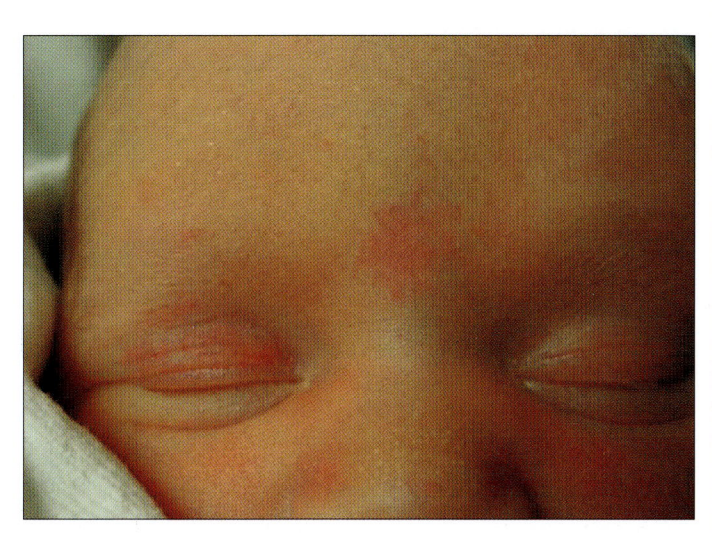

2.4 A salmon patch in a neonate.

Port wine stain

Clinical presentation
Port wine stain is a vascular malformation which presents as a deep red/purple vascular patch, present at birth, most often unilateral on the face; however, any site can be affected (**2.5**).

Differential diagnosis
Salmon patch is paler, and occurs on the nape of the neck, forehead, and eyelid. Infantile haemangiomas will grow larger in the first 4 weeks of life. Other vascular and lymphatic malformations are usually associated with soft tissue swelling.

Management
Port wine stains persist and darken throughout life, and cause considerable psychological morbidity. They may rarely be associated with other abnormalities, e.g. lesions affecting the trigeminal area may be associated with ocular or intracranial involvement leading to glaucoma, epilepsy, and developmental delay (Sturge–Weber syndrome). Referral should be made in the first few months of life for assessment for associated conditions, and consideration for treatment with pulsed dye laser, if available.

Lymphangioma circumscriptum

Clinical presentation
This uncommon lymphatic malformation presents at birth with a cluster of papules varying in colour from clear to straw coloured to deep purple, which resemble frogspawn (**2.6**). There may be associated soft tissue swelling.

Differential diagnosis
Other vascular birthmarks should be distinguished by colour or early proliferation.

Management
Lymphangioma persist and may enlarge throughout life. Surgical removal is difficult because there is a deep component. If weeping and crusting is a problem, CO_2 or Erb YAG laser may give symptomatic relief.

Congenital melanocytic naevus

Clinical presentation
Congenital melanocytic naevi are palpable brown lesions with some variation in pigment within them, seen in 1–2% of infants at birth (**2.7**; see Chapter 4, **4.20–4.22**). Most are small (<1.5 cm) or medium sized (1.5–20 cm); a few may cover large areas of the body surface. They persist lifelong and may become more raised and develop coarse hairs within them as the child gets older.

Differential diagnosis
Congenital melanocytic naevi are generally darker brown than other pigmented birthmarks.

Management
Management of congenital melenocytic naevi must consider risk of malignancy and cosmetic appearance. Risk of malignancy with small- and medium-sized lesions is considered to be <5%, so prophylactic excision is not routinely recommended. Excision may be considered for cosmetic reasons. Change within a congenital naevus should prompt referral for consideration of biopsy. Large congenital melanocytic naevi are extremely complex to manage and require specialist assessment.

Café au lait macule

Clinical presentation
These are tan coloured, evenly pigmented nonpalpable lesions up to around 10 cm in size, presenting at birth or in the first few years of life, most often on the trunk and limbs (**2.8**).

Differential diagnosis
Congenital melanocytic naevi are generally darker in colour, and may be palpable.

Management
Lesions persist throughout life but are not usually a cosmetic problem; therefore, treatment is not required. If >5 *café au lait* macules are present, there is a high chance (up to 95%), that the patient has neurofibromatosis, so the patient should be referred for further assessment.

2.5 A port wine stain affecting the trigeminal area.

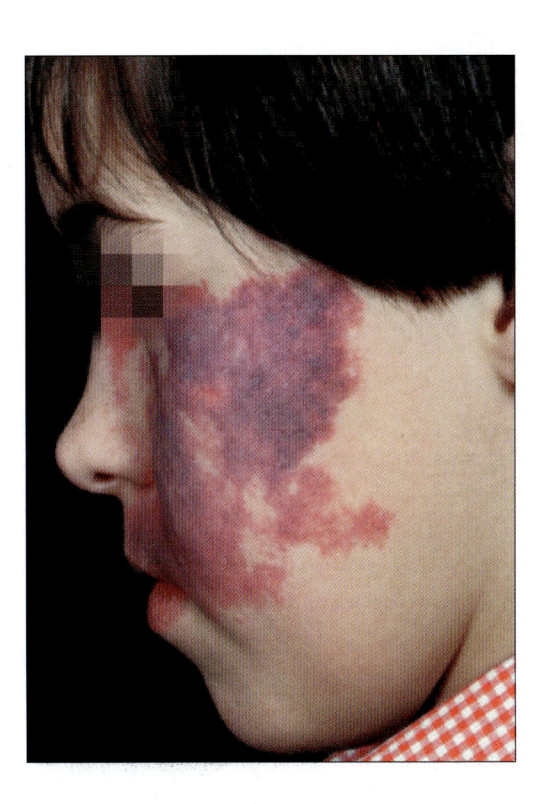

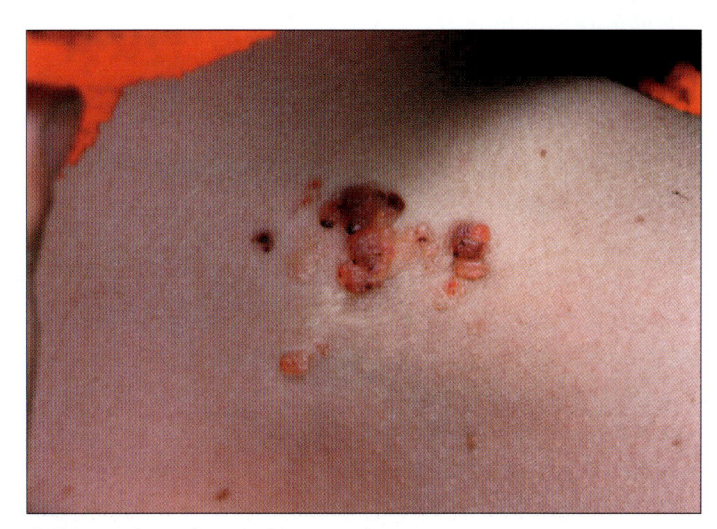

2.6 Lymphangioma circumscriptum.

2.7 A large and a small congenital melanocytic naevus.

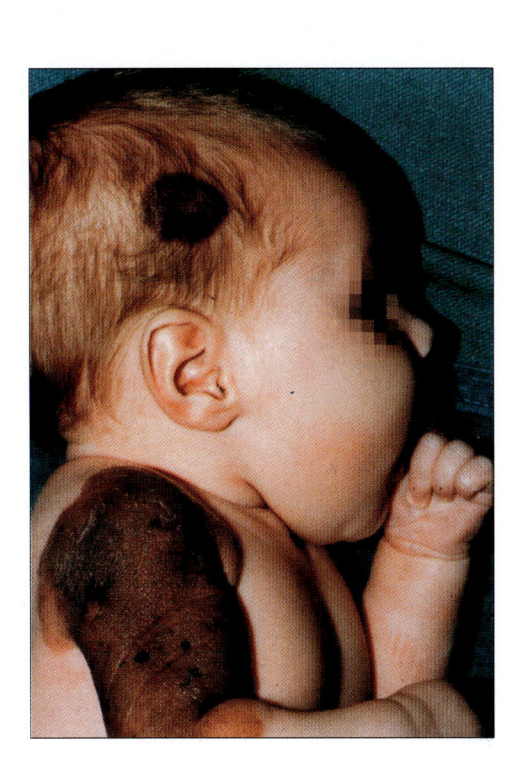

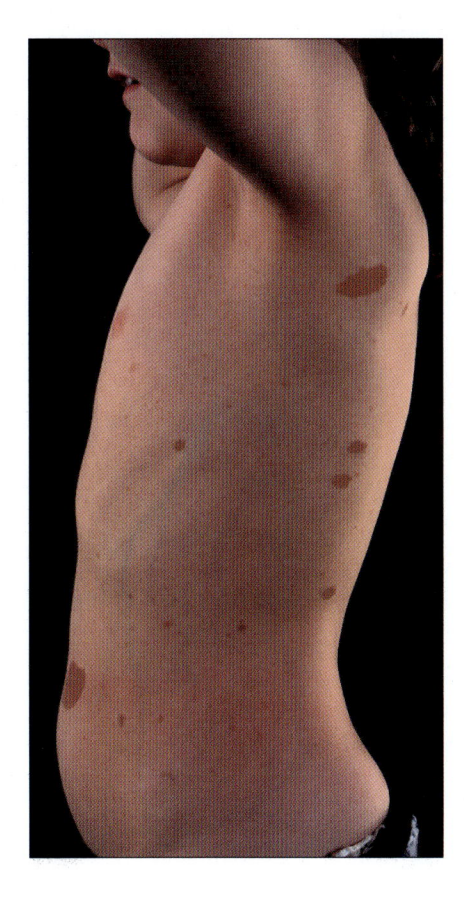

2.8 Café au lait patches in a child with neuro-fibromatosis.

Mongolian blue spot

Clinical presentation
This is a large blue patch on the lower back, commonly seen in oriental babies at birth (**2.9**).

Differential diagnosis
Bruising, which may be mistaken for child abuse.

Management
Lesions generally disappear in the first few years of life. No treatment is necessary.

Sebaceous naevus

Clinical features
This is an uncommon yellowish papule or plaque, present at birth, which often presents as a hairless area on the scalp (**2.10**).

Differential diagnosis
Trauma from forceps/ventouse delivery; aplasia cutis.

Management
Surgical removal can be considered if they are a cosmetic problem. There is a small increased risk of basal cell carcinoma in adult life.

Epidermal naevus

Clinical presentation
Children present with a linear brown or skin coloured warty plaque, which may be present at birth or develop in the first few years of life. They are of variable size, from 1–2 cm to the length of a limb (**2.11**), and will often extend during early childhood. Occasionally, epidermal naevi are multiple and may be associated with other abnormalities.

Differential diagnosis
Other birthmarks are distinguished by lack of linear pattern. Lichen striatus is an inflammatory linear condition that appears in later childhood and resolves in months to years.

Management
Epidermal naevi persist for life. Treatment, if needed, is by surgical removal or laser, but scarring or recurrence may occur.

Aplasia cutis

Clinical presentation
Aplasia cutis is a developmental abnormality with an area of absence of skin. It presents as an ulcerated red area present on the scalp at birth, which heals with a scar, within which the hair does not grow (**2.12**).

Differential diagnosis
Sebaceous naevus has a warty surface and the skin is intact; trauma from forceps/ventouse during delivery.

Management
Surgical excision of the scar can be considered, if it is a cosmetic problem.

Paediatric dermatoses

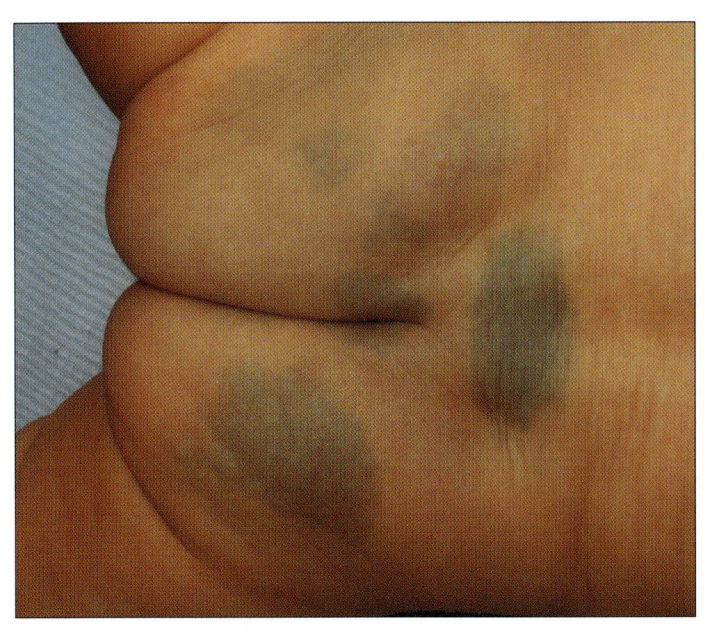

2.9 Mongolian blue spot.

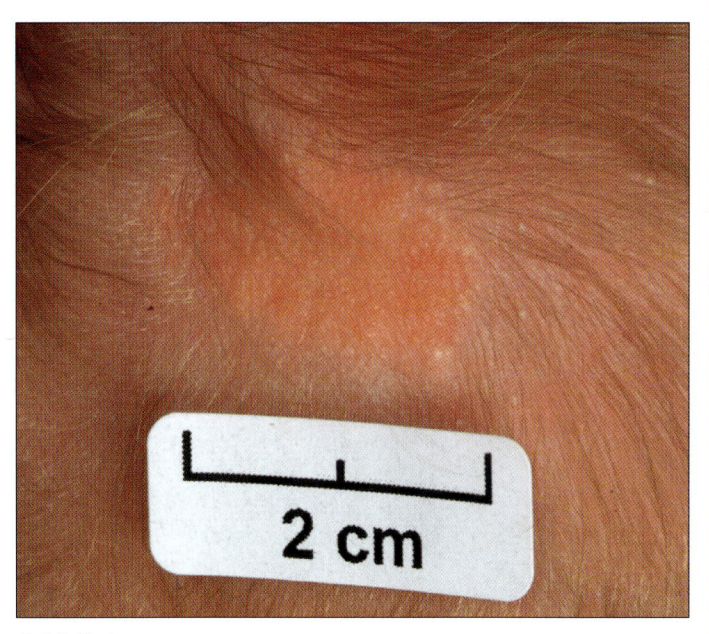

2.10 Sebaceous naevus.

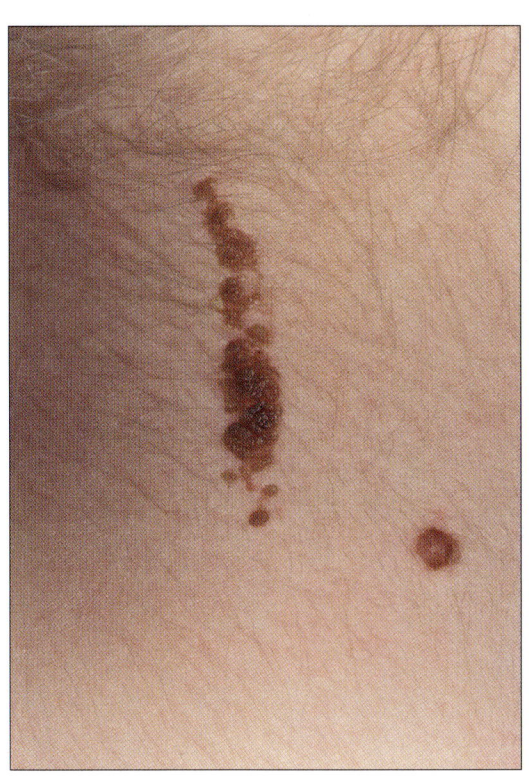

2.11 A linear epidermal warty epidermal naevus.

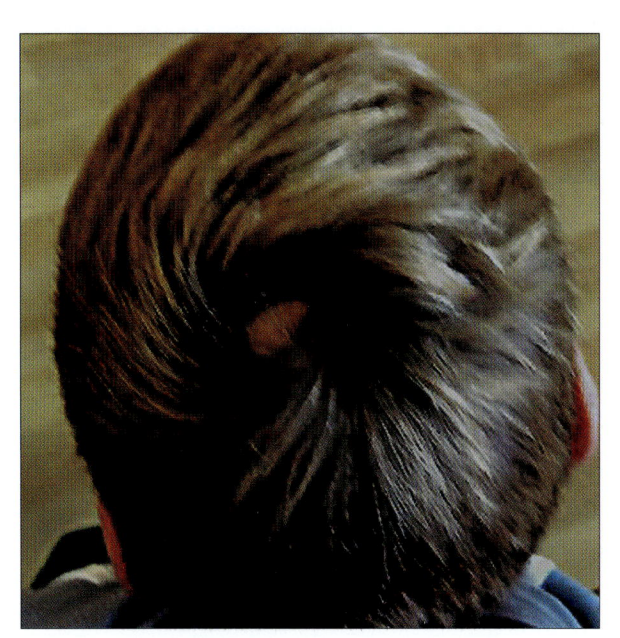

2.12 Aplasia cutis results in a localized bald patch on the scalp.

Other childhood lesions

Pilomatricoma

Clinical presentation
Pilomatricoma is a benign adnexal tumour which presents in childhood as a firm, solitary 0.5–3 cm blue-red nodule most commonly on the face (**2.13**). It grows slowly over months and may calcify.

Differential diagnosis
Pilomatricomas can be mistaken for epidermal cysts or dermoid cysts, but are distinguished by bluish colour and firmer texture.

Management
These lesions should be surgically excised.

Pyogenic granuloma

Clinical presentation
Pyogenic granuloma is a benign vascular tumour which often follows minor injury to the skin. It presents as a bright red, shiny 'wet' nodule, most commonly on the face or fingers, which bleeds easily on minor trauma (see Chapter 4, **4.41**).

Differential diagnosis
Appearance is characteristic.

Management
Treatment is with currettage or electrodesication.

Xanthogranuloma

Clinical presentation
Xanthogranuloma is a rare benign tumour of histiocytes which presents in early childhood as an orange/yellow nodule (**2.14**). It resolves spontaneously in 1–5 years. Occasionally, multiple lesions occur. There is a rare association with neurofibromatosis and juvenile leukaemia.

Differential diagnosis
Xanthogranulomas may mimic mastocytomas, but are distinguished by absence of wealing.

Management
Treatment is not required because xanthogranulomas undergo spontaneous resolution.

Mastocytosis

Clinical presentation
Collections of mast cells may form a solitary lesion, called a mastocytoma, or may develop throughout the skin as a rash called urticaria pigmentosum (**2.15**). Approximately 50% of all cases of mastocytosis occur in children, generally before 2 years of age.

A mastocytoma presents as a red/brown nodule, which produces wealing if the lesion is rubbed (Darier's sign). Urticaria pigmentosum presents as a rash composed of hundreds of pale brown macules predominantly over the trunk. Often, parents have noticed wealing after pressure or a hot bath.

Differential diagnosis
Solitary mastocytomas and urticaria pigmentosum can be distinguished from other lesions and rashes by their distinctive pale brown colour and presence of wealing on rubbing.

Management
Mastocytomas resolve spontaneously over 2–3 years. No treatment is needed. Urticaria pigmentosum shows slower resolution, with around 50% clear by adolescence. Troublesome wealing can be treated with antihistamines. Patients with urticaria pigmentosum should avoid drugs which release histamine, e.g. aspirin, codeine, as they can precipitate severe urticaria and systemic effects.

Paediatric dermatoses 21

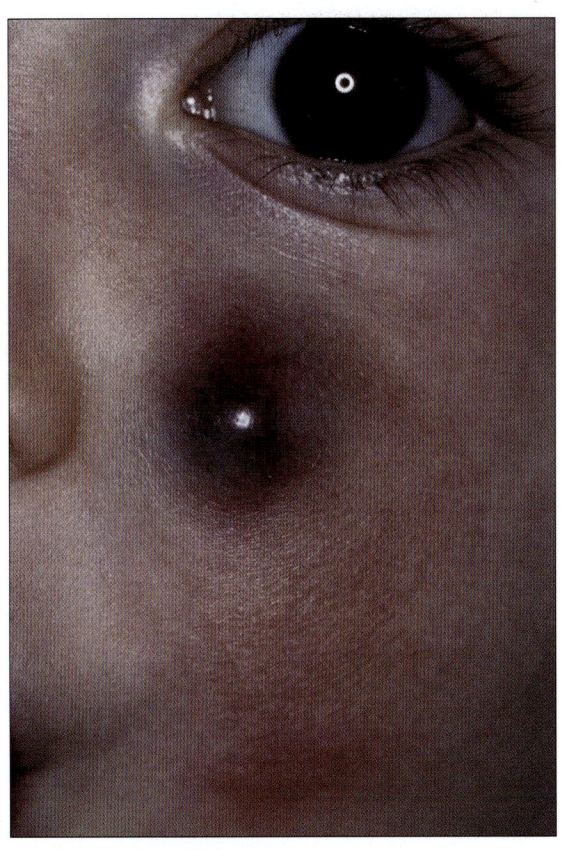

2.13 Pilomatricoma.

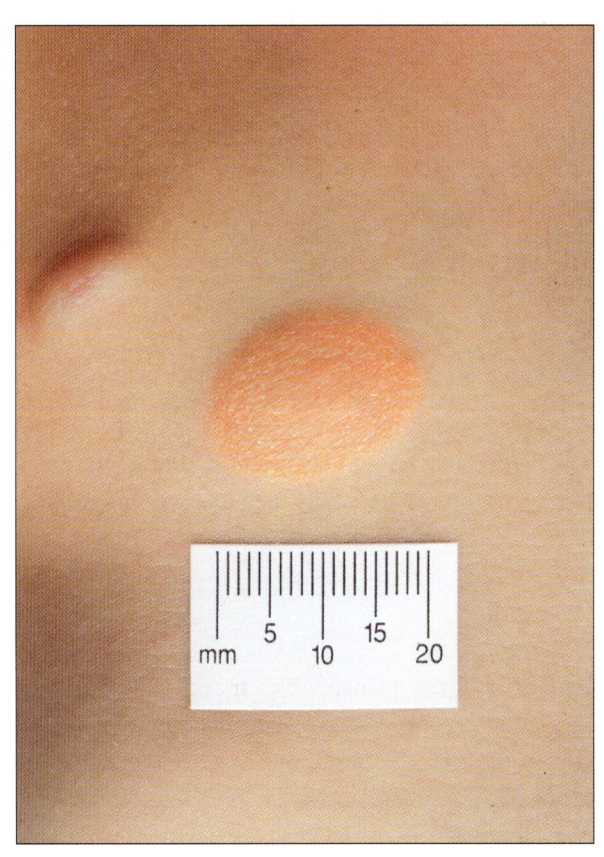

2.14 Xanthomgranuloma.

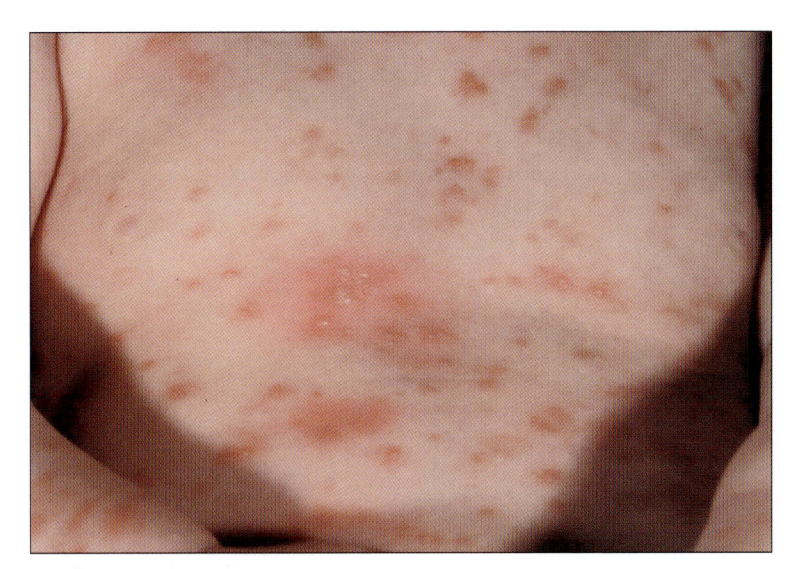

2.15 Urticaria pigmentosum.

22 Paediatric dermatoses

Granuloma annulare
Clinical presentation
Granuloma annulare is an inflammatory disorder of the skin which presents as an annular ring of smooth, skin-coloured or pink coalescing papules with central clearing (**2.16**). Lesions are often solitary, but may be multiple, and most commonly affect the dorsum of the feet.

Differential diagnosis
Granuloma annulare is frequently misdiagnosed as ringworm, but is easily distinguished by lack of scale.

Management
There is no effective treatment for granuloma annulare. Spontaneous resolution generally occurs over months to years.

2.16 Granuloma annulare.

Spider naevus
Clinical presentation
Pre-adolescent children present with a red papule on the face, made up of a central arteriole with peripheral vessels radiating from it (**2.17**). Pressure on the arteriole will cause blanching. May be solitary, or two or three may be present. In children, there is not usually an association with liver disease.

Differential diagnosis
The appearance is characteristic.

Management
Spider naevi will tend to resolve by the teenage years, so treatment is not generally necessary. Very large lesions can be treated with cautery or pulsed dye laser, if available.

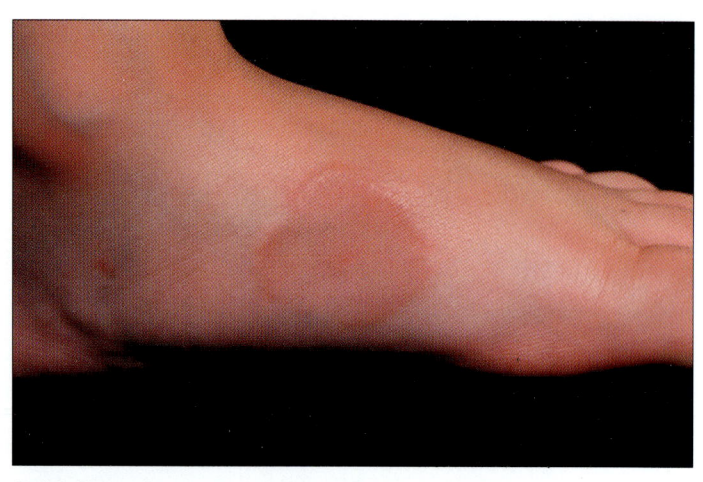

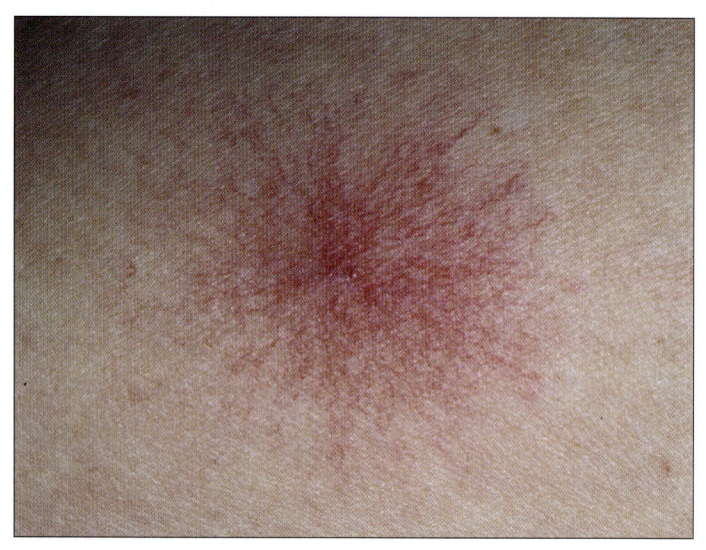

2.17 Spider naevus.

Paediatric dermatoses

RASHES

Neonatal and infantile rashes

Miliaria
Clinical presentation
Miliaria rubra is an eruption of erythematous papules and vesicles 1–4 mm in diameter, affecting the face, upper trunk, and flexures. It is common in the neonatal period, and lesions may occur in crops (**2.18**). Miliaria crystallina is much less common, and comprises a widespread eruption of thin walled 1–2 mm vesicles without erythema, occurring in the first 2 weeks of life. In both conditions the infant is well.

Differential diagnosis
Erythema toxicum neonatorum is diffuse erythema with occasional papules, seen in 50% of newborns in the first few days of life. Herpes simplex and staphylococcal infections cause pustular/vesicular rashes in an unwell child.

Management
These conditions are self-limiting over a few weeks.

Irritant nappy rash
Clinical presentation
This is a bright red, glazed, confluent erythema affecting the convex surfaces of the nappy area which are in contact with the urine and faeces. Erosions and ulcers can occur when severe (**2.19**). Groin flexures are spared.

Differential diagnosis
Irritant nappy rash, which does not respond to simple treatment, should be reassessed with consideration of rarer causes of rash in the nappy area (*Table 2.2*).

Management
Frequent changing of the nappy is advised, with application of a barrier cream.

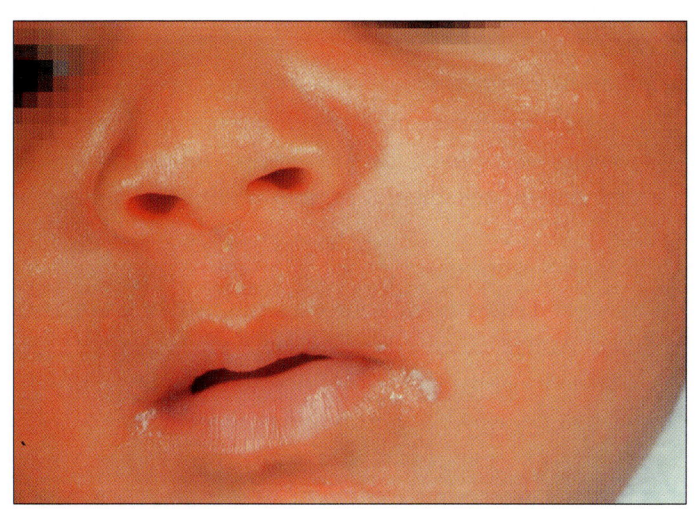

2.18 Miliaria rubra.

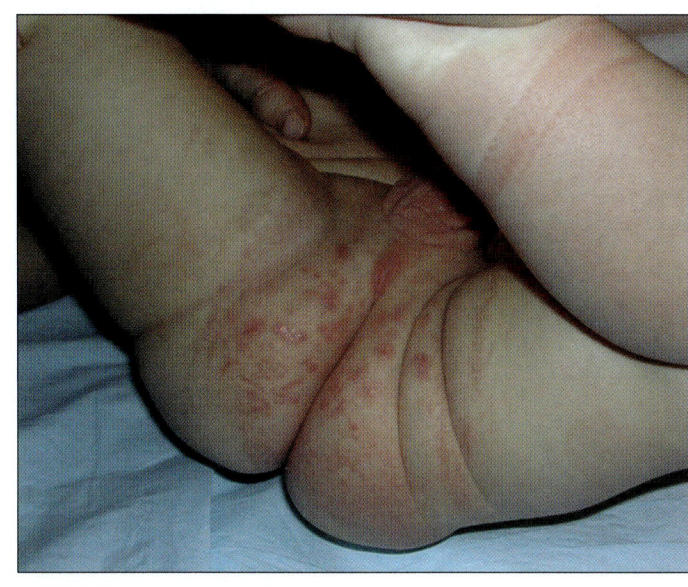

2.19 Irritant nappy rash.

24   Paediatric dermatoses

Seborrhoeic dermatitis

Clinical presentation
A bright red, confluent, nonitchy eruption of the nappy area, sometimes also involving the scalp, face, and trunk, occurring in infants under 3 months (**2.20**).

Differential diagnosis
Psoriasis and seborrhoeic dermatitis can look very similar in infancy. Atopic eczema is itchy, and associated with dry skin. Irritant nappy rash is confined to the convex surfaces and is painful. *Candida* infection has characteristic satellite papules (**2.21**). Langerhans cell histiocytosis is a very rare, more papular, brownish eruption of the groin and scalp, which progresses over weeks to months (**2.22, 2.23**).

Management
This condition is self-limiting over weeks to months. Combination therapy with a cream containing 1% hydrocortisone and an antifungal can improve the appearance.

Atopic eczema in infancy

Clinical presentation
Atopic eczema in infancy usually presents after 4 weeks of age as a dry, scaly, erythematous rash affecting the face, scalp, and sometimes the trunk and limbs (**2.24, 2.25**). The rash is poorly demarcated, blending into normal skin. It is itchy and causes distress to the child. There is usually a family history of eczema, asthma, or hay fever.

Differential diagnosis
Seborrhoeic dermatitis is brighter red, affects the nappy area and is nonitchy. Ichthyosis is present at, or soon after, birth as a dry scaly skin, without a rash. Scabies is a generalized papular rash, including palms, soles, and genitals, of sudden onset, without associated dry skin.

Management
Emollients can be used to relieve dry skin. Mild topical steroid can be applied to red areas in bursts of up to 7 days when needed.

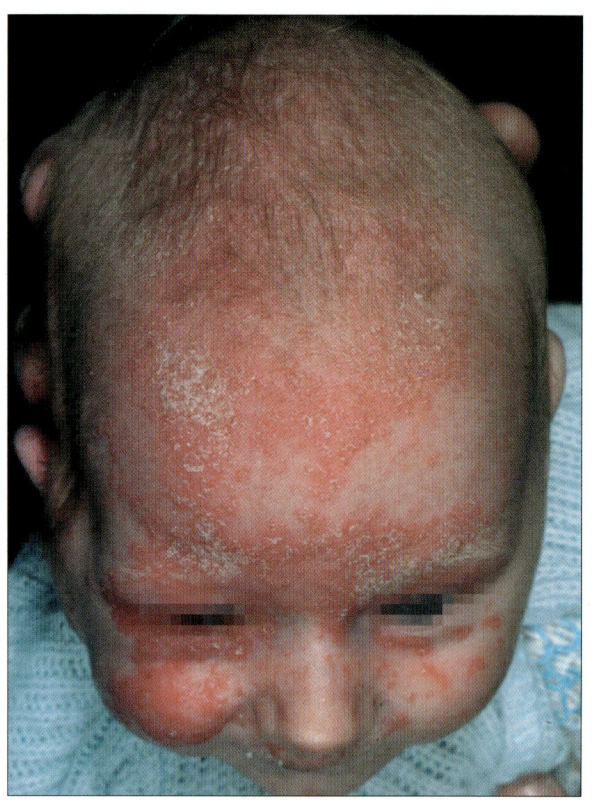

2.20 Infantile seborrhoeic dermatitis.

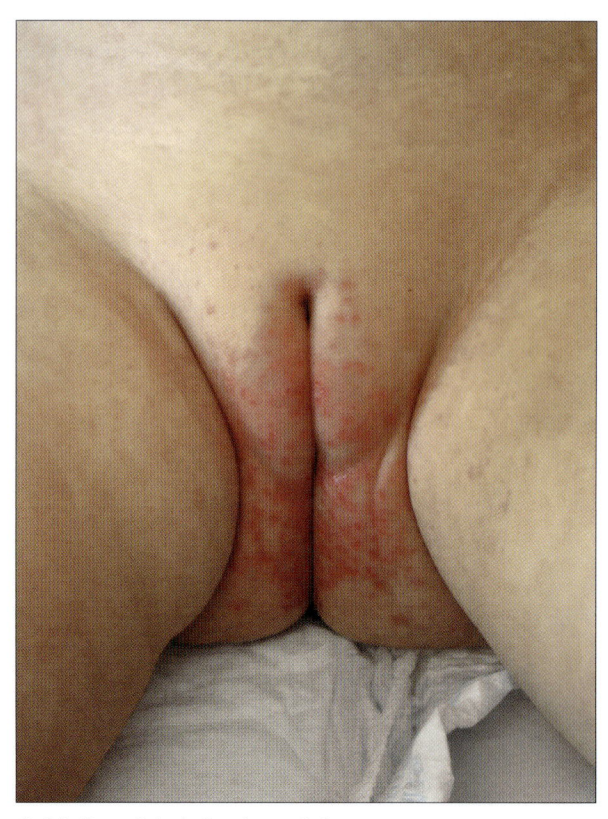

2.21 *Candida* infection of the nappy area.

Paediatric dermatoses 25

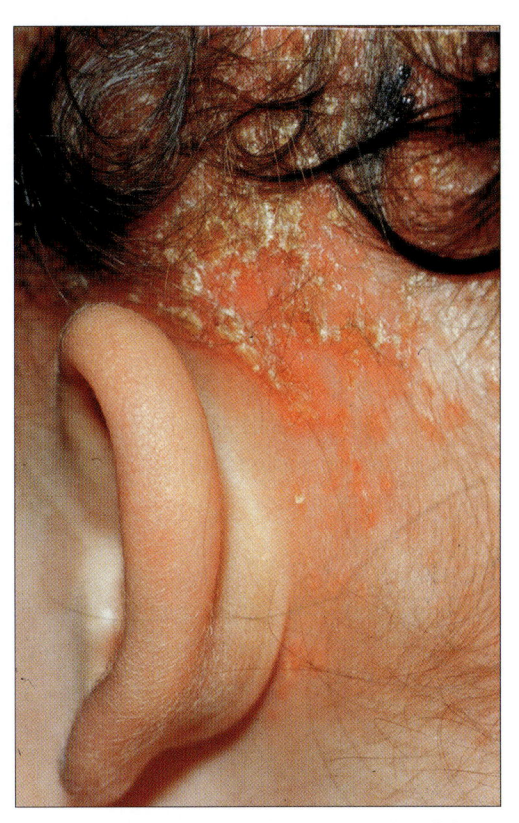

2.22 Langerhans cell histiocytosis of the scalp resembling seborrhoeic dermatitis.

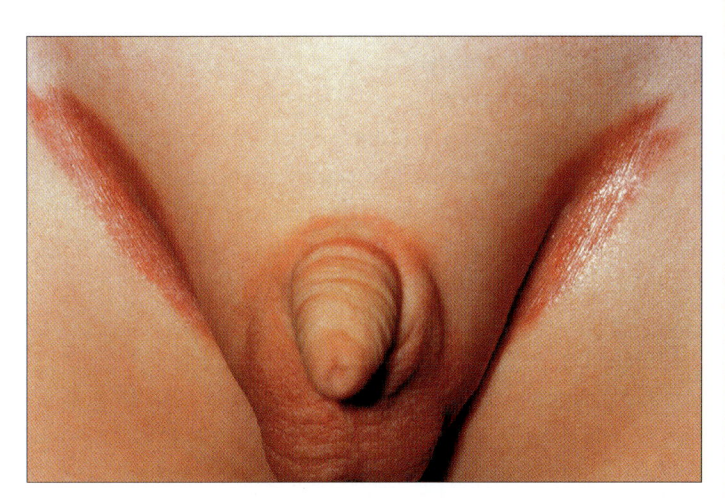

2.23 Langerhans cell histiocytosis of the groin resembling psoriasis.

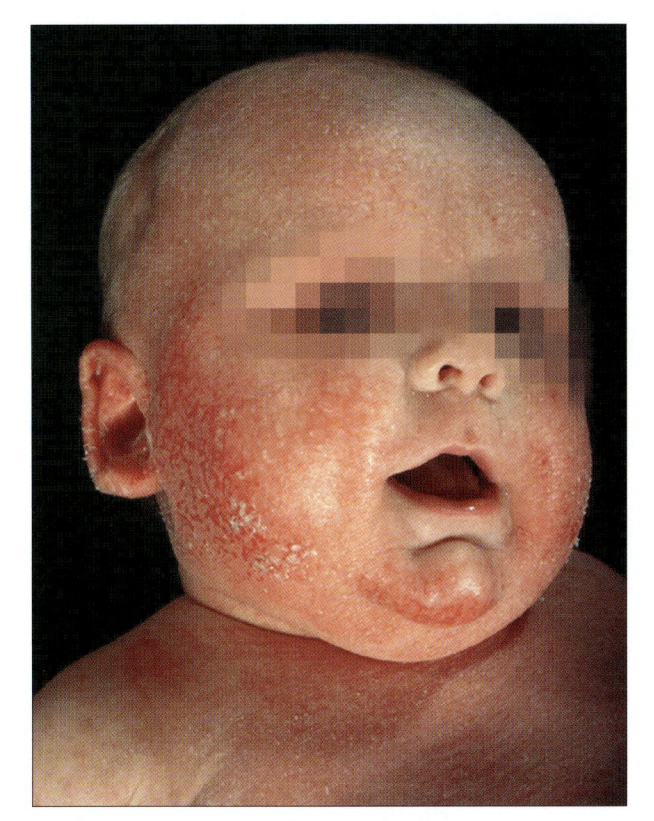

2.24 Atopic eczema affecting the face.

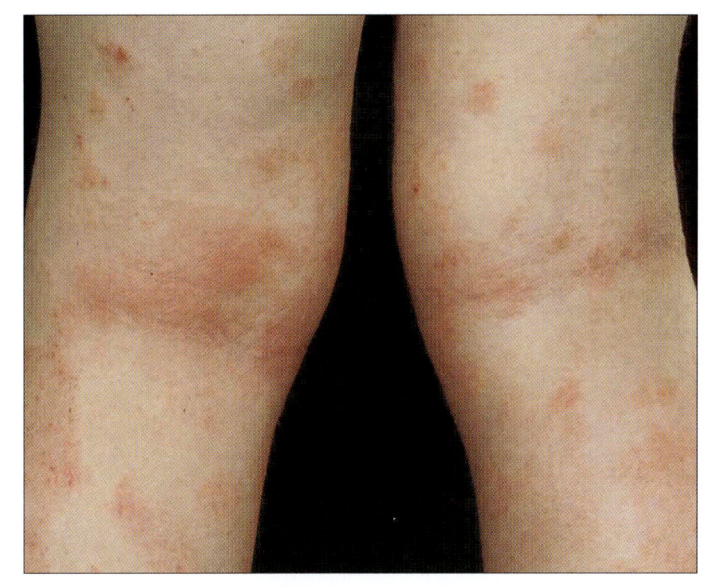

2.25 Atopic eczema affecting the knee flexures.

Psoriasis in infancy

Clinical presentation
Infants present with a salmon pink, well demarcated, scaly erythema often affecting the nappy area (**2.26, 2.27**); the scalp, face, and trunk may also be involved (**2.28**). It is usually nonitchy and not too distressing for the child. There may be a family history of psoriasis.

Differential diagnosis
Irritant nappy rash is localized to concave skin in contact with urine and faeces. Seborrhoeic eczema is less well demarcated, and responds more easily to treatment.

Management
Nappy psoriasis can be difficult to treat. It usually requires a topical steroid of at least moderate strength.

Ichthyosis

Clinical presentation
Ichthyosis is a genetic condition in which the skin fails to shed normally, resulting in a build up of adherent scale. The most common type, ichthyosis vulgaris (autosomal dominant), causes fine white scaling which becomes apparent in the first year of life, and spares the flexures (**2.29**). The rarer X-linked ichthyosis may affect all areas of the body with large, fish-like scales. Other, very rare subtypes may be associated with erythema and sparse hair.

Differential diagnosis
Atopic eczema causes erythema and characteristically involves the flexures. However, atopic eczema coexists in 50% of patients with ichthyosis vulgaris, so distinction can be difficult.

Management
Simple emollients can be used to hydrate the skin. Referral is recommended for genetic advice/testing in severe cases.

Epidermolysis bullosa

Clinical presentation
Abnormal blistering occurs due to skin fragility. The commonest type, epidermolysis bullosa simplex (autosomal dominant), presents with blisters of the feet (**2.30**). It may be mild with onset after the child starts to walk, and is often exacerbated by heat. Other, more severe forms, present in infancy with widespread blistering and scarring.

Differential diagnosis
Epidermolysis bullosa simplex is distinguished from simple friction blisters by extent and severity of blistering, and by family history.

Management
Patients with suspected epidermolysis bullosa should be referred for accurate diagnosis. The charity DebRA (www.debra.org.uk) will provide education, nursing input, and genetic testing for patients with all forms of epidermolysis bullosa.

Infantile acne

Clinical presentation
Infants present with papules, pustules, and comedones (blackheads and whiteheads) on the central cheeks. It usually occurs in boys aged 3–24 months (**2.31**).

Differential diagnosis
Eczema and impetigo can present with a red face, but comedones only occur in acne.

Management
Infantile acne tends to resolve by 5 years. Treatment may be needed to prevent scarring. Topical benzoyl peroxide, antibiotics, and retinoids can be used. Oral tetracyclines are contraindicated, but oral erythromycin may be helpful.

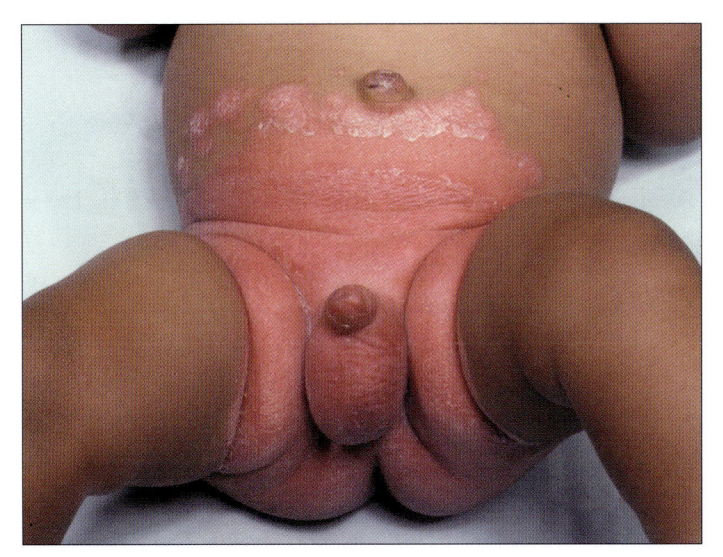

Paediatric dermatoses 27

2.26 Nappy psoriasis.

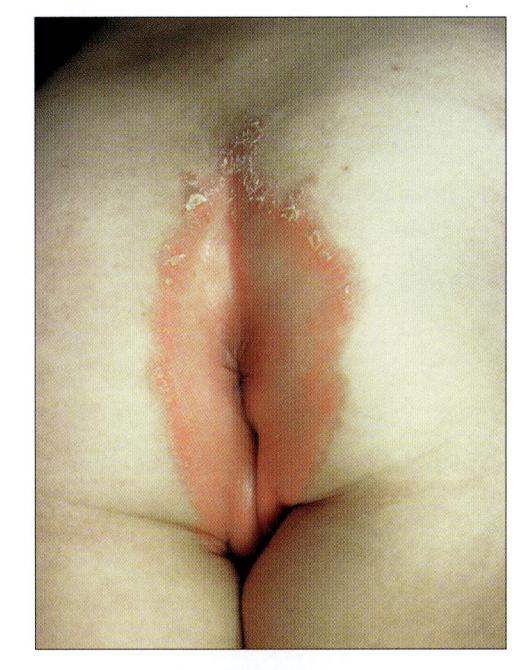

2.27 Perianal psoriasis.

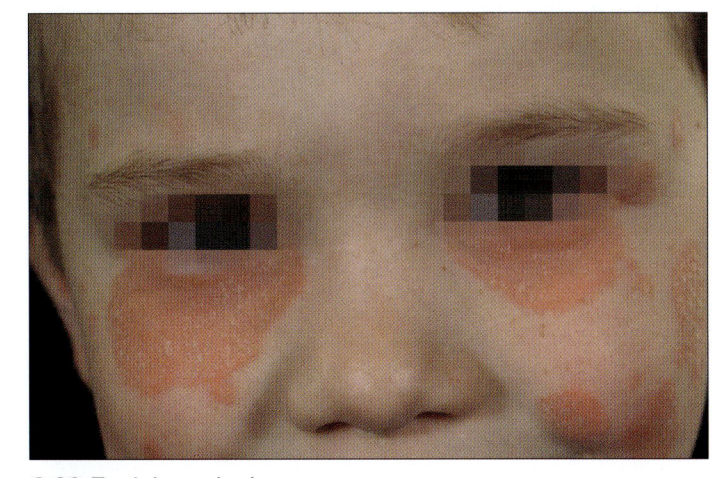

2.28 Facial psoriasis.

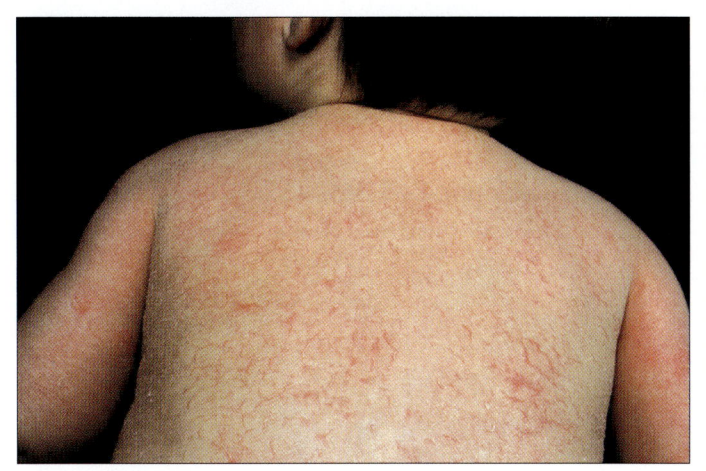

2.29 Ichthyosis vulgaris.

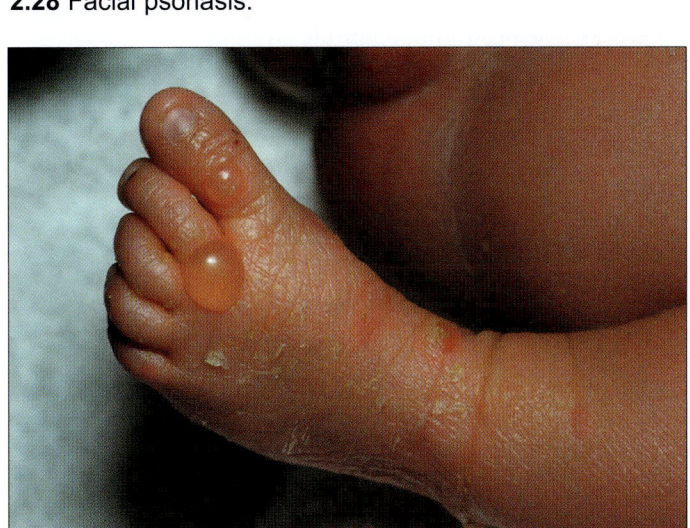

2.30 Epidermolysis bullosa simplex.

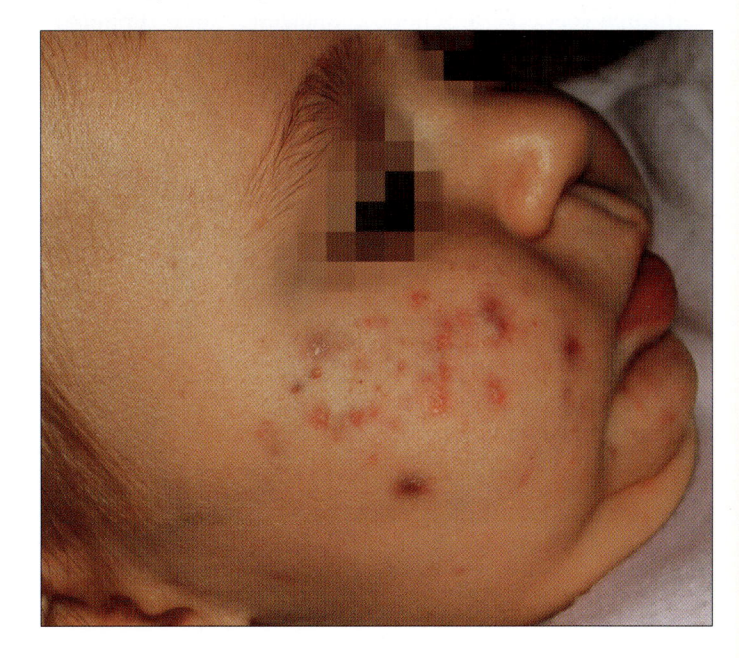

2.31 Infantile acne.

Childhood rashes

Toxic erythema
Clinical presentation
This is a term used to describe an acute, morbilliform, erythematous eruption due to drugs, virus, or bacteria (**2.32**). The child is often mildly unwell. Spontaneous resolution occurs over 1–2 weeks, followed by desquamation.

Differential diagnosis
Toxic erythema needs to be distinguished from specific dermatological diseases and viral infections.

Management
Simple emollients and antihistamines can give symptomatic relief. Suspected drugs should be stopped.

Staphylococcal scalded skin syndrome (SSSS)
Clinical presentation
SSSS is a serious but treatable, toxin mediated reaction to staphylococcal infection. Infants and young children present with sudden onset of fever, skin tenderness, and erythema with denudation or blistering of skin, often accentuated in the flexures (**2.33**).

Differential diagnosis
The main differential diagnosis is toxic epidermal necrosis which is a type of severe drug eruption.

Management
Antistaphylococcal antibiotics, analgesia, and supportive skin care should be given as a matter of urgency. Hospital admission is required in all but the mildest cases.

Henoch–Schönlein purpura (HSP)
Clinical presentation
A purpuric rash develops predominantly over the lower limbs and buttocks, most commonly in children aged 4–7 years (**2.34**). This is an allergic vasculitis, and may be precipitated by an upper respiratory tract infection. There may be associated abdominal or renal involvement. Most children have self-limiting disease over 4–6 weeks, but relapses can occur.

Differential diagnosis
HSP must be distinguished from meningococcal septicaemia

Management
Treatment consists of symptomatic relief and skin care. Systemic steroids are given if there is significant abdominal or renal involvement, but benefit is uncertain.

Pityriasis rosea
Clinical presentation
Pityriasis rosea consists of a rash of fine, scaly, pale pink plaques typically in a fir tree distribution over the trunk (**2.35**). A history of a single, 'herald' patch 1–2 weeks earlier can usually be obtained. Pityriasis rosea is probably due to an unidentified viral infection. It typically lasts 4–6 weeks before gradually resolving.

Differential diagnosis
Pityriasis rosea can mimic guttate psoriasis.

Management
No treatment is generally required.

Paediatric dermatoses 29

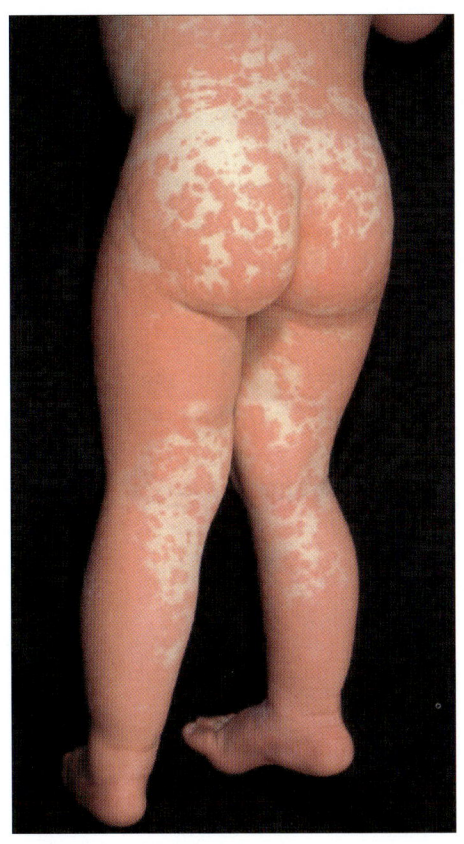

2.32 Toxic erythema.

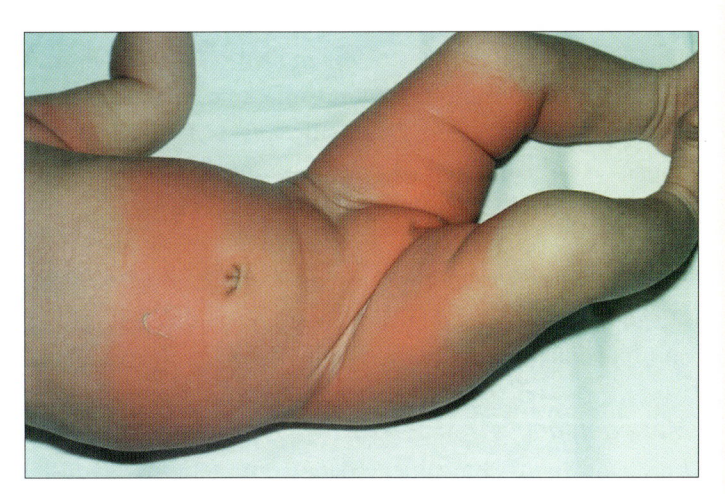

2.33 Staphylococcal scalded skin syndrome.

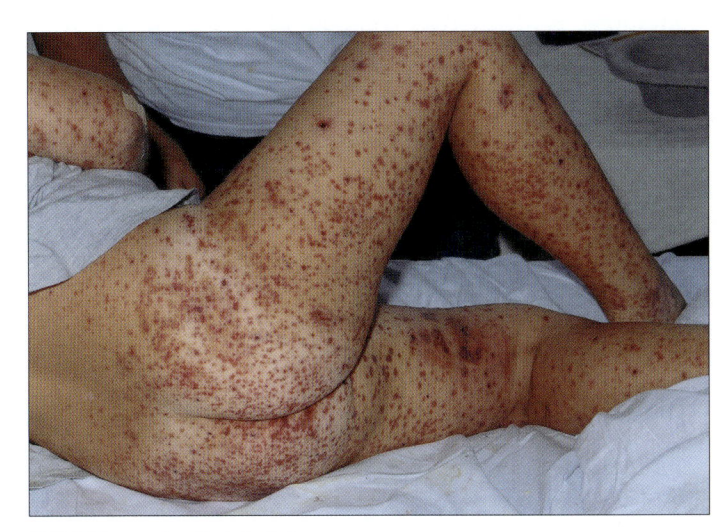

2.34 Henoch–Schönlein purpura.

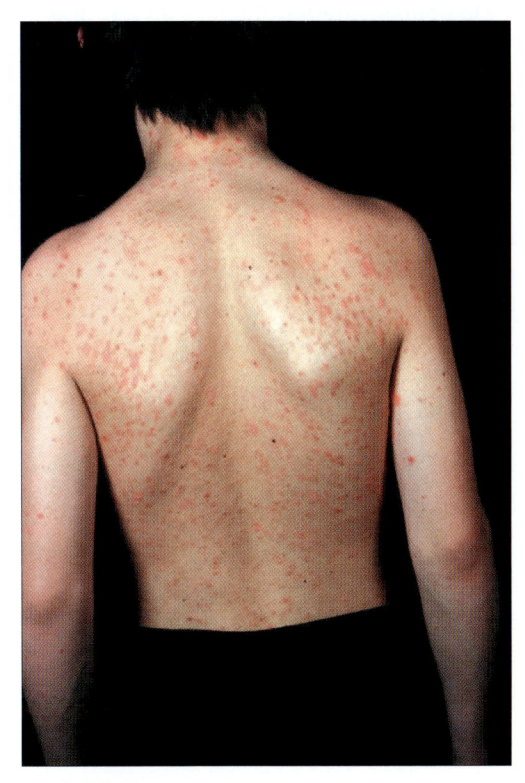

2.35 Pityriasis rosea.

Keratosis pilaris

Clinical presentation

This condition presents with rough skin on the upper arms due to follicular plugs of keratin, sometimes with associated erythema (**2.36**); it less frequently affects the cheeks and thighs. The condition is very common, often runs in families, and is frequently not noticed by patients.

Differential diagnosis

Diagnosis is usually straightforward from the distribution and follicular pattern.

Management

Frequently no treatment is required. The condition tends to improve in the summer and as the patient gets older. Emollients may make the skin feel smoother.

Vitiligo

Clinical presentation

Patients present with well-defined depigmented (white) nonscaly patches, often in a symmetrical pattern on the face, trunk, or limbs (**2.37**).

Differential diagnosis

Pityriasis versicolour (trunk) and pityriasis alba (face) have a scaly surface, and are less pale and well-defined. In postinflammatory hypopigmentation, there is a clear history of preceding inflammation. Naevus depigmentosum is a form of hypopigmented birthmark, which is stable throughout life.

Management

Vitiligo may remain stable, partially resolve, or progress over months to years. A trial of potent topical steroid is worthwhile in the early stages. Light therapy can be helpful. Referral should be offered for cosmetic camouflage.

Pityriasis alba

Clinical presentation

Multiple, poorly defined hypopigmented patches occur in this condition on the cheeks in children, often appearing after a sunny holiday (**2.38**).

Differential diagnosis

Pityriasis alba should be distinguished from vitiligo and postinflammatory hypopigmentation.

Management

Reassurance that the pigment will return to normal is usually sufficient. Sun protection may prevent recurrence.

Chronic bullous disease of childhood

Clinical presentation

Children present with groups of blisters, often occurring in rings on the face, trunk, and genitals, starting at age 3–5 years. The blisters are nonitchy. This is a rare, autoimmune condition.

Differential diagnosis

Blisters may occur in several skin conditions (*Table 2.1*). Diagnosis of chronic bullous disease of childhood can be confirmed by the appearance of a linear band of IgA on biopsy immunofluorescence. In the genetic group of conditions epidermolysis bullosa, blistering occurs from infancy at sites of trauma. In papular urticaria, a cluster of bites and blisters occur, which quickly heal. In dermatitis herpetiformis, blisters are intensely itchy, and occur on the extensor surfaces of limbs and buttocks, usually in older children or adults (**2.39**).

Management

Oral dapsone will usually control the blistering until it resolves spontaneously over a few years.

Paediatric dermatoses 31

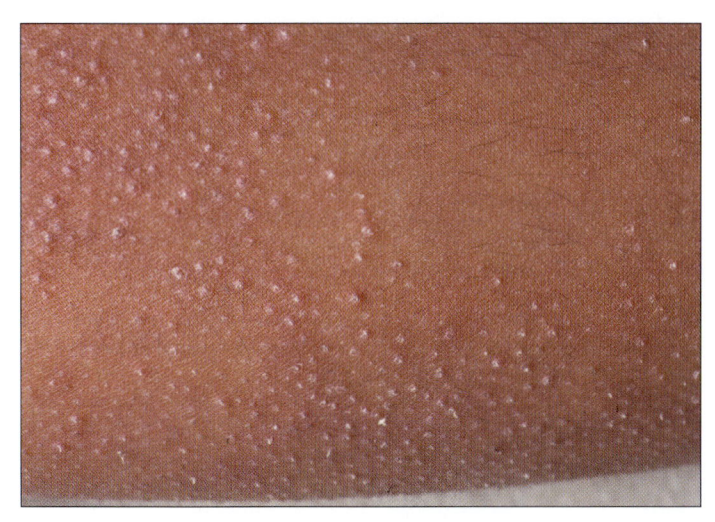

2.36 Keratosis pilaris.

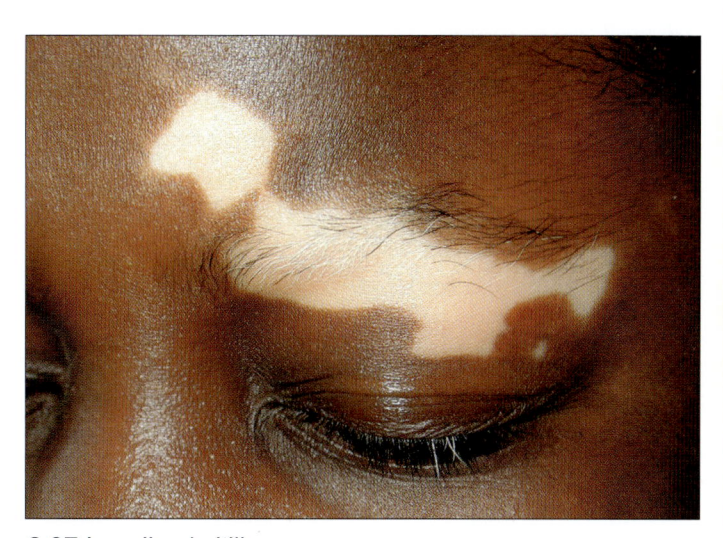

2.37 Localized vitiligo.

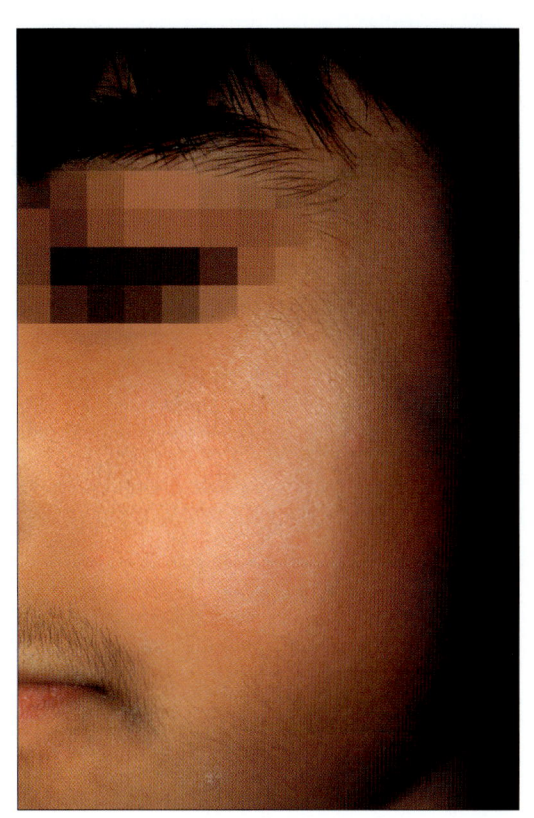

2.38 Pityriais alba.

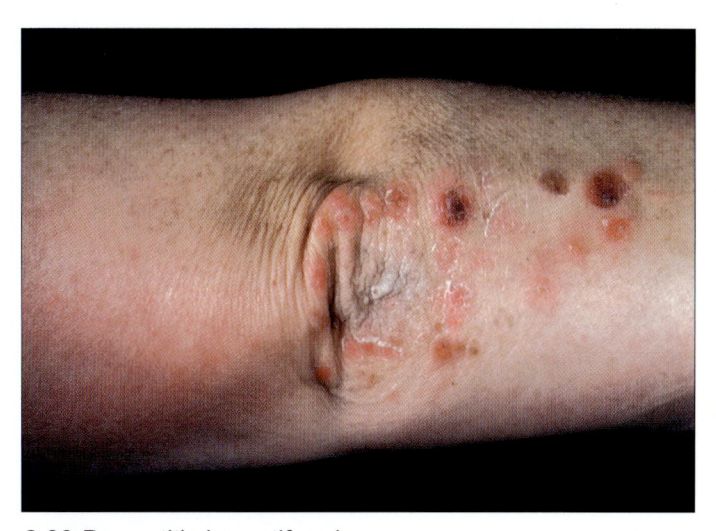

2.39 Dermatitis herpetiformis.

32 Paediatric dermatoses

Juvenile plantar dermatosis (JPD)
Clinical presentation
This is a common condition affecting prepubertal children. They complain of painful, itchy feet; examination shows glazed erythema, hyperkeratosis, and fissuring affecting the anterior third of the sole (**2.40**). The condition lasts months to years with intermittent flares.

Differential diagnosis
JPD should be differentiated from pitted keratolysis, which is a corynebacter infection causing maceration of the forefoot; tinea pedis, which is concentrated in the toe webs; and allergic contact dermatitis, which affects the whole sole.

Management
JPD is helped by reducing sweating with measures such as avoiding occlusive footwear, and wearing cotton socks. Emollients may give symptomatic relief.

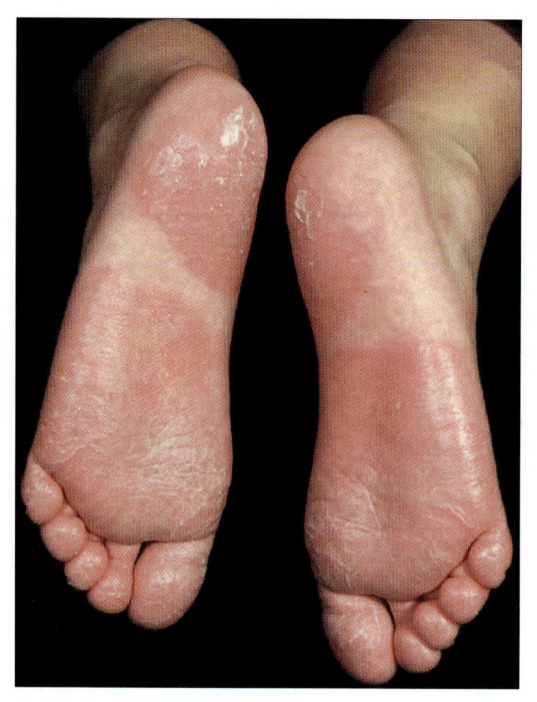

Striae
Clinical presentation
Adolescent children may develop linear, atrophic, purple/red striae on the lower back or inner thighs due to disruption of connective tissue during a period of rapid growth (**2.41**).

Striae may also be due to excess topical steroid use, or, very rarely, Cushing's disease or genetic connective tissue abnormalities.

Differential diagnosis
Appearance is characteristic.

Management
There is no effective treatment. Severe striae or atypical sites should be referred for exclusion of underlying disease.

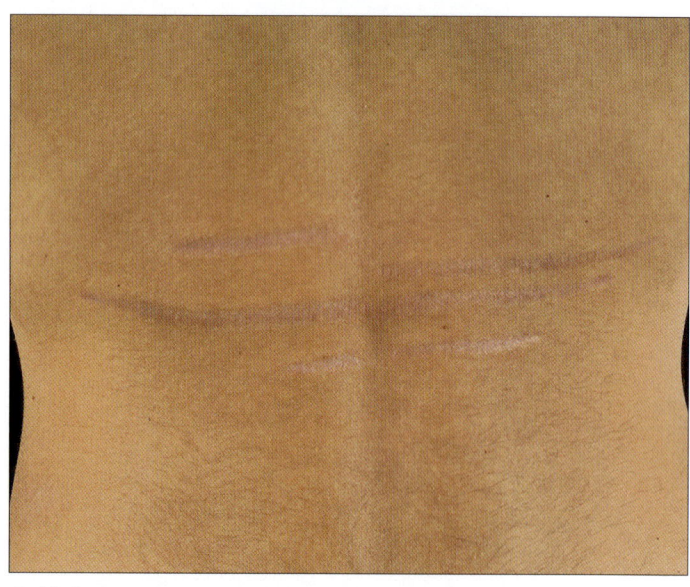

2.40 Juvenile plantar dermatosis.

2.41 Striae due to rapid growth in adolescence.

Further reading

Harper J, Oranje A, Prose N (eds) (2005). *Textbook of Paediatric Dermatology* (2nd edn). Blackwell Scientific, Oxford.

Spitz JL (2005). Genodermatoses. A Clinical Guide to Genetic Skin Disorders, 2nd edn. Lippincott Williams & Wilkins, Philadelphia.

Verbov J (1988). *Essential Paediatric Dermatology*. Clinical Press, Bristol.

Chapter 3

Widespread rashes

Georgina E Elston, MRCP and Graham A Johnston, FRCP

Introduction

In order to diagnose a rash correctly, a history and examination are necessary. An experienced dermatologist may be able to take one look at a rash and come up with a diagnosis but, for the less experienced, the history, distribution, configuration, and morphology of the rash will point to the correct diagnosis or differential.

Urticaria

Introduction

Urticaria is characterized by an acute eruption of recurring, pruritic papules and plaques (**3.1**). It is often self-limiting, but in many patients becomes chronic and relapsing where it can greatly impair quality of life.

Clinical presentation

An urticarial rash consists of weals: pruritic, raised, oedematous papules and plaques, usually erythematous with a pale centre. Scaling is always absent. An important clinical clue is that individual lesions appear on any part of the skin within a few minutes and will have resolved within 24 hours, although new lesions may be appearing elsewhere on the skin. Another clue to the diagnosis is if the patient is dermographic (although not demonstrable in all cases) (**3.2**). A firm, but gentle, scratch of the skin with an orange stick will produce a linear weal within 5–10 minutes. Rarely, the condition is associated with angio-oedema where there can be swelling of the lips, tongue, and around the eyes (**3.3**).

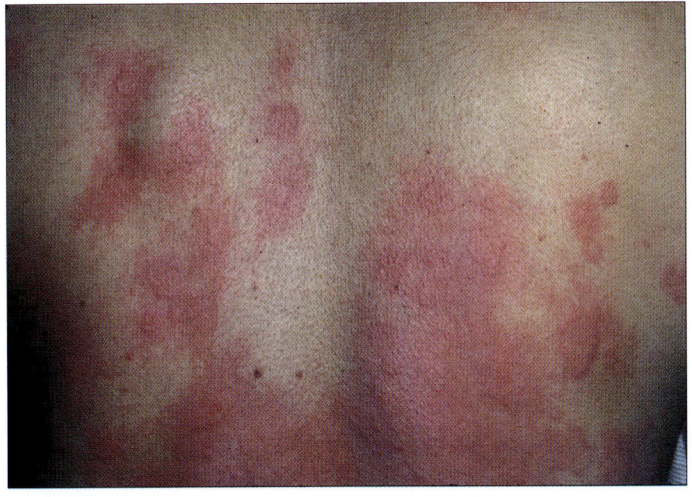

3.1 Chronic idiopathic urticaria on the back.

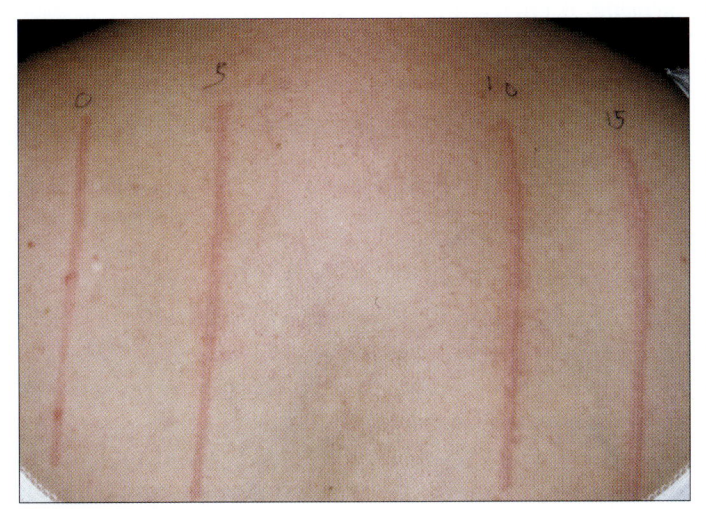

3.2 Dermographism.

34　Widespread rashes

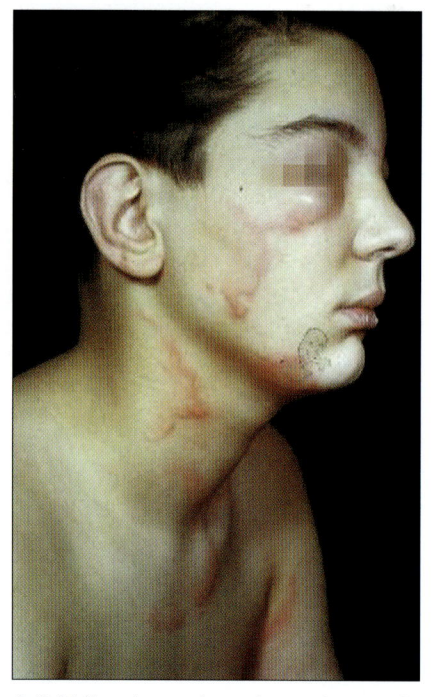

3.3 Urticaria and angio-oedema of the face.

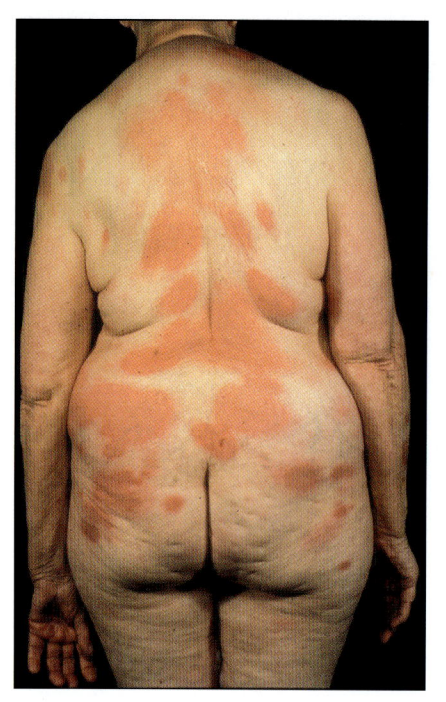

3.4 Fixed drug eruption from temazepam.

Histopathology
A biopsy is not usually indicated for diagnostic purposes, as the features are nonspecific, with oedema and a mixed dermal inflammatory infiltrate. However, histology can exclude the possibility of urticarial vasculitis.

Differential diagnosis
Drug reactions should be considered if there is a history of new drugs preceding the rash (**3.4**). In urticarial vasculitis, lesions persist for more than 24 hours and resolve with bruising. Contact urticaria should be considered if local applications of products preceded the rash (**3.5**). Papular urticaria is possible if there is a history of contact with mosquitoes, bed bugs, or fleas (are their pets scratching too?) (**3.6**, **3.7**).

Management
Acute urticaria, normally triggered by drugs, food, or infections has a good prognosis, resolving in less than 1 month. Treatment is symptomatic with high-dose antihistamines.

Chronic urticaria lasts longer than 6 weeks and may continue for many years in some cases. It is idiopathic in the vast majority of cases and investigations are not indicated. Again treatment is with single or combination high-dose

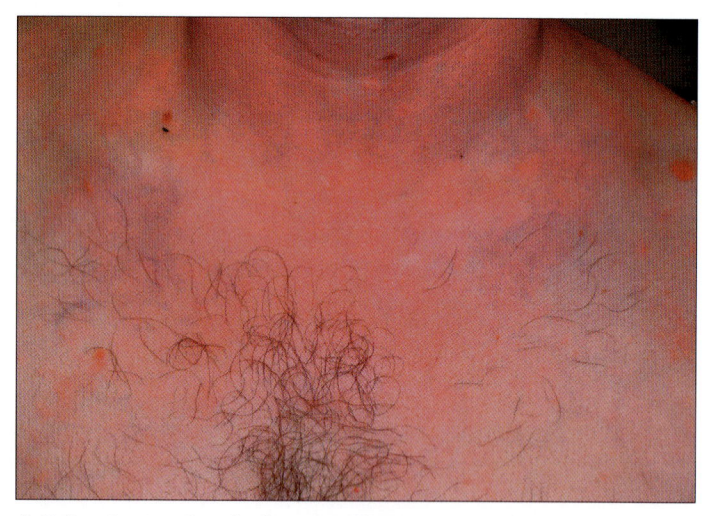

3.5 Contact urticaria from perfume.

antihistamines and avoidance of associated triggers (which may include pressure, sun exposure, and exercise, although there is usually no history of a trigger). Addition of H_2 blockers such as cimetidine as well as the tricyclic antidepressant doxepin can also be helpful.

Widespread rashes

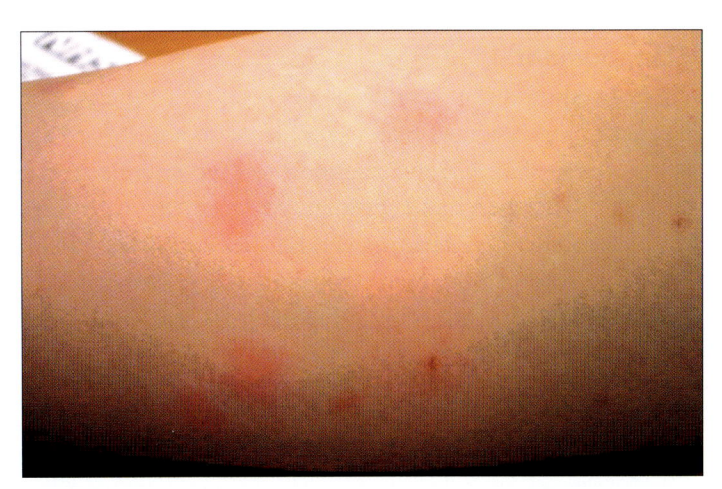

3.6 Papular urticaria on the arm. Note the close proximity of the lesions 'breakfast, lunch and tea' for the flea!

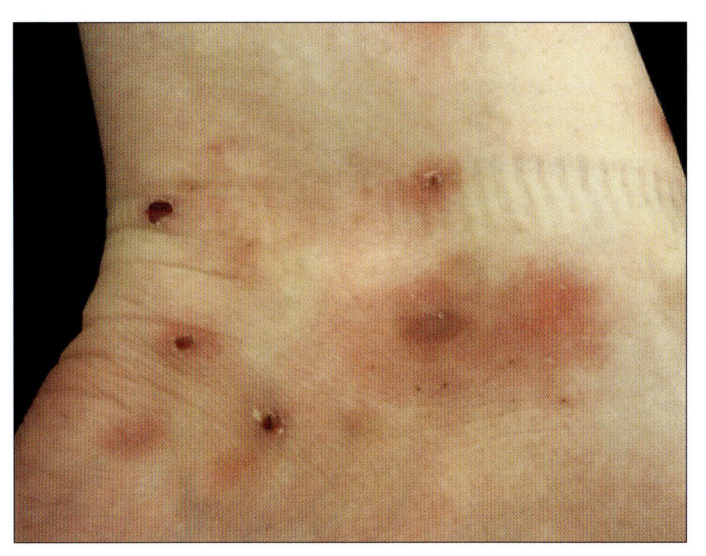

3.7 Excoriated papular urticarial lesions on the ankle.

Erythroderma

Introduction
Erythroderma is an acute and serious medical condition that can make patients feel shivery and unwell. Patients should be admitted to hospital for close monitoring and treatment.

Clinical presentation
Erythroderma simply means red skin with involvement of over 90% of the skin surface area. The skin is angry, inflamed, and hot to touch. Usually there is a surface scale, which may be fine or coarse (**3.8–3.10**). The skin is not always itchy. Patients become acutely unwell with fever,

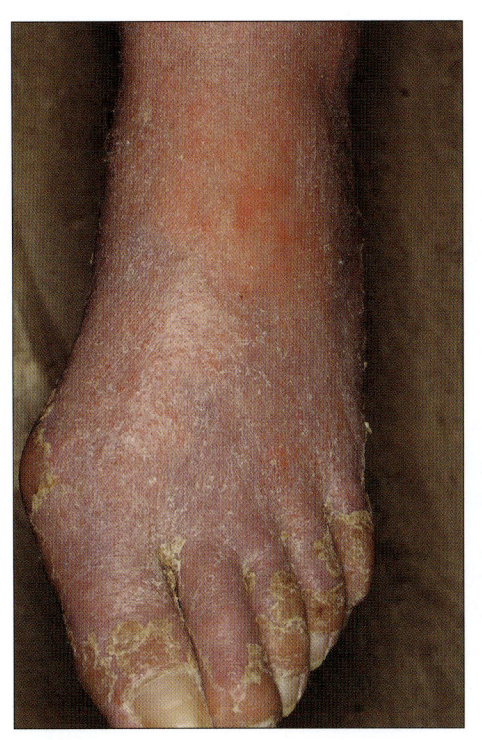

3.8 Erythrodermic cutaneous T-cell lymphoma (Sezary's syndrome).

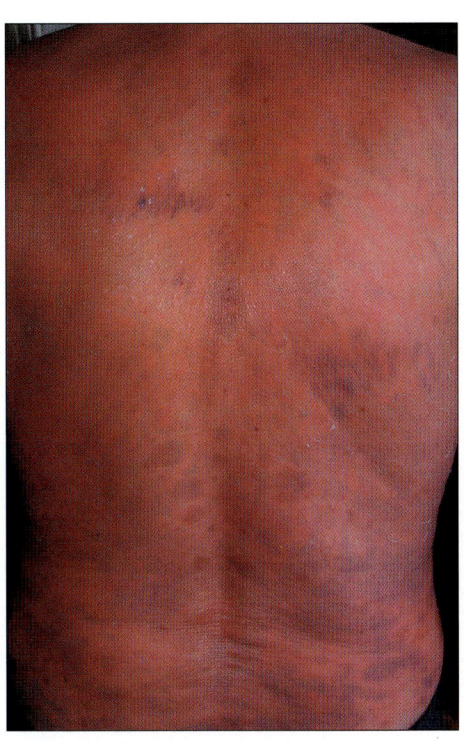

3.9 Erythrodermic psoriasis.

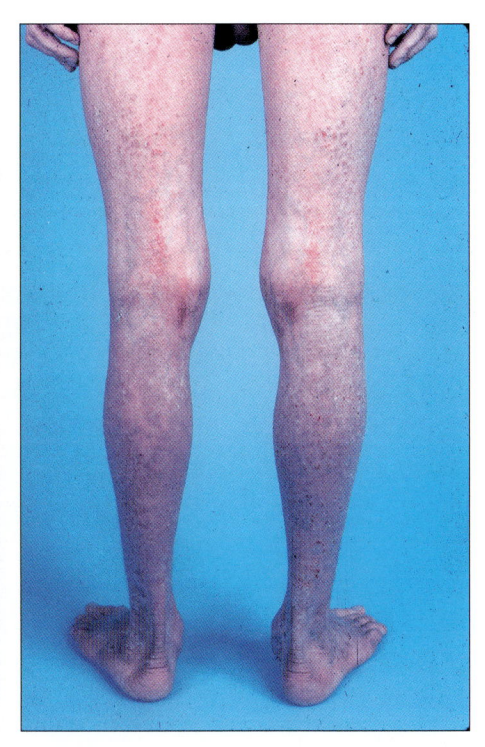

3.10 Erythrodermic atopic eczema.

36 Widespread rashes

shivering, malaise, and lethargy due to the considerable loss of heat, fluid, and protein from their inflamed skin. Palmo-plantar involvement is common, with hyperkeratosis and fissuring. Nails can exhibit onycholysis or may even shed. Hair loss can occur with scalp involvement. Patients become dehydrated and hypothermic as a result of insensible fluid loss from the skin. Peripheral oedema develops due to low albumin and high output cardiac failure. Lymphadenopathy may be found but should alert one to the possibility of cutaneous lymphoma.

Histopathology
A biopsy may be nonspecific in the early stages but can help differentiate psoriasis and eczema. The presence of eosinophils would lead to a careful inquiry about drugs including nonprescribed medication.

Differential diagnosis
There are four main causes of erythroderma:
- Psoriasis (**3.9**).
- Eczema (**3.10**).
- Drug reaction (**3.11**).
- Cutaneous lymphoma (mycosis fungoides) (**3.8**).

Less common causes include pityriasis rubra pilaris and seborrhoeic dermatitis. Clues to the cause include a pre-existing dermatosis or recent changes of medication. Consider lymph node biopsy and CT/MRI imaging if lymphoma is suspected.

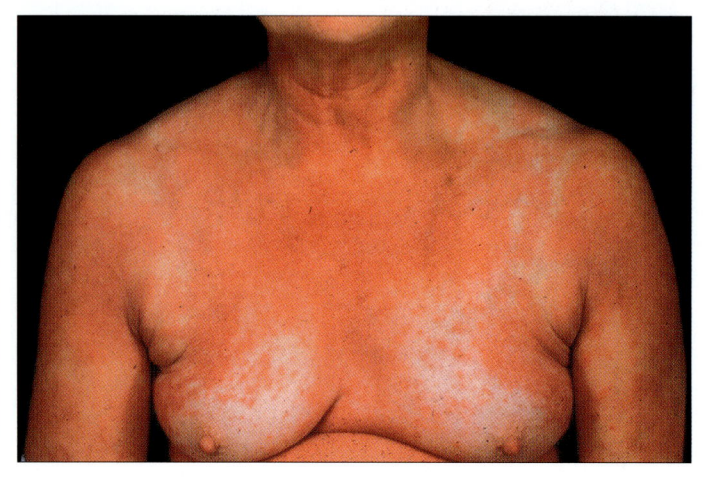

3.11 Erythrodermic drug reaction from prednisolone.

Management
Patients should be admitted to hospital. Liberal and frequent application of bland emollients should be applied to the whole skin. Careful attention to fluid and electrolyte balance is needed, and protein replacement with high calorie/protein supplements should be considered. This condition can be life threatening, particularly in the elderly, who may develop infections, hypothermia, and associated high output cardiac failure.

Atopic eczema

Introduction
Atopic eczema usually presents in childhood and settles spontaneously by the teenage years. In some patients atopic eczema persists into adult life or can start for the first time in adulthood. Asthma and hay fever are commonly associated with this condition or may be found in first-degree relatives.

Clinical presentation
The clinical features include generalized xerosis (dry skin) and red, itchy, patches and plaques of dry, scaly skin with overlying excoriations (**3.10, 3.12**). More chronic disease presents with thickening of the skin with accentuation of the surface markings (lichenification) (**3.12**). This is a consequence of continual scratching. In patients with darker skin there will also be hyperpigmentation at the site of the eczema. The distribution usually includes the popliteal and antecubital fossae but may involve any site (**3.12–3.14**). White dermographism is a clue to the diagnosis, being a white line produced after gentle scratching of the skin. Palmo-plantar involvement often presents with erythema, vesicles, scaling, and painful fissures.

Histopathology
Intercellular oedema (spongiosis) is the hallmark of eczema. Intraepidermal vesicles associated with a lymphocytic infiltrate are also seen. In more chronic disease, psoriasiform hyperplasia occurs.

Differential diagnosis
Seborrhoeic and discoid dermatitis need to be considered. Patch testing is helpful if the history is suggestive of allergic contact dermatitis. In scabies, which is often complicated by an infected eczema, look for the presence of burrows, particularly with genital involvement.

Management

Emollients should be applied regularly to the dry skin and used as soap substitutes. Topical steroids are the mainstay of treatment and the strength needed varies depending on the site, severity, and chronicity of the eczema. Ointments are preferable to creams in the majority of cases where the skin is dry and scaly. Calcinuerin inhibitors are useful alternatives to steroids for facial eczema. They should not be used if patients get recurrent herpes infections, and patients should avoid direct sunlight. Oral steroids are sometimes required for severe flares of eczema and are preferred in short courses.

Coal tar is now less commonly used but remains useful as it has anti-inflammatory properties and comes in the form of pastes, creams, bandages, shampoos, and bath additives. Bandaging is a useful way to intensify the effect of topical agents while preventing further damage by scratching. Sedative antihistamines can help patients to sleep at night but are best used intermittently. Cyclosporin is of proven use in severe chronic eczema but is only licensed for short-term use in the UK. Phototherapy can benefit patients when used in addition to other therapy, but the total lifetime dose is limited.

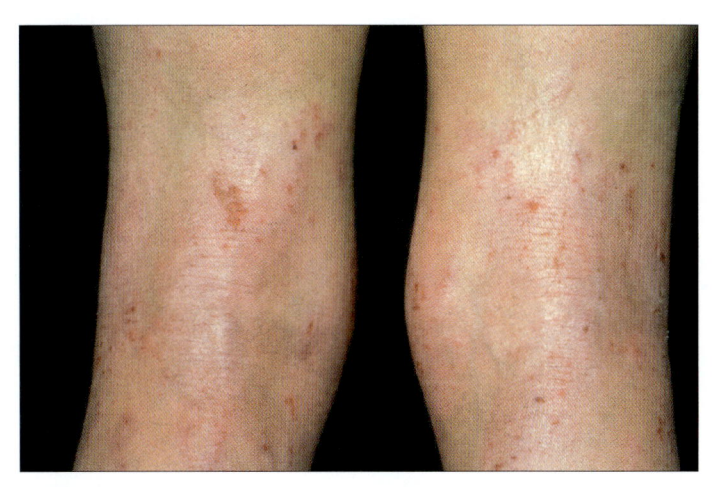

3.12 Flexural eczema in the popliteal fossae.

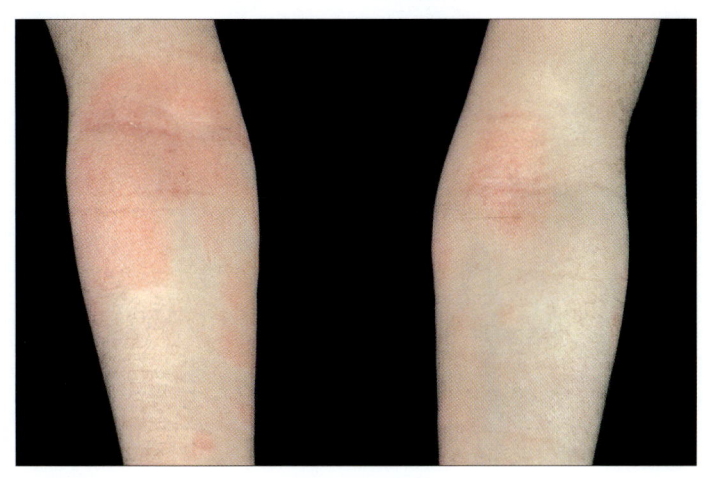

3.13 Flexural eczema in the cubital fossae.

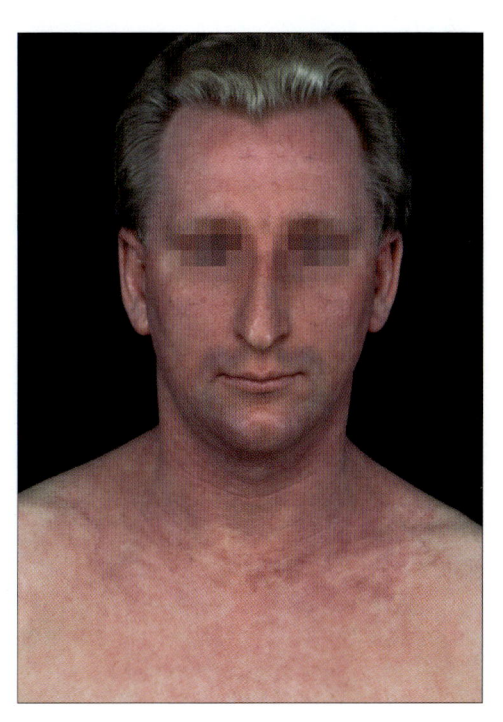

3.14 Facial atopic eczema.

Discoid eczema

Introduction
Discoid eczema is also known as nummular eczema, which simply describes the coin shaped plaques.

Clinical presentation
Intensely itchy, erythematous, dry, scaly, papules and vesicles coalesce into well-defined annular plaques, which can be several centimetres in diameter. Golden crusting due to secondary infection with *Staphylococcus aureus* is common (**3.15**). Lesions typically occur over the legs at first but may be scattered over the trunk, arms, and hands. Excoriations and lichenification may be evident. It is mainly seen in elderly males where it is not associated with atopy and IgE levels are usually normal. It is also seen in some young adults.

Histopathology
The typical eczematous feature, spongiosis, is seen with acanthosis of the epidermis.

Differential diagnosis
In psoriasis, scale predominates and vesicles are absent; look for clues at other sites such as nail changes or scalp involvement. In tinea corporis lesions are flatter with a fine scale. A skin scraping is often useful (**3.16**). In primary impetigo lesions are flat, superficial, and painful rather than itchy. A skin swab is helpful in guiding treatment (see Chapter 9).

Management
Discoid dermatitis is typically unresponsive to standard topical corticosteroids. A combination of super-potent steroid and antibiotic is often needed, and systemic steroids are sometimes required in widespread cases. It can run a chronic course.

3.15 Discoid eczema on the arms.

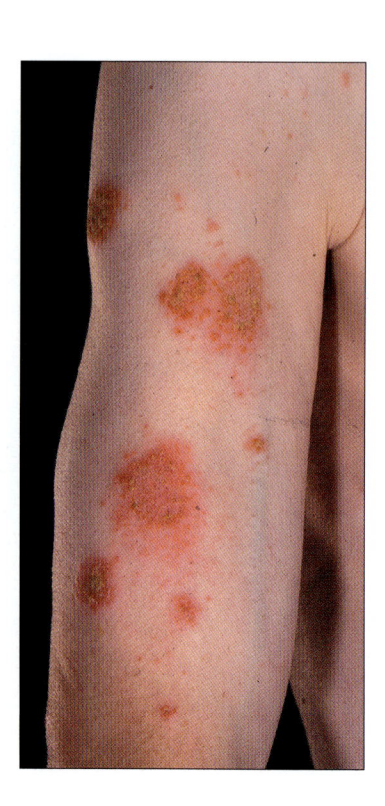

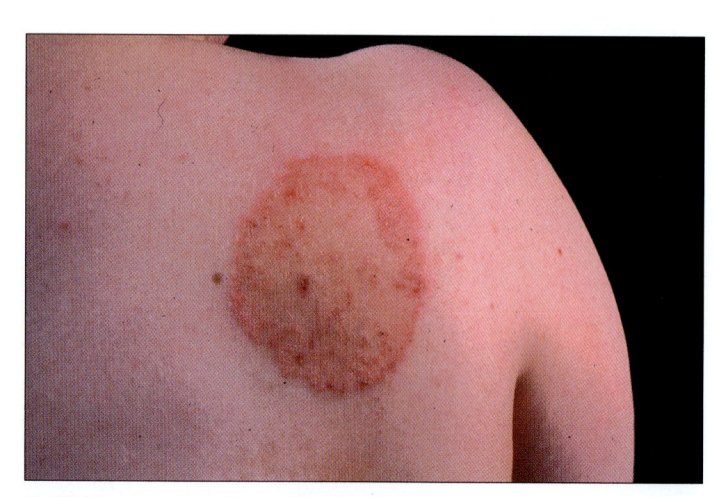

3.16 Tinea corporis on the back.

Psoriasis vulgaris

Introduction
Psoriasis is a chronic inflammatory condition affecting 2% of the population. It can have widespread involvement of the skin, nails, and joints and patients can feel very self-conscious about their appearance and constant scaling.

Clinical presentation
Psoriasis occurs in many guises. Chronic plaque psoriasis typically produces well-demarcated papules and plaques with a salmon-pink base and overlying silvery scale (**3.17**, **3.18**). The extensor aspects of the elbows and knees are frequently affected sites as well as the scalp and lower back (**3.19**, **3.20**). This common presentation is relatively easy to diagnose. However, psoriasis can affect other areas of the skin including face, palms and soles, flexor areas, and nails, all showing very different clinical features and making the correct diagnosis more challenging (**3.21**, **3.22**). The clinical features and possible differential diagnoses can be seen in

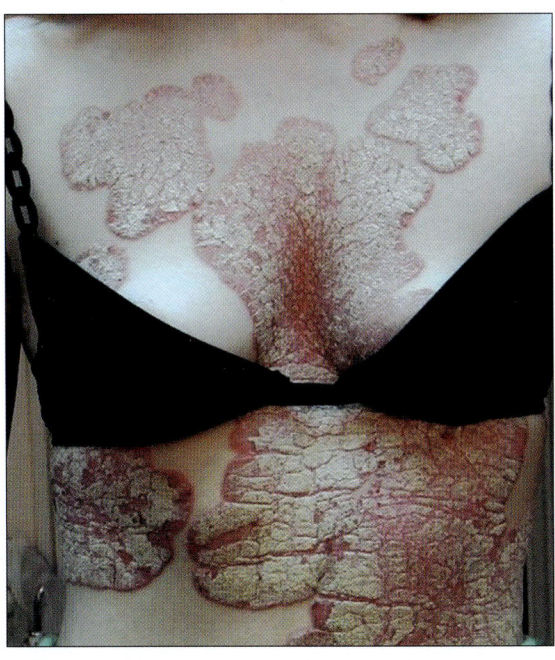

3.17 Chronic plaque psoriasis on the trunk.

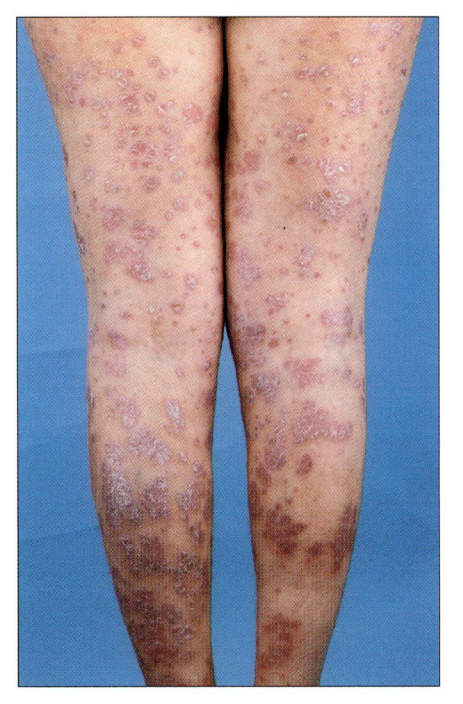

3.18 Widespread chronic plaque psoriasis on the legs.

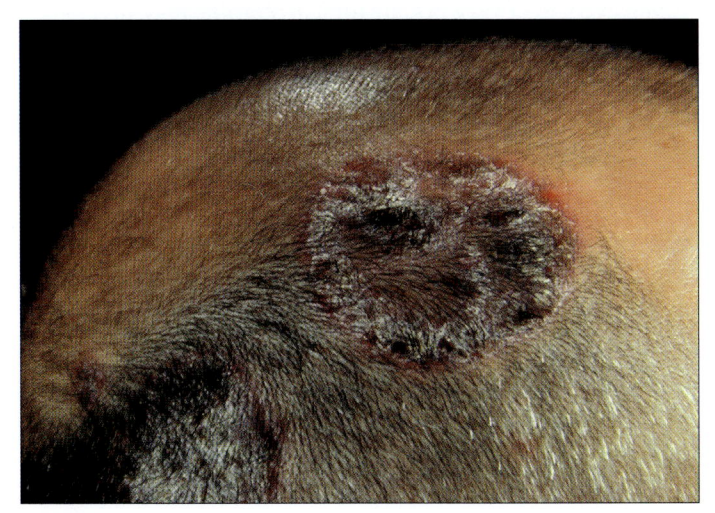

3.19 Scalp psoriasis.

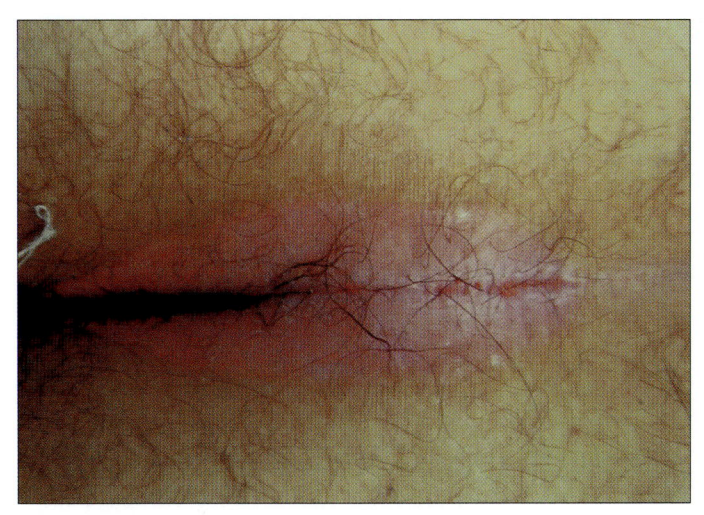

3.20 Perianal and natal cleft psoriasis.

40 Widespread rashes

3.21 Distal interphalangeal psoriatic arthritis. Notice the psoriatic nail changes.

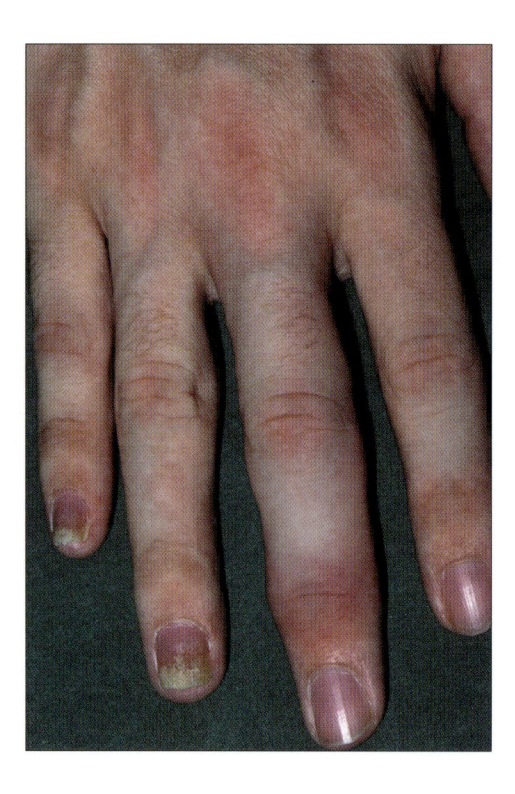

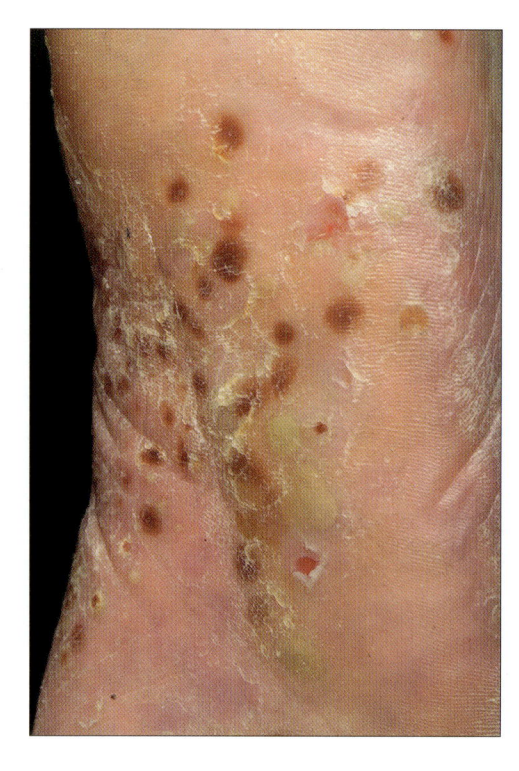

3.22 Localized pustular psoriasis of the sole of the foot.

Table 3.1. Clues to the diagnosis include a positive family history of psoriasis, scalp involvement, and nail changes.

Triggers known to exacerbate psoriasis include trauma (Koebner's phenomenon), streptococcal infections (especially in guttate psoriasis), stress, and drugs such as beta-blockers, lithium, antimalarials, nonsteroidal anti-inflammatory drugs, and ACE inhibitors. Roughly 5% of patients with psoriasis will develop an associated psoriatic arthropathy. There are five different types that may often overlap (*Table 3.2*).

Histopathology
In the epidermis, parakeratosis (nuclei retained in the stratum corneum) and acanthosis (thickening) are seen. Dilated capillary loops are seen in the elongated dermal papillae. A T-lymphocytic infiltrate in the upper dermis and epidermis forms microabscesses (of Munro) in the stratum corneum.

Differential diagnosis
Differential diagnoses are listed in *Table 3.1*.

Management
Topical treatments
Emollients are safe and easy to use. They can sooth and hydrate the skin and may have an antiproliferative effect in psoriasis. They remain an important treatment in all types of psoriasis including erythroderma.

Vitamin D analogues are mainly used for chronic plaque psoriasis. They can irritate the skin and should therefore not be used in more inflammatory disease. The creams and ointments do not stain skin or clothes and do not smell, making this a more acceptable treatment to patients.

Mild to moderate topical steroids can be used on flexural and facial areas. Moderate to potent steroids can be used on affected areas of the trunk and limbs. Very potent steroids should be limited to areas on the palms, soles, and scalp. Extensive use of very potent topical steroids may precipitate acute generalized pustular psoriasis. Systemic steroids should be avoided altogether as they may produce a rebound phenomenon on reducing or stopping treatment.

Dithranol is an effective treatment but can stain skin and clothing. Low concentrations of 0.1% are used initially as it can be an irritant to the skin. Increasing concentrations are used every few days as tolerated. A short-contact preparation is available for patients to use at home.

Coal tar preparations have anti-inflammatory properties and also reduce the scale of psoriasis. Preparations can be made in concentrations from 1–10%. The treatment is messy and smelly and is generally applied under bandages although some 'cleaner' preparations are available which are more practical for home use.

Table 3.1 Clinical features and differential diagnoses of psoriasis

	Clinical features	Differential diagnosis
Plaque psoriasis	Bilateral, relatively symmetrical involvement commonly affecting the extensor aspects of elbows, knees, sacrum, and umbilicus. Involvement on any other area may also occur	Lichen simplex chronicus; tinea corporis; discoid eczema; mycosis fungoides
Guttate psoriasis	Disseminated small round papules appear over the body, often precipitated by a streptococcal tonsillitis	Pityriasis rosea; secondary syphilis
Flexural psoriasis	Red shiny, nonscaly well-defined plaques in the axillae, groins, submammary, perineal, and natal cleft areas. Fissures can be seen deep in the skin folds	Candida; intertrigo; tinea cruris; erythrasma
Palmo-plantar psoriasis	Acral involvement can be very difficult to differentiate from eczema with scaling, erythema, and fissures. Vesicles are absent in psoriasis	Palmo-plantar dermatitis; palmo-plantar keratoderma
Scalp psoriasis	There can be diffuse involvement of the scalp or discrete red plaques with a thick adherent scale	Seborrhoeic dermatitis; scalp eczema; lichen simplex chronicus
Psoriatic nails	Pitting, onycholysis (separation of the nail from the nail bed), hyperkeratosis, and oil spot (yellow-brown spot seen under the nail plate) may be seen	Tinea unguium; yeast infection of nail plate
Pustular psoriasis	This may be localized (e.g. to the palms and soles [3.22]) or may be generalized – von Zumbusch. Multiple sterile pustules occur in waves. Patients are often very unwell with a fever and are prone to dehydration, hypothermia, and sepsis, which may prove fatal	Pustular drug eruption; folliculitis; bullous impetigo
Erythrodermic psoriasis	Erythematous skin involving the majority of the skin. Patients can also be unwell with loss of heat, protein, and fluids from the inflamed skin	Causes of erythroderma such as: eczema; drug reaction; cutaneous lymphoma

Keratolytics such as salicylic acid can be helpful, particularly for thick scaly scalps, palms, or soles. Tazarotene is a topical retinoid. This can irritate the skin, especially the flexures, and should be avoided in pregnancy.

Systemic treatments

Systemic treatments should be reserved for severe, resistant, complicated, and unstable psoriasis. Phototherapy can be useful for extensive disease including guttate psoriasis but does not help genital or scalp psoriasis. Ultraviolet B (UVB) lamps are used to irradiate the skin several times a week and produce a response that can often be prolonged. PUVA (ultraviolet A light with oral psoralen) enhances the therapeutic effect of the radiation. Due to the increased risks of skin cancer, the total amount of phototherapy used in a patient's lifetime is limited. Other side-effects include burning, tanning, and ageing of the skin.

Methotrexate is an effective and relatively safe treatment. Once established on treatment patients can continue for many years. Side-effects include myelosuppression,

Table 3.2 Types of psoriatic arthritis

Type	Clinical features
Distal interphalangeal joint involvement (3.21)	Predominantly the distal interphalangeal joints are affected
Mono- or oligoarthropathy	The commonest form associated with psoriasis – asymmetrical
Rheumatoid arthritis-like	A symmetrical polyarthritis as seen in rheumatoid arthritis but the patient is seronegative
Ankylosing spondylitis-like	May involve spine and/or sacroiliac joints, with or without peripheral arthropathy
Arthritis mutilans	A rare and destructive arthritis with telescoping of the fingers and toes due to gross osteolysis

hepatotoxicity, and teratogenicity. Both male and female patients should use adequate contraception during, and for 6 months after treatment. Regular monitoring of full blood count, liver function tests, and urea and electrolytes should take place throughout treatment. Liver biopsy should be considered after a total cumulative dose of 1.5 g has been taken, to rule out liver fibrosis.

Cyclosporin is highly effective with a swift onset of action but long-term use is limited due to its nephrotoxicity. Regular monitoring of serum creatinine is required. Other side-effects include hypertension, which should be monitored, and there is an increased risk of developing lymphoma with prolonged treatment.

Acitretin is a systemic retinoid and must therefore not be used in pregnancy. Its teratogenic risk persists up to 2 years after stopping treatment and so is not the treatment of choice in women of childbearing age. It flattens down psoriatic plaques particularly when used in conjunction with PUVA. Common side-effects include dry lips and hair thinning. Less commonly, serum triglycerides may become raised. These should be monitored along with renal and liver function.

Fumaric acid esters are licensed for use outside the UK. They are indicated in severe chronic stable plaque psoriasis. Side-effects include abdominal cramps and diarrhoea along with flushing and headaches. These are dose-dependent. Lymphopenia is commonly seen and treatment should be reduced or withdrawn if levels are less than $0.5 \times 10^9/l$. Hepatotoxicity and nephrotoxicity have been reported.

Scabies

Introduction

Scabies is an intensely itchy dermatosis caused by the mite *Sarcoptes scabiei*. The infestation occurs at all ages, but particularly in children. Scabies is highly contagious and person-to-person spread occurs via direct contact with the skin. Scabies is transmitted by close personal contact. Infants and children are therefore particularly liable to infection. Outbreaks can occur among the elderly in nursing homes and can be transmitted to nursing staff. Transmission between adults is often by sexual contact.

Clinical presentation

A history of itching in several members of the family over the same period is almost pathognomonic. Pruritus is the hallmark of scabies, regardless of age. In adults, scabies is characterized by intractable pruritus (worse at night) and with lesions in the web spaces, fingers, flexor surfaces of the wrists, and genital areas. The most common presenting lesions are papules, vesicles, pustules, and nodules. The pathognomonic sign is the burrow; a short, wavy, scaly, grey line on the skin surface. These burrows are most easily found on the hands and feet, particularly in the finger web spaces, thenar and hypothenar eminences, and on the wrists (3.23–3.25). In men, itchy papules on the scrotum and penis are pathognomonic. Definitive diagnosis relies on microscopic identification of mites or eggs from skin scrapings of a burrow.

Management

Permethrin 5% dermal cream is the treatment of choice for scabies in the UK, Australia, and the USA. It is the most effective topical agent, is well tolerated, and has low toxicity. Malathion should be used as second choice. Children should be given aqueous preparations because alcoholic lotions sting and can cause wheeze. Lindane is less effective than permethrin. It has been withdrawn in many countries because of reports of aplastic anaemia and concerns about potential neurotoxicity. Benzyl benzoate is irritant and should not be used in children. Treatment of contacts should take place on the same days as treatment of the patient to avoid reinfection.

After successful treatment to kill the scabies mite, itching can persist for up to 6 weeks as the eczematous reaction settles down. Patients can be treated as for regular eczema with emollients and topical steroids with or without topical antibiotics, depending on the clinical presence of secondary infection with *Staphylococcus aureus*.

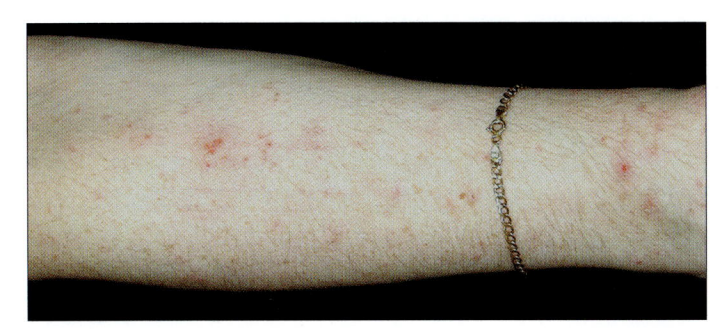

3.23 Scabies rash on the forearm.

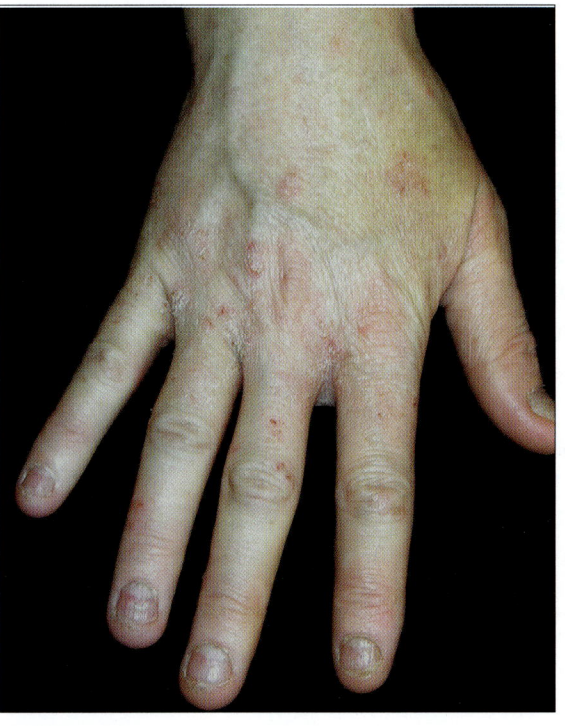

3.24 Scabies rash on the back of the hand with burrows visible in the finger webs.

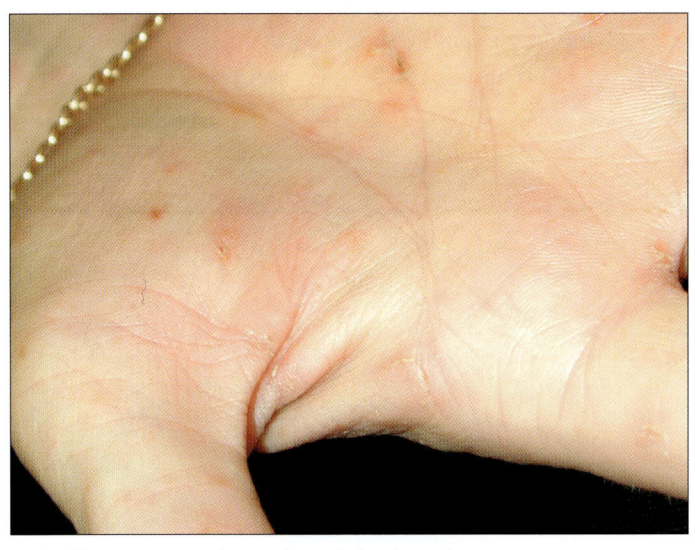

3.25 Burrows on the palm of the hand.

Erythema multiforme

Introduction
Erythema multiforme (EM) is an acute, self-limiting mucocutaneous disorder of variable severity and is commonest in adolescents and young adults. It is usually divided into major and minor forms. Classically, all forms of EM are thought to represent different points in a spectrum of disease severity and are simply divided into minor and major depending on whether there is mucosal involvement, when the eponym Stevens–Johnson syndrome is used.

Clinical presentation
The minor form classically presents with indurated annular lesions with central clearing (target lesions) on the palms and soles but these may occur at any site (**3.26, 3.27**). This often develops following an infectious illness and presents little diagnostic difficulty in adults. Lesions appear over 7–14 days and resolve spontaneously. The development of lesions at the site of prior trauma to the skin (the isomorphic phenomenon) is well recognized.

The major form implies more extensive skin involvement and lesions can coalesce with development of central blisters. Mucosal involvement occurs and conjunctival involvement may lead to keratitis and corneal ulceration. In EM major pulmonary symptoms, often with X-ray changes, are common. These may be attributed to an antecedent upper respiratory tract infection, typically *Mycoplasma pneumoniae*.

The two main causes are drugs (including sulphonamides, allopurinol, and phenytoin), and infection, particularly herpes simplex and mycoplasma. Frequently no cause is identified. Recurrent EM suggests recurrent infection with herpes simplex.

Histopathology
Typical histological changes include variable degrees of a perivascular lymphohistiocytic inflammatory infiltrate, dermal oedema, and basal cell vacuolation, which can be very marked, together with keratinocyte necrosis.

Differential diagnosis
Target lesions are characteristic of EM. Among the differential diagnoses to be considered are: bullous impetigo (see Chapter 9); primary herpes simplex infection (see Chapter 9); immuno-bullous disorders (**3.28, 3.29**); and cutaneous lupus (see Chapter 6).

Bullous impetigo can be identified by a positive microbacterial swab. Herpes simplex virus (HSV) *per se* or as an antecedent trigger for the development of EM is an important differential diagnosis. If mucosae are involved, then immunobullous disorders such as pemphigus vulgaris or mucous membrane pemphigoid should be considered. Immunobullous disorders can be excluded by histopathological examination, plus direct immunofluorescence, and the presence of circulating anti-epidermal antibodies. Lupus is excluded not only histologically but, more importantly, by the absence of antinuclear antibodies and antibodies to the extractable nuclear antigens.

Management
EM is a self-limiting condition and simply needs treating symptomatically. Eye involvement should prompt a referral to ophthalmology. If the condition becomes recurrent secondary to recurrent HSV, then long-term prophylactic aciclovir could be used.

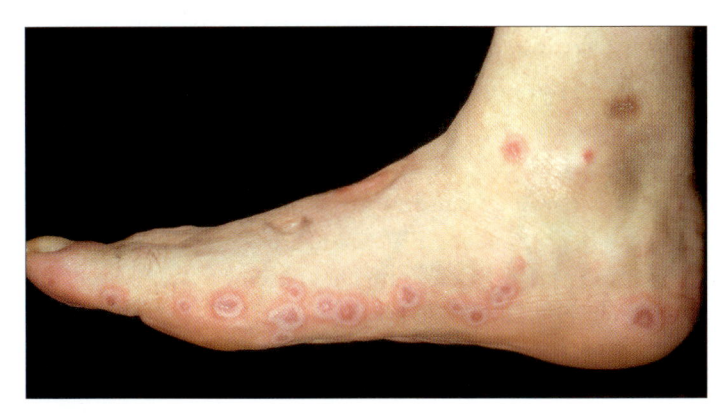

3.26 Erythema multiforme on the foot.

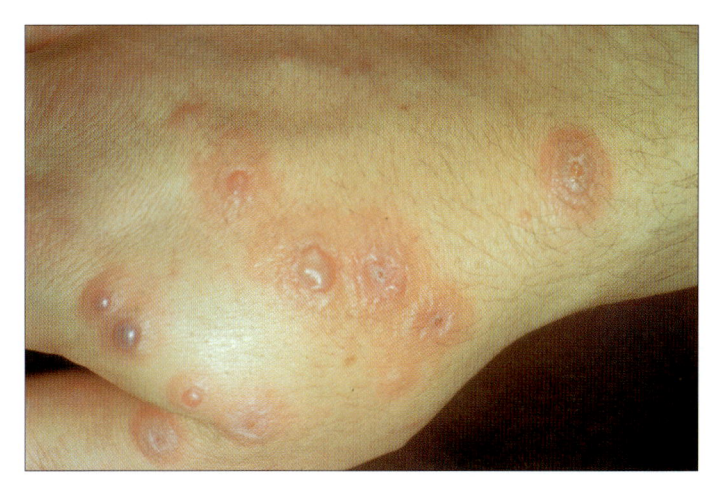

3.27 Erythema multiforme on the hand.

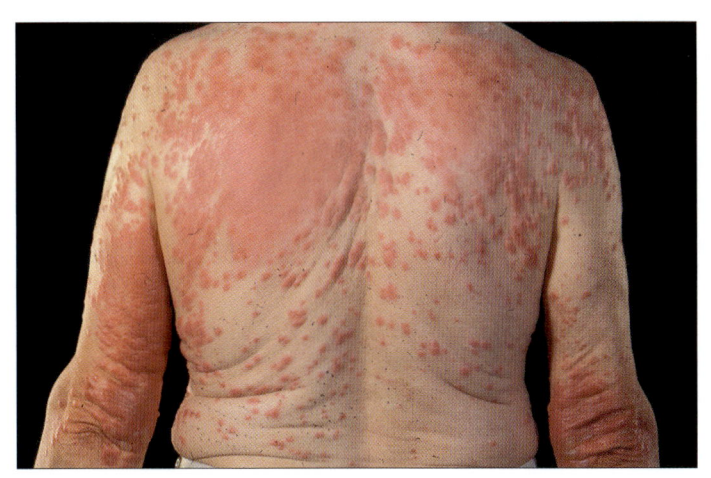

3.28 Widespread bullous pemphigoid on the trunk and arms.

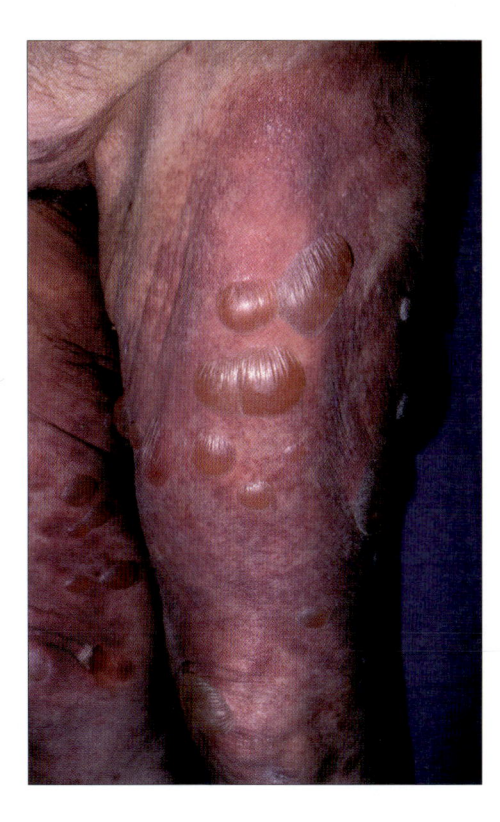

3.29 Bullous pemphigoid on the thigh.

Further reading

Johnston GA (2004). Treatment of bullous impetigo and the staphylococcal scalded skin syndrome in infants. *Expert Rev Anti Infect Ther* **2**:439–446.

Johnston GA, Sladden MJ (2005). Scabies: diagnosis and treatment. *BMJ* **331**:619–622.

Lebwohl MG, Berth-Jones J, Coulson IM, Heymann W (eds) (2006). *Treatment of Skin Disease: Therapeutic Strategies for the Dermatologist.* (2nd edn). Mosby, London.

Sladden MJ, Johnston GA (2004). Common skin infections in children. *BMJ* **329**:95–99.

Sladden MJ, Johnston GA (2005). Current options for the treatment of impetigo in children. *Expert Opin Pharmacother* **6**:2245–2256.

Wakelin SH (2002). *Handbook of Systemic Drug Treatment in Dermatology.* Manson Publishing, London.

Walker GJA, Johnstone PW (2000). Interventions for treating scabies. Cochrane Database of Systematic Reviews **3**:CD000320. DOI:10.1002/14651858.CD000320.

Chapter 4

Skin tumours

Vishal Madan, MBBS, MD, MRCP and John T Lear, MD, MRCP

Introduction

Tumours in the skin can be conveniently divided into benign or malignant. Recognition of which group a particular tumour falls into is paramount. Benign tumours tend to be slow growing, symmetrical lesions (**4.1**) whereas malignant ones usually grow faster and keep growing and will expand in a haphazard manner, so will often be asymmetrical (**4.2**). The history and the ABCDE system (Chapter 1) of examining tumours will help in making a diagnosis.

Nonmelanoma skin cancers

Nonmelanoma skin cancers (NMSC), which include basal (BCC) and squamous cell cancers (SCC), are the most common human cancers. Because of their relatively low metastatic rate and relatively slow growth, these are frequently underreported. The high prevalence and the frequent occurrence of multiple primary tumours in affected individuals make NMSCs an important but underestimated public health problem.

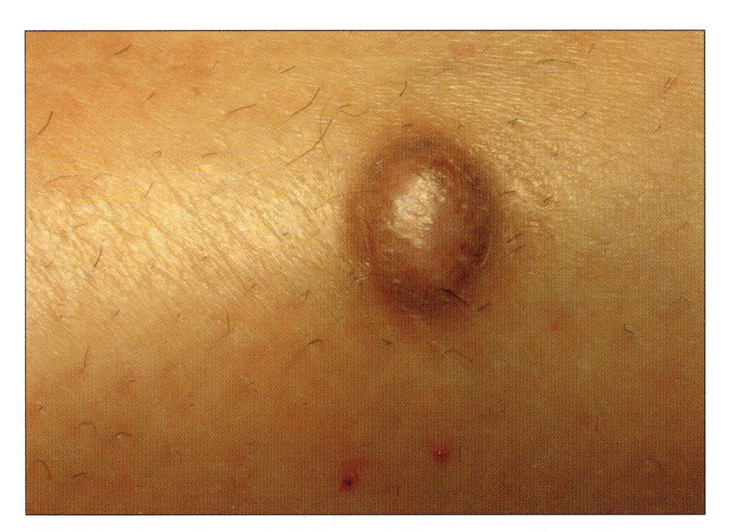

4.1 A benign pigmented dermatofibroma on the shin.

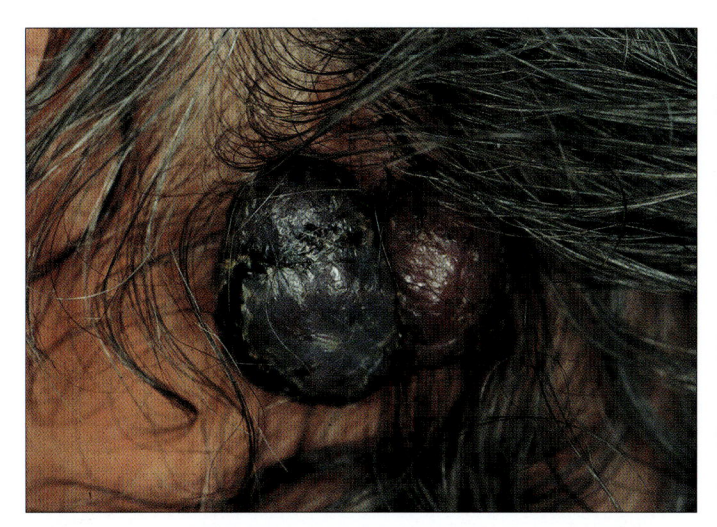

4.2 Nodular melanoma of the scalp. This was a rapidly growing tumour that was asymmetrical and ulcerating and had a very poor prognosis.

Skin tumours

The recognition of premalignant skin lesions and conditions is important, as early treatment may allow prevention of the malignant process. It may also allow for these lesions and conditions to be followed carefully and any malignancy that develops may be recognized and treated at an early stage. This chapter deals with such premalignant skin lesions and conditions and the tumours that may develop if these are left undiagnosed or untreated.

Actinic (solar) keratosis

Introduction
These are focal areas of abnormal proliferation and differentiation occurring on chronically ultraviolet (UV) irradiated skin, and appear as circumscribed, hyperkeratotic lesions carrying a variable but low (0.025–16%) risk of progression to invasive SCC[1]. Their presence is an important indicator of excessive UV exposure and increased risk of NMSC.

Risk factors for the development of actinic keratoses include excessive (lifetime) exposure to UV or ionizing radiation, radiant heat or tanning beds in individuals with fair skin, blond hair, and blue eyes, low latitude, working outdoors, light skin, history of sunburn, immunosuppressive therapy for cancers, inflammatory disorders, and organ recipients[2].

Clinical presentation
The lesions are asymptomatic papules or macules with a dry, rough, adherent yellow or brownish scaly surface (4.3, 4.4) that are better recognized by palpation than by inspection. Diagnosis is usually made clinically. The lesional size varies from 1 mm to over 2 cm and the usual sites of involvement are the sun-exposed sites such as the face, scalp, and dorsa of hands of middle-aged or elderly patients. Left untreated, these lesions often persist but regression may follow irritation of the individual lesion.

Differential diagnosis
Differentiation from early SCC may sometimes be difficult, especially for smaller lesions. Other differentials include viral warts, seborrhoeic keratoses, and discoid lupus erythematosus.

Management
Sun avoidance and sunscreen use should be advised. For limited numbers of superficial lesions, cryotherapy is the treatment of choice and gives excellent cosmetic results. If the clinical diagnosis is doubtful, larger lesions can be curetted and the specimen can be assessed histopathologically. Excision is usually not required except where diagnostic uncertainty exists.

Topical treatments with 5-fluorouracil cream, diclofenac gel and imiquimod cream[3] offer the benefit of treating early lesions and those covering large areas, but with a varying degree of erythema and inflammation. Topical 6-aminolevulinic acid-based photodynamic therapy, chemical peels, cryotherapy, and dermabrasion are other techniques used in the treatment of actinic keratoses.

4.3 Multiple keratotic lesions on the back of the hands and forearms. Most were actinic keratoses and the larger lesions were intraepithelial carcinomas.

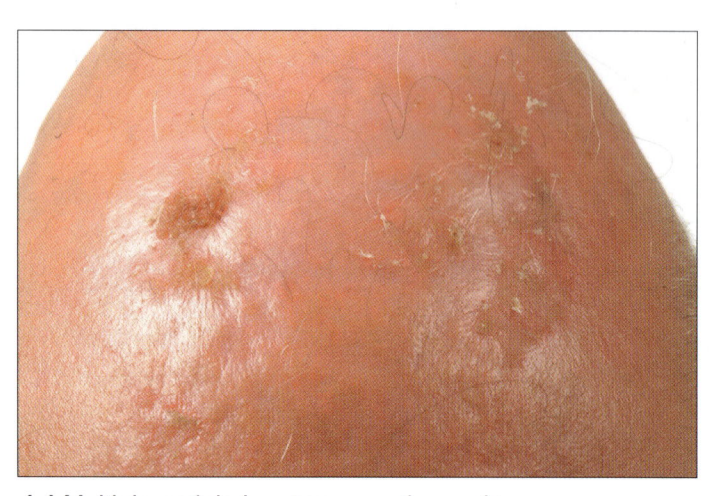

4.4 Multiple actinic keratoses on the scalp.

Intraepithelial carcinomas (IEC, Bowen's disease)

Introduction
Also known as squamous cell carcinoma *in situ*, these are usually solitary, slowly enlarging erythematous lesions on sun-exposed and nonexposed sites, with a small potential for invasive malignancy. UV irradiation is an important cause, especially in white populations. Arsenic exposure (ingestion of trivalent inorganic arsenic) seems important in the development of lesions in populations consuming contaminated water[4]. Radiation and viral agents have also been implicated, although a combination of these factors may be involved in some patients.

Clinical presentation
Lower legs of elderly women are most frequently involved. Individual lesions are asymptomatic, discrete, slightly scaly, erythematous plaques with a sharp but irregular or undulating border (4.5). Hyperkeratosis or crust may sometimes form, but ulceration is a marker of development of invasive cancer (4.6). Actinic damage of the surrounding skin is usually present.

Differential diagnosis
Conditions from which Bowen's disease must be differentiated include lichen simplex, psoriasis, and actinic keratoses.

Management
As with actinic keratoses, the treatment options include destructive measures like curettage and cautery, cryotherapy and surgical excision for larger lesions; delayed wound healing following destructive treatments may be an issue. Topical treatments include 5-fluorouracil and imiquimod. Topical 5-aminolaevulinic acid-based photodynamic therapy (ALA-based PDT) is also an established treatment for Bowen's disease.

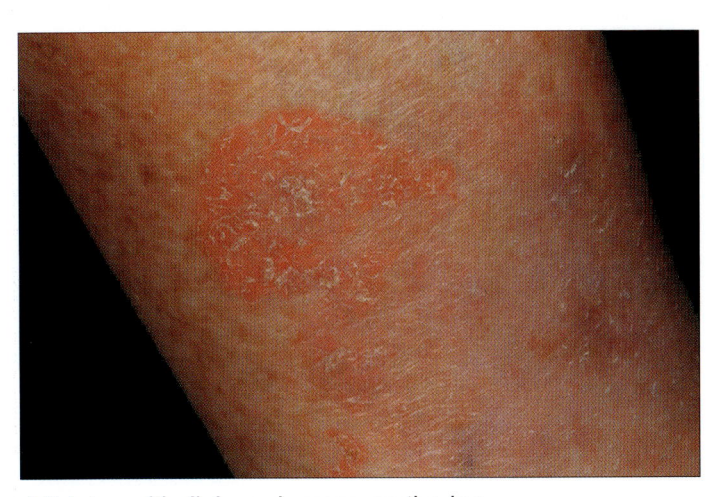

4.5 Intraepithelial carcinomas on the leg.

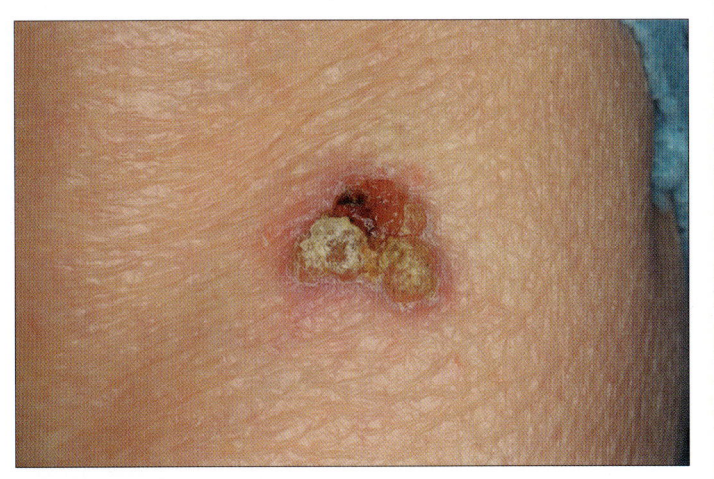

4.6 IEC developing features of invasion – ulcerating granulation tissue appearance with hyperkeratosis.

Cutaneous horn

Introduction
Cutaneous horns (cornu cutaneum) are uncommon lesions consisting of keratotic material resembling that of an animal horn. These may arise from a wide range of benign, premalignant, or malignant epidermal lesions.

Clinical presentation
The diagnosis is made clinically. The lesion is a hard yellow-brown horn that occurs typically in sun-exposed areas, particularly the face, ear, nose, forearms, and dorsum of hands (4.7). Even though over 60% of cutaneous horns are benign, the possibility of skin cancer should always be kept in mind[5]; inflammation and induration indicate malignant transformation.

Differential diagnosis
The primary diagnosis may be a viral wart, molluscum contagiosum, keratoacanthoma, actinic or seborrhoeic keratosis.

Treatment
Although the underlying disorder may be clinically evident, surgical excision and histopathological analysis are indicated to rule out any malignant transformation.

Disseminated superficial actinic porokeratosis

Introduction
Disseminated superficial actinic porokeratosis (DSAP) is an uncommon autosomal dominant chronic disorder of keratinization, characterized by multiple superficial keratotic lesions surrounded by a slightly raised keratotic border. SCC development within lesions of porokeratosis has been described, as has its association with immunosuppression. Sun exposure and immunosuppression are known triggers to the development of these lesions, which are also inherited as an autosomal dominant trait.

Clinical presentation
The lesions appear on sun-exposed areas as slightly raised keratotic rings, which expand outwards, with the skin within the ring being atrophic and hyperpigmented.

Differential diagnosis
The outward expansion and sharp rim of the lesion distinguish it from other skin lesions (4.8).

Management
Cryotherapy with liquid nitrogen is the standard treatment although 5-fluorouracil is also used.

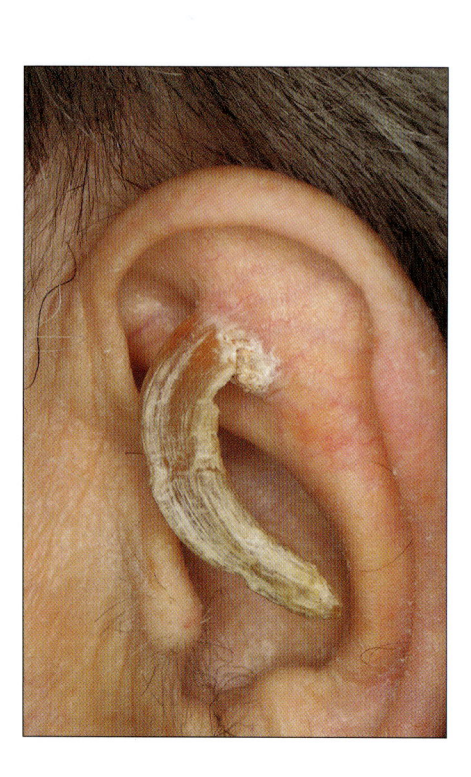

4.7 A cutaneous horn. The presence of a marked shoulder at the base of the horn can be a sign of malignancy.

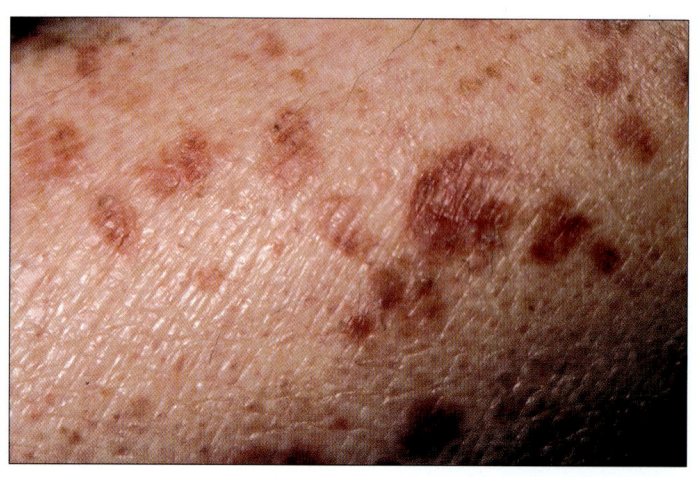

4.8 Disseminated superficial actinic porokeratoses on the leg.

Skin tumours

Erythroplasia of Queyrat

Introduction
Erythroplasia of Queyrat is a carcinoma *in situ* that mainly occurs on the glans penis, the prepuce, or the urethral meatus of elderly males. Up to 30% progress to invasive squamous cell carcinoma. The condition usually occurs in fair-skinned individuals but may also occur in dark subjects. Human papilloma virus infection has been implicated. Although histologically indistinguishable from Bowen's disease, clinically and epidemiologically this is a separate entity.

Clinical presentation
The commonest site of involvement is the glans penis of uncircumcised men, although it may also occur on the shaft or scrotum or vulva in females. The lesion is a solitary, sharply defined, discrete, nontender, erythematous plaque with erosive or slightly scaly surface (see Chapter 7).

Differential diagnosis
Erythroplasia of Queyrat must be differentiated from psoriasis, eczema, lichen planus, Zoon's balanitis, fixed drug eruption, and extramammary Paget's disease.

Management
To prevent functional impairment and mutilation of the vital structure, treatment modalities of choice include 5-fluorouracil, imiquimod, and microscopically controlled surgery (Moh's). Progression to invasive SCC is the norm in untreated cases.

Radiation-induced keratoses

Introduction
Chronic diagnostic, therapeutic, or occupational radiation exposure may result in radiodermatitis, radiation-induced keratoses, or radiation-induced malignancy. Ionizing radiation used in the treatment of internal malignancies, cutaneous malignancies, benign skin tumours, or benign inflammatory dermatoses may induce radiation keratoses. The potential for malignant change is proportional to the radiation dose.

Clinical presentation
Chronic radiodermatitis, which usually precedes the development of radiation keratoses, produces cutaneous features similar to those of chronic sun exposure (4.9). Radiation-induced keratosis has morphological and histopathological similarities to actinic keratosis, although elastotic changes and vascular obliteration may be more marked in radiation keratosis.

Management
The available treatment options include curettage, electrodessication, and excision.

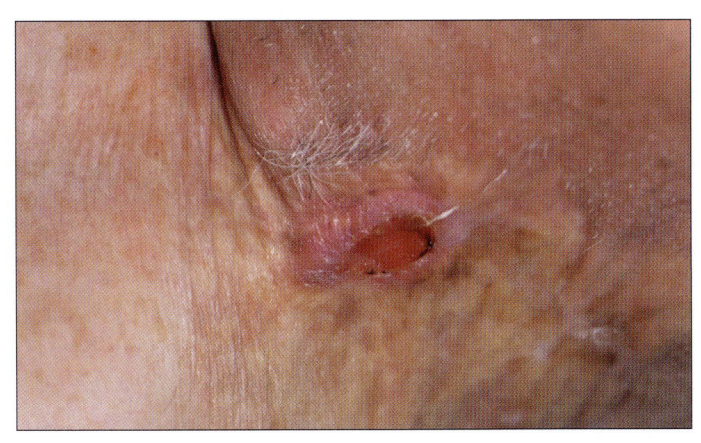

4.9 Radiodermatitis.

Arsenical keratoses

Introduction
These are arsenic-induced corn-like keratoses, most commonly occurring over the palms and soles. The lesions may progress to SCC in 5% or less of the patients. Exposure to arsenicals may be industrial, medicinal, or from consumption of contaminated well water. In addition to arsenic-related skin diseases including keratosis, Bowen's disease, BCC, and SCC, there is also an increased risk of some internal malignancies.

Clinical presentation
Numerous corn-like areas of hyperkeratosis occur over the palmar and/or plantar skin. In addition to these lesions, patients may have other cutaneous manifestations of chronic arsenicosis, including macular hyperpigmentation, multiple superficial BCC, and Bowen's disease. Inflammation, induration, rapid growth and ulceration signify malignant transformation.

Differential diagnosis
Viral warts, Darier's disease, lichen planus, and familial punctate palmar/plantar keratosis may cause diagnostic difficulties.

Management
Keratolytic ointments, cryotherapy, curettage, and oral acitretin have their advocates. Periodic examination for cutaneous or visceral malignancies should be performed.

Basal cell carcinoma

Introduction
This is the most common malignant tumour affecting humans. The low malignant and metastatic potential of this tumour makes it an underestimated health problem, although the associated morbidity can be significant. The incidence of BCC continues to rise and the age of onset has decreased, owing to habits and lifestyles leading to increased sun exposure. The incidence is increasing by ~10%/year worldwide, indicating that the prevalence of this tumour will soon equal that of all other cancers combined[6]. Furthermore, 40–50% of patients with one or more lesions will develop at least one more within 5 years.

UV radiation is the major aetiological agent in the pathogenesis of BCC. However, though exposure to UV is essential, its relationship with risk is unclear and epidemiological studies suggest its quantitative effect is modest. Recent studies suggest that intermittent rather than cumulative exposure is more important[7]. The relationship between tumour site and exposure to UV is also unclear. The distribution of lesions does not correlate well with the area of maximum exposure to UV in that BCCs are common on the eyelids, at the inner canthus, and behind the ear, but uncommon on the back of the hand and forearm. Thus, though exposure to UV is critical, patients develop BCC at sites generally believed to suffer relatively less exposure. The basis of the different susceptibility of skin at different sites to BCC development is not known.

The concept of genetic susceptibility to BCC is complex as genes may influence susceptibility as well as tumour numbers, rate of appearance, and site. Candidate genes may be selected from those involved in DNA repair, defence against oxidative stress, immune modulation, tanning, and other related biochemical activities. Some of the better studied genes include p53, cytochrome P450s (CYP), CYP2D6, and glutathione S-transferases (GST) with the GSTM1 null genotype predisposing to BCC, probably due to its role in defence against UV-induced oxidative stress[8,9]. Somatic and germ line mutations in *PTCH* gene and disrupted expression of the human homologues of *Hh* (*sonic hedgehog*; *SHH*), *Ptc* (*PTCH* and *PTCH2*), *Smo* (*SMOH*), and *Ci* (*GLI*) have been demonstrated in BCC tumourigenesis.

Clinical presentation
Nodular BCC
This is the most common clinical variant, representing approximately 60% of all BCC. The lesion is a translucent, pink or red, well-defined papule or nodule with surface telangiectasia (**4.10**). As the lesion enlarges, ulceration may occur which may then be diagnosed as nodulo-ulcerative variant, or may slowly progress to reach a large size destroying the underlying tissue, an appearance that is referred to as 'rodent ulcer' (**4.11**). Even with larger destructive lesions, the diagnosis can be made by examining the ulcer edges which are elevated, translucent and telangiectatic (**4.12**). Variable amounts of pigmentation may be present which may be confused with melanocytic lesion.

Superficial BCC

This variant is more commonly seen over truncal skin. The lesion is flat, erythematous or pink, with an irregular outline and thread-like margin (**4.13**). Surface scale, central atrophy and pigmentation may be additional features.

Morphoeic or sclerodermiform BCC

As suggested in the name, the lesion resembles a plaque of morphoea. The dense underlying fibrosis gives the lesion its indurated feel; the lesion is ivory coloured with the presence of superficial telangiectasia (**4.14**). Ulceration is uncommon and recurrence rate after treatment high.

Cystic BCC

In addition to the above-mentioned common variants of BCC, cystic degeneration of the BCC may occur which may give the lesion its blue-grey cystic appearance (**4.15**).

4.10 Nodular BCC.

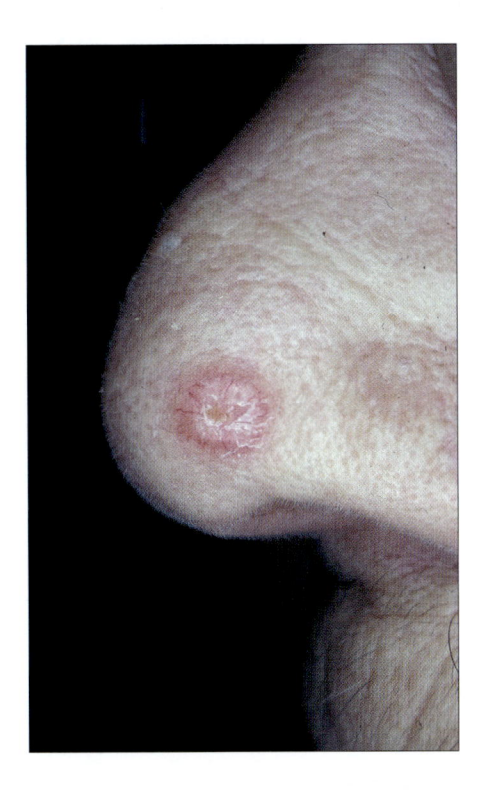

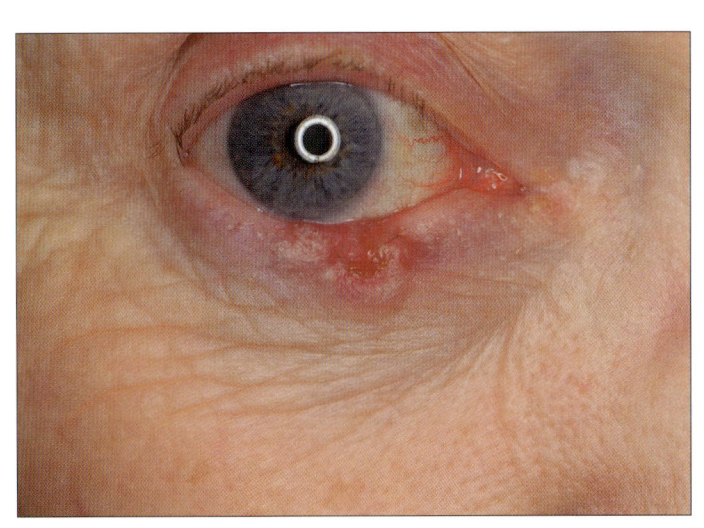

4.11 A small rodent ulcer (nodulo-ulcerative BCC) on the lower eyelid.

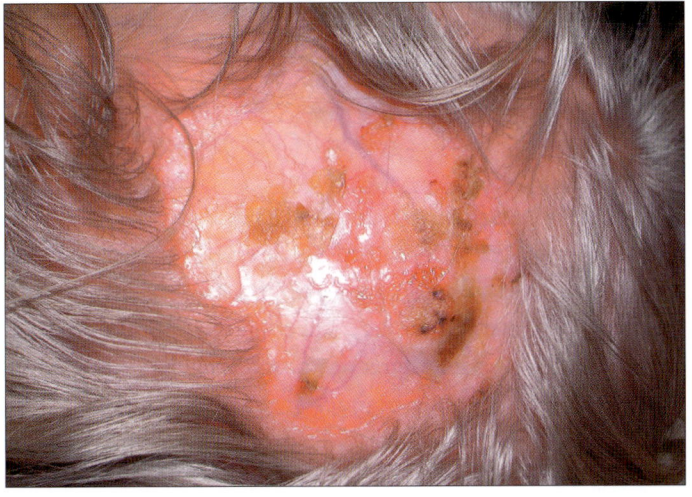

4.12 A large rodent ulcer of the scalp.

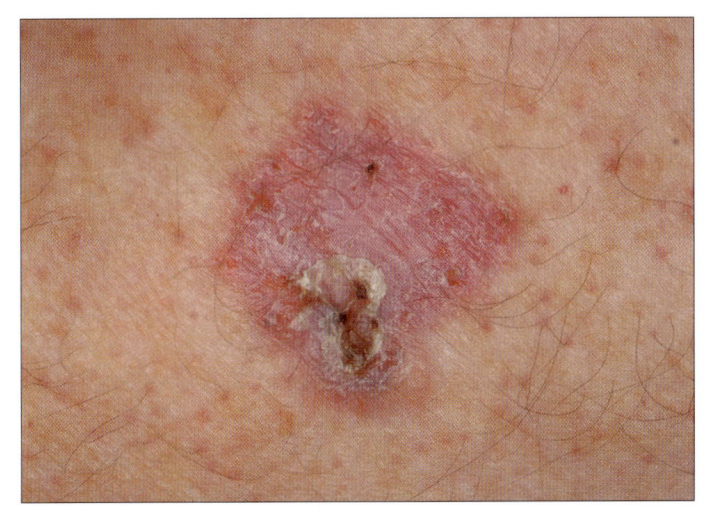

4.13 A superficial BCC on the back.

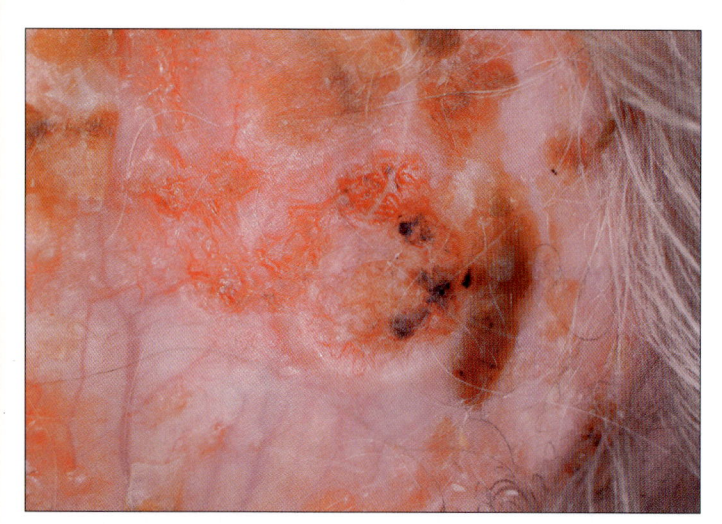

4.14 A morphoeic BCC.

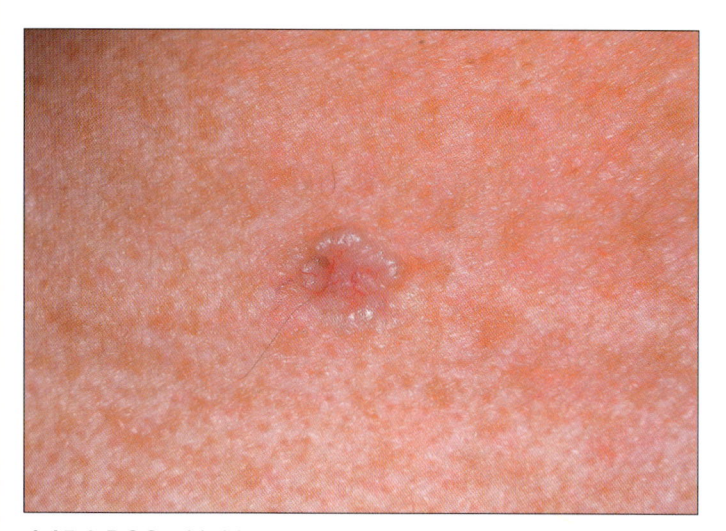

4.15 A BCC with blue-grey cystic degeneration and telangiectasia.

Management
Various tumour characteristics dictate the choice of therapy. These include tumour site, size, clinical subtype, and the ability to define tumour margins. Patients' age, coexisting medical problems, and previous treatments are also important. Destructive therapies include curettage and cautery, cryotherapy, lasers, surgical excision, and Moh's micrographic excision. Moh's excision is the treatment of choice for recurrent, morphoeic, large and nodular BCCs with ill-defined margins and for lesions at high-risk sites like nasolabial folds, nose, and periocular regions. Photo-dynamic therapy and imiquimod are newer modalities which have been explored in the management of BCC with promising results.

Squamous cell carcinoma

Introduction
SCC is the second commonest skin cancer after BCC. Early diagnosis and treatment of SCCs are important to avoid metastasis and tissue destruction as these cancers are more invasive and have a higher metastatic spread compared to BCCs.

Although ultraviolet radiation is the most important risk factor in the genesis of both SCCs and BCCs, there is a proportionately greater effect of increasing sun exposure on the risk of developing SCC. Chronic irritation, inflammation, and injury to the skin can predispose to malignant SCC. Examples include complicated scars from frostbite, electrical injury, chronic sinuses or fistulas, chronic osteomyelitis, chronic stasis dermatitis, and scars following various cutaneous infections. The most often reported dermatoses complicated by cancer are discoid lupus erythematosus, scarring variants of epidermolysis bullosa, genital lichen sclerosus et atrophicus, its variant balanitis xerotica obliterans, and lichen planus. Photochemotherapy (PUVA) increases the risk of developing SCC and this correlates with the cumulative dose of ultraviolet A. As discussed above, arsenic is an important chemical carcinogen implicated in the development of SCC; patients who have received a renal transplant have a 50 to 250-fold increased risk of developing this tumour. Various syndromes are associated with SCC development, including xeroderma pigmentosum, albinism, Muir–Torre syndrome, KID (keratosis, icthyosis, deafness), and Werner syndrome.

As with BCC, several candidate susceptibility genes have been identified in the pathogenesis of SCC. Amongst others these include *p53*, *p63*, *RAS*, *CDKN2A*, and *MC1R*. Human papilloma virus infection, immunosuppression, and DNA repair enzyme defects are other mechanisms which appear to play an active role in SCC pathogenesis.

Clinical presentation
SCC usually develops on sun-exposed sites on the background of photodamaged skin; the most common sites are back of hands, upper face, lower lip, and pinna. The skin around the lesion has signs of photodamage and the lesion itself may be a nodule, plaque, or an ulcerated and tumid area (**4.16–4.18**). A common feature of all SCC lesions is induration, which is usually the first sign of malignancy. The margins of the tumour are ill defined, indicating spread

Skin tumours

beyond the visible limits. Not uncommonly, the lesion is papillomatous with a superficial adherent crust. Ulcerated or eroded tumour is revealed on removal of the crust.

Differential diagnosis
Keratoacanthomas (**4.19**) are self-healing lesions which resemble SCCs clinically and histologically. They are best excised, as the diagnosis is often difficult to make.

Management
As with BCCs the choice of treatment depends upon the tumour and patient characteristics. Complete excision or destruction of the primary tumour and prevention of metastasis is the aim of treatment, which for smaller (<1 cm) and slow-growing well-differentiated tumours may be accomplished using destructive therapies like cryotherapy, curettage, cauterization, and laser ablation. For larger lesions (>1cm), surgical excision is the standard treatment. Moh's micrographic surgery is the treatment of choice for high-risk tumours.

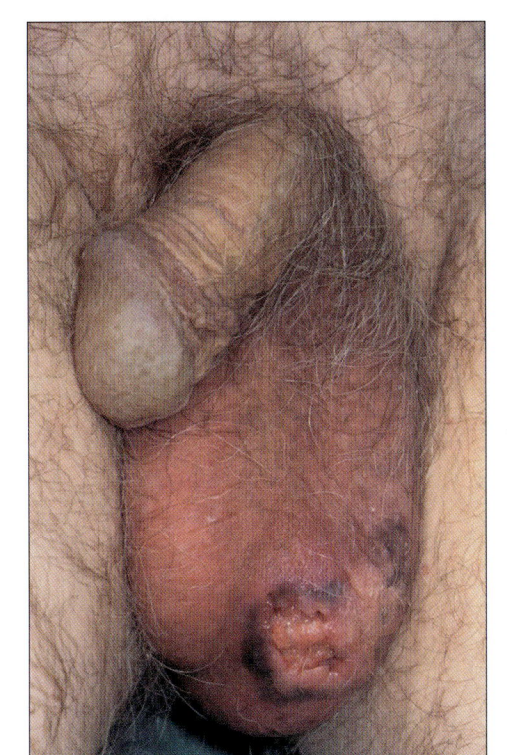

4.16 Ulcerating SCC of the side of the nose.

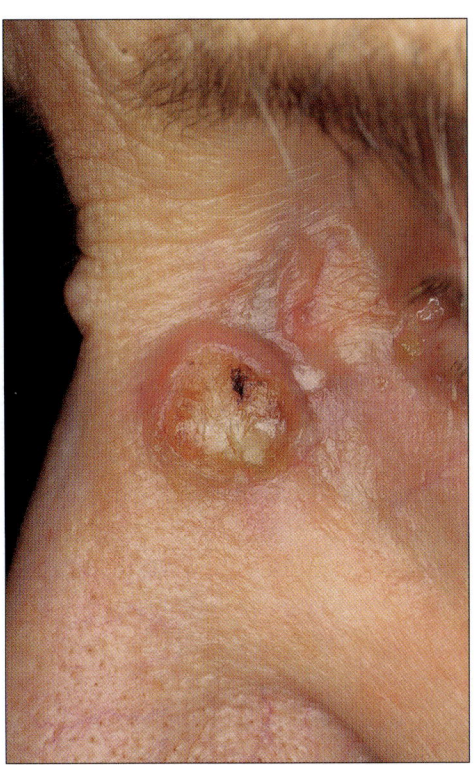

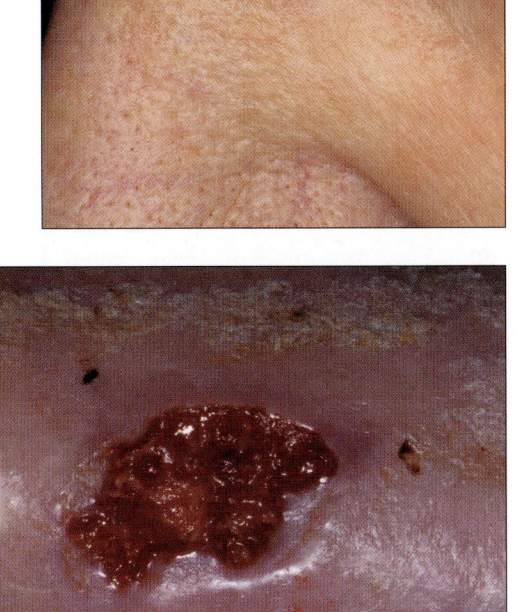

4.17 SCC of the scrotum.

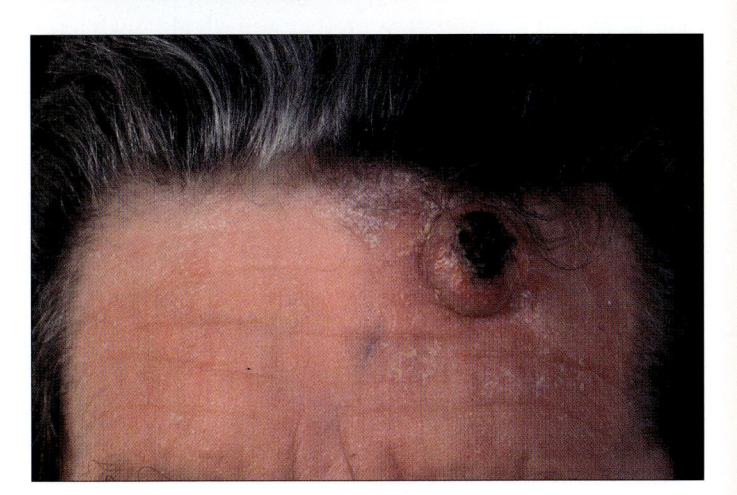

4.18 Ulcerating SCC of the shin.

4.19 Keratoacanthoma of the forehead.

MELANOMA AND MELANOMA PRECURSORS

The incidence of melanoma continues to rise, perhaps due to the emphasis on early recognition and diagnosis. As the leading killer skin disease, early diagnosis is critical as it influences survival. For patients with thin (0.75 mm) primary melanoma, the 5-year survival rate is nearly 100%; 5-year survival for those with advanced disease at diagnosis is extremely poor. Clearly therefore, early diagnosis of this skin tumour cannot be stressed enough. At present the only available effective tool for early diagnosis of melanoma is clinical evaluation and identification of thin or early melanomas using the ABCDE system (Asymmetry, Border irregularity, Colour variegation, and Diameter ≥6 mm Enlargement).

Most early melanomas have:
- Asymmetry – the two halves of the lesion are not similar.
- Border irregularity – most melanomas have irregular borders.
- Colour variability – variegation in colour within the lesion is noted in most melanomas. This however, may not be true in amelanotic melanomas.
- Diameter – most melanomas are identified when they reach a diameter of ≥6 mm.
- Enlargement – malignant tumours continue to grow.

Melanomas arise either from pre-existing melanocytic lesions (30%) or normal skin (70%).

Melanoma precursors

Congenital melanocytic naevi (CMN)
Introduction
These are pigmented lesions present at birth although a few (tardive) may appear later in life. These lesions may be precursors of malignant melanoma, regardless of their size. The lesions form between the fifth and twenty-fourth week of gestation. The dysregulated growth of melanoblasts/melanocytes occurs as a result of error in the neuroectoderm. Also, the melanoblasts' migration to the leptomeninges and integument is dysregulated.

Clinical presentation
CMNs are homogenous brown pigmented lesions with well demarcated borders, mammilated surface and, sometimes, hypertrichosis (**4.20–4.22**). Although most congenital melanocytic lesions are regular and symmetric, some, especially large ones, may be asymmetric and irregular, with varying pigmentation and may therefore simulate melanoma. The lesions are classified depending upon the size: those less than 1.5 cm are called small, 1.5–19.9 cm medium, and those 20 cm or more in greatest diameter are known as giant CMNs. Patients with large lesions are at an increased risk of developing melanomas although the risk varies with size, depth of penetration, surface features, and homogeneity of the lesions.

Management
Most CMNs do not progress to melanomas; therefore, routine excision of these lesions is not indicated. Treatment of these lesions is tailored for the individual patient, with careful consideration of the pros and cons of anaesthesia, surgery, and postoperative cosmetic considerations. Prophylactic excision of large lesions with atypical features, nodularity, or thickening should be considered.

Dysplastic (Clark's) naevus
Introduction
Dysplastic naevi are markers of increased risk of development of malignant melanoma. These are acquired, pigmented, clinicopathological entities which develop *de novo* or from CMNs and represent disordered proliferation of atypical melanocytes. There is increasing evidence that suggests that families and individuals with multiple dysplastic naevi are prone to developing malignant melanoma, and that this may be due to a dominantly inherited gene. Several candidate susceptibility genes for melanoma and dysplastic naevi have been described including tumour suppressor gene *p16/cyclin dependent kinase 2A*, oncogene *CDK4*, and a tumour suppressor gene *p19*. Defective DNA repair systems for UV-induced DNA damage and microsatellite instability are other mechanisms thought to be responsible for the genesis of these lesions.

Clinical presentation
The clinical distinction between dysplastic naevus and malignant melanoma can be very difficult. The lesions are round, oval or ellipsoid macules usually ≥5 mm with indistinct margins and are brown, tan, pink, or red in colour with colour variegation (**4.23–4.27**). Unlike CMNs, these develop later in life and do not undergo spontaneous resolution.

Skin tumours 57

Management

This remains challenging and for lesions that are changing in size, colour, shape, and pigmentation pattern, is usually excision. Photographs of the lesions and, in cases of multiple naevi, the whole body, should be taken for surveillance, which may reduce the need for excision of lesions for histopathological analysis and help in the identification of early malignant melanomas. Patients with familial and sporadic dysplastic naevi should be followed regularly at 3 and 6 monthly intervals, respectively. Sun avoidance should be advised and sunscreen use advocated.

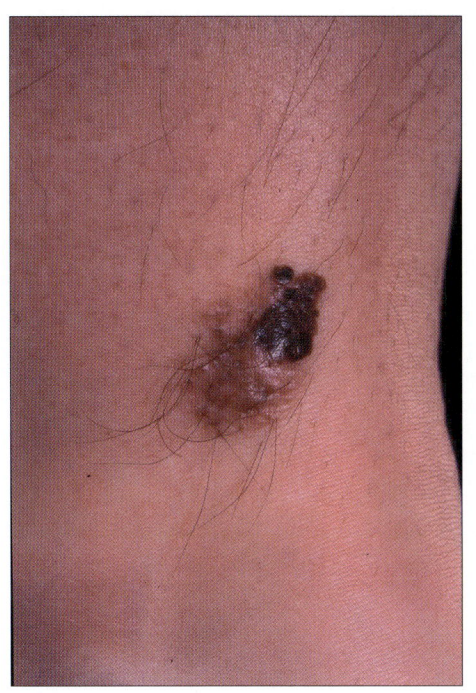

4.20 Melanoma developing in a congenital melanocytic naevus of the ankle.

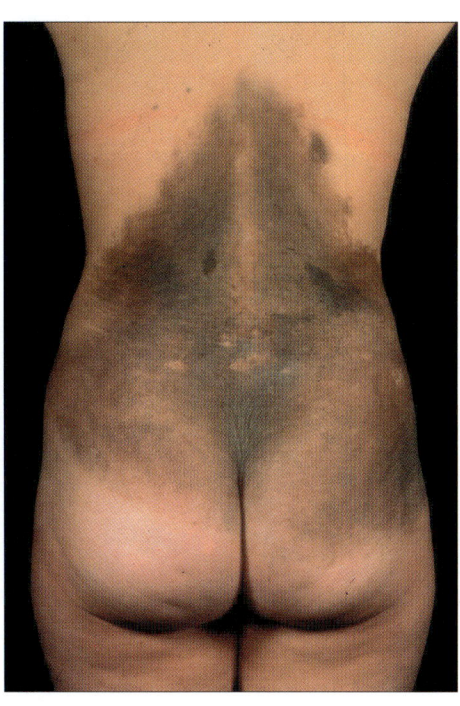

4.21 Large bathing trunk congenital melanocytic naevus.

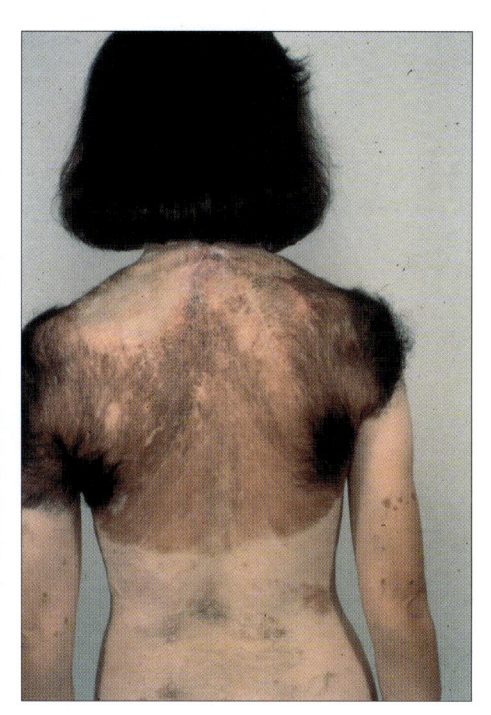

4.22 Melanoma and in-transit secondaries in a large CMN.

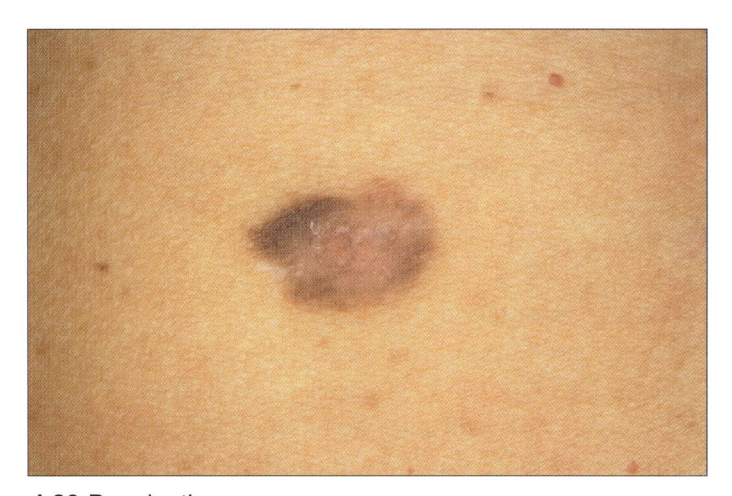

4.23 Dysplastic naevus.

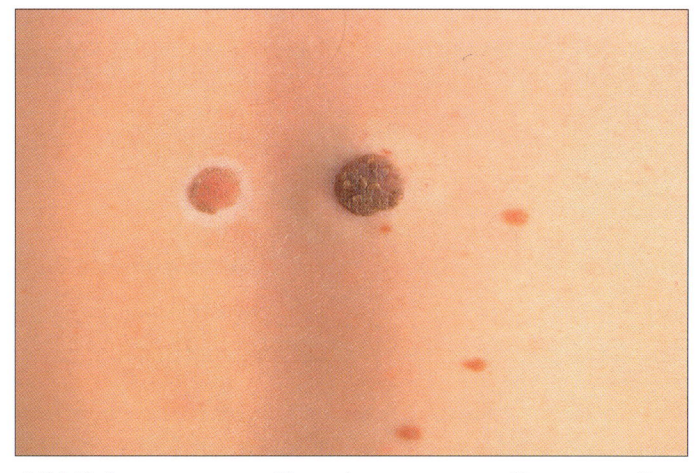

4.24 Halo naevus, papillomatous naevus with surrounding local anaesthetic and 4 junctional naevi on the back.

58 Skin tumours

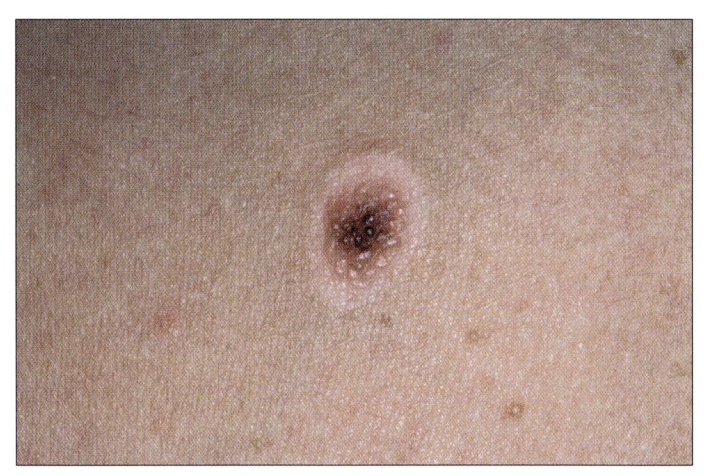

4.25 Halo naevus. These are benign lesions where the mole disappears leaving a depigmented patch.

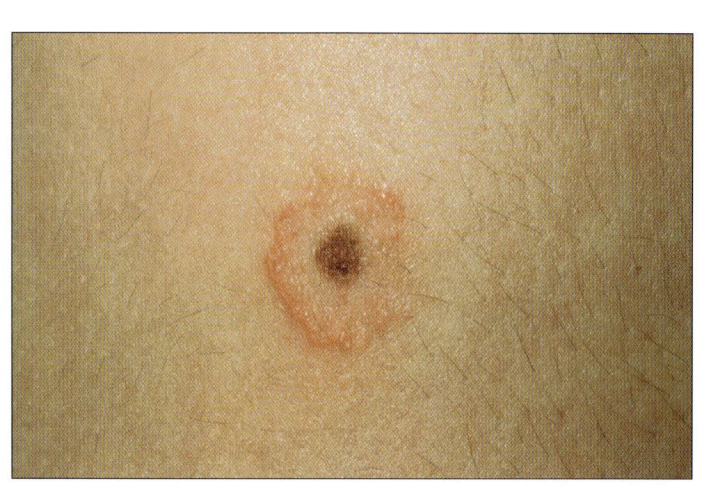

4.26 Meyerson's naevus – a benign mole surrounded by eczematous inflammation.

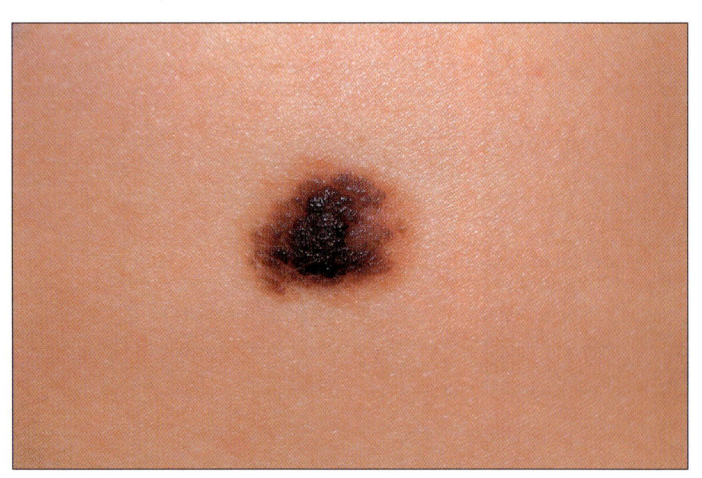

4.27 A compound melanocytic naevus.

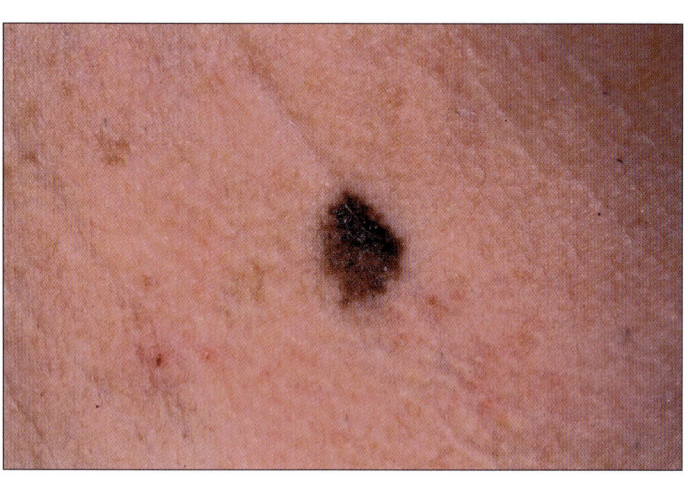

4.28 An early lentigo maligna.

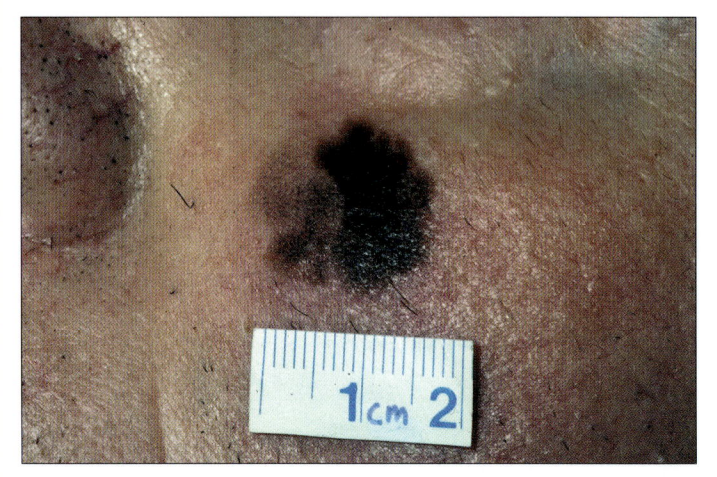

4.29 A more extensive lentigo maligna.

Lentigo maligna (melanoma in situ)

Introduction
This is the precursor lesion of lentigo maligna melanoma. The same factors are involved as described for malignant melanoma and dysplastic naevi.

Clinical presentation
Lesions are always present on sun damaged skin of older patients, with a slow progression to lentigo maligna melanoma. The individual lesion is a flat, brown-black macule of variable size, with irregular but sharply defined borders, on a background of sun damaged skin (**4.28, 4.29**).

Skin tumours 59

Management

Factors such as site and size of lesion and patient comorbidities influence the treatment modality undertaken. Surgical excision is the treatment of choice to obtain clinical and histological clearance, but many other modalities have been used with variable success. Moh's micrographic surgery is associated with the lowest recurrence rate at 4–5%, but conventional surgery, cryotherapy, and radiotherapy also yield good results, with recurrence rates in the order of 7–10%[10]. Other options include laser ablation and topically applied imiquimod.

Malignant melanoma

Superficial spreading melanoma

The commonest form comprising 70% of all melanomas. This presents as a uniformly elevated dark brown to black plaque with marked variegation in colour (**4.30–4.32**) and may be associated with regional lymphadenopathy. Usual sites of occurrence include the upper back and legs.

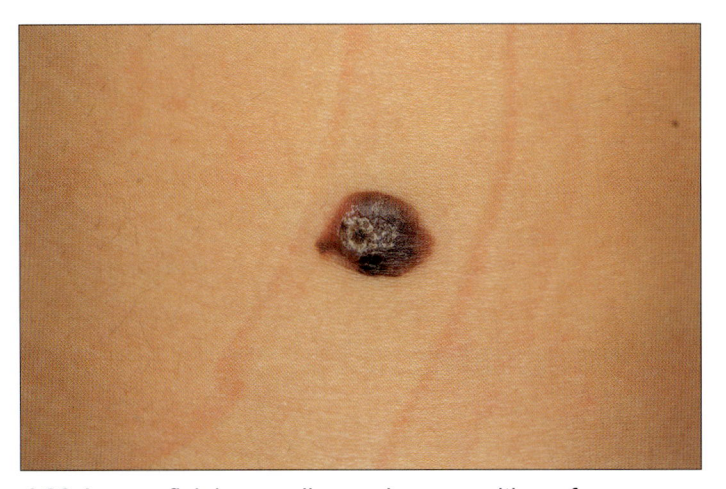

4.30 A superficial spreading melanoma with surface ulceration.

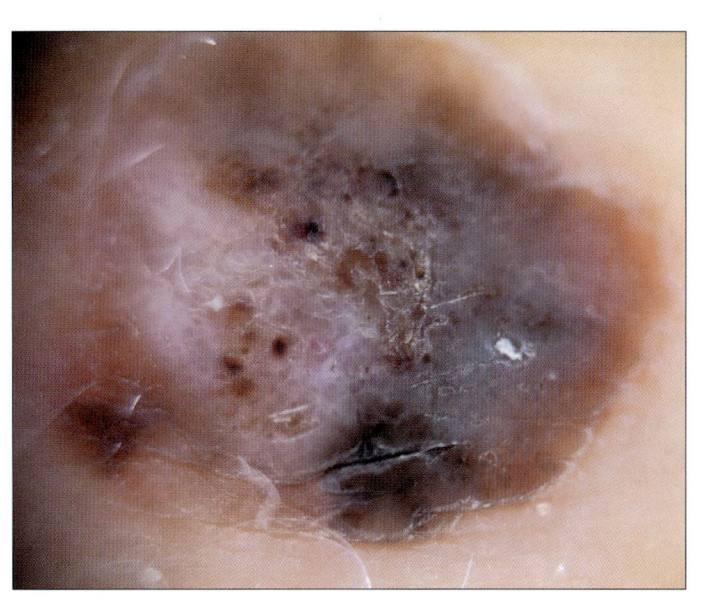

4.31 Dermatoscopic findings of **4.30**.

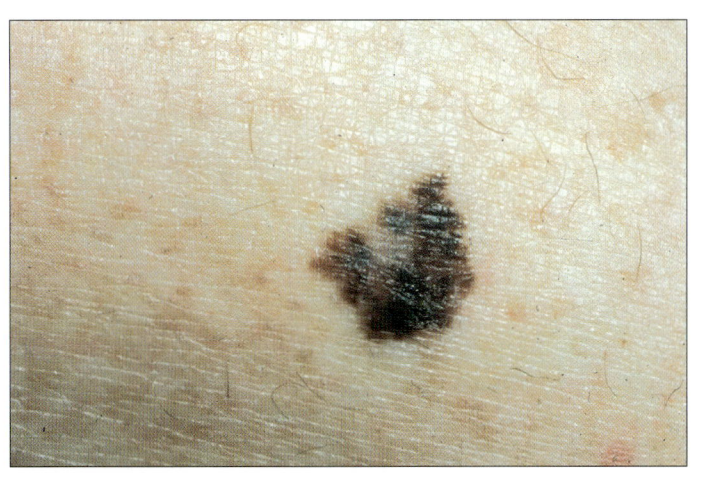

4.32 Superficial spreading melanoma with regression.

60 Skin tumours

Nodular melanoma
The second most common form of malignant melanoma. This form tends to involve the dermis at a relatively early stage, in contrast to others that tend to remain confined to the epidermis. The lesion differs from other variants in being a uniformly dark blue, brown, or black coloured nodule with smooth margins and a rapid progression (**4.33, 4.34**).

Lentigo maligna melanoma
This lesion develops from lentigo maligna. In contrast to lentigo maligna, which is a uniformly flat macule, this is a flat patch or macule with focal areas of papules or nodules and variegation in colour (**4.35**).

Acral lentiginous melanoma
These are more common in brown-skinned individuals. It involves the palms, soles, finger or toenail bed, and mucocutaneous skin of the mouth, genitalia, or anus.

On the palm and sole skin, these appear as irregularly pigmented slow growing macules (**4.36, 4.37**), which later develop papules or nodules in the vertical growth phase. The subungual lesions involve the nail matrix and extend to cause nail ulceration and eventual destruction as a result of involvement of the nail bed and nail plate (**4.38, 4.39**).

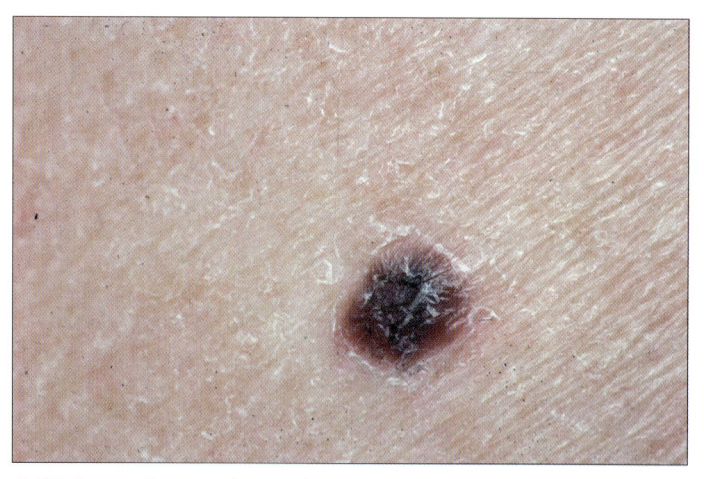

4.33 An early nodular melanoma.

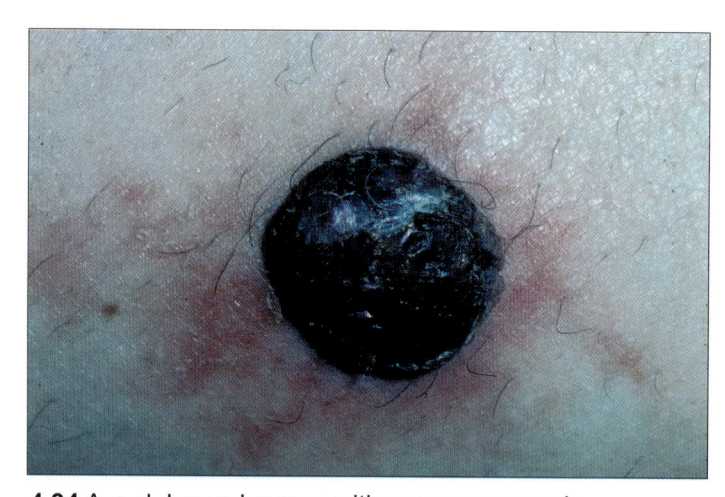

4.34 A nodular melanoma with a poor prognosis.

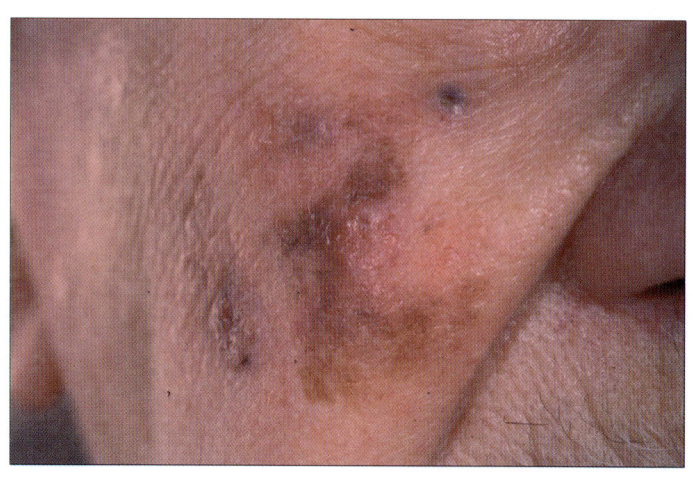

4.35 A lentigo maligna melanoma and a coincidental senile comedone.

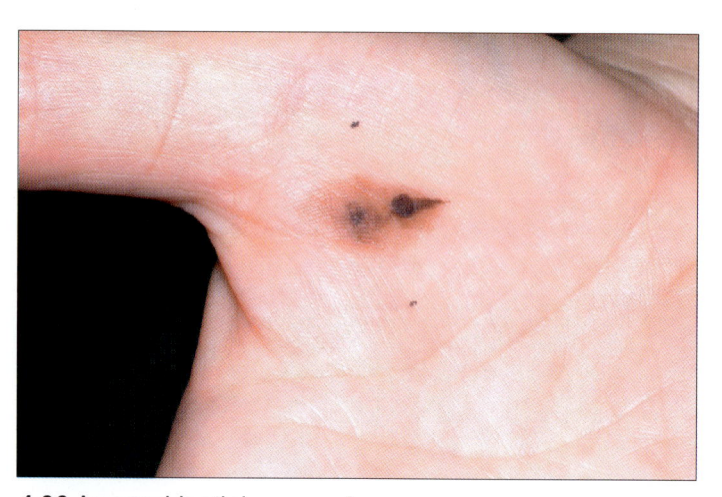

4.36 An acral lentiginous melanoma.

Desmoplastic melanoma

This is an uncommon histological variant of melanoma, with a dermal fibroblastic component and a high incidence of local recurrence and nodal metastases, requiring early aggressive surgery. It is most commonly seen on sun-damaged skin of the head and neck. The lesions may be variegated lentiginous macules or a dermal nodule. Absence of pigmentation commonly leads to a delay in diagnosis.

Verrucous melanoma

Verrucous naevoid malignant melanoma is a recently described variant of malignant melanoma that may be confused both clinically and histologically with SCC or benign exophytic lesions[11]. It is considered as a variant of superficial spreading melanoma characterized by an exophytic papilliferous growth pattern.

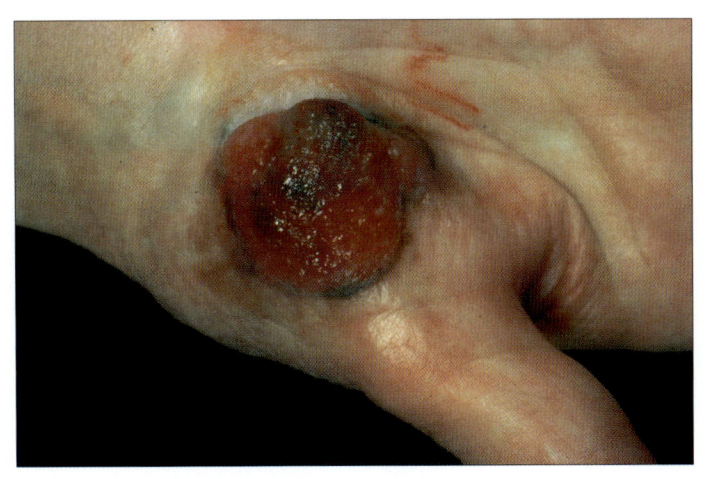

4.37 A more advanced acral lentiginous melanoma.

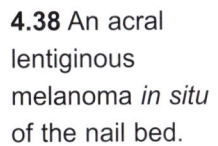

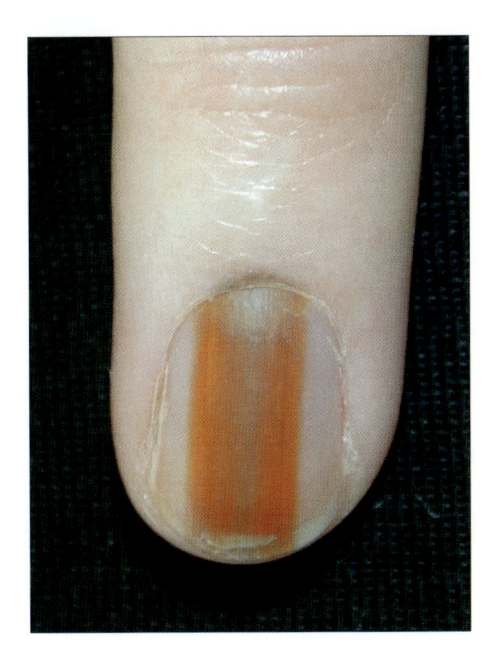

4.38 An acral lentiginous melanoma *in situ* of the nail bed.

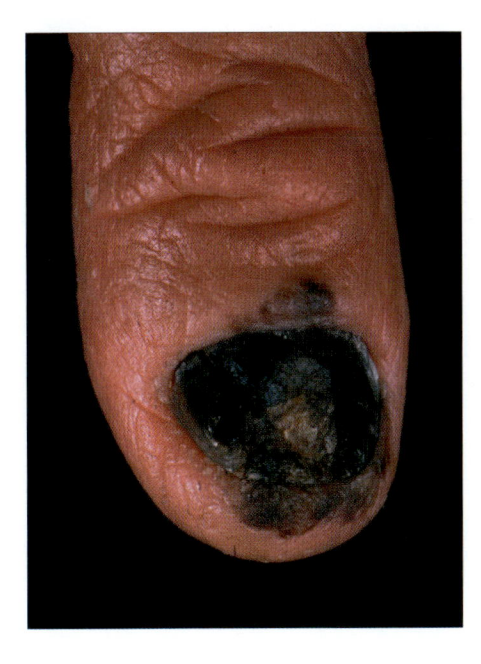

4.39 An acral lentiginous melanoma of the thumb with Hutchinson's sign (proximal spread of pigmentation).

Skin tumours

Differential diagnosis
Differential diagnosis of malignant melanoma includes: haemangioma, pyogenic granuloma, pigmented seborrhoeic wart, and senile comedone (**4.40–4.43**).

Management of melanoma
Surgical excision with margins based on Breslow thickness forms the cornerstone of treatment of malignant melanoma. The British Association of Dermatologists in their published guidelines for management of patients with malignant melanoma[12] recommends the margins listed in *Table 4.1* to be included in the excision of malignant melanoma lesions.

At present, sentinel lymph node biopsy is a staging and prognostic tool. Adjuvant therapy in the form of chemotherapy, immunotherapy, or vaccine therapy may be considered for patients with thick primary tumours and positive lymph nodes as these have a high risk of recurrent disease. Patients with primary melanomas should be closely followed, every 2–3 months for the initial 3 years, for signs of recurrent disease. Finally, patients should carry out regular skin self-examinations and they should be encouraged to use sunscreens and other sun avoidance measures.

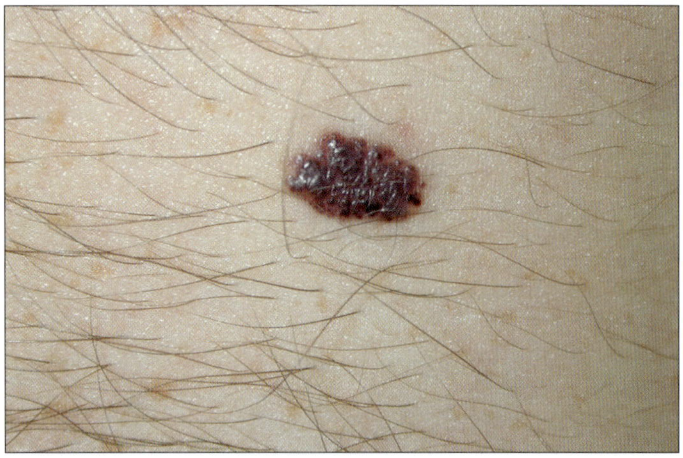

Table 4.1 Margins recommended in the excision of malignant melanoma lesions

Breslow thickness	Margin
In situ	0.2–0.5 cm
<1 mm	1 cm
1–2 mm	1–2 cm
2.1–4 mm	2–3 cm
>4 mm	2–3 cm

4.40 Thrombosed haemangioma.

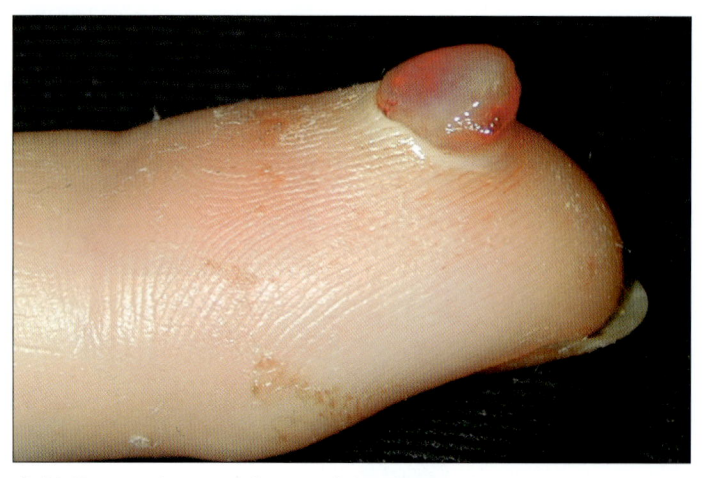

4.41 Pyogenic granuloma of the finger tip.

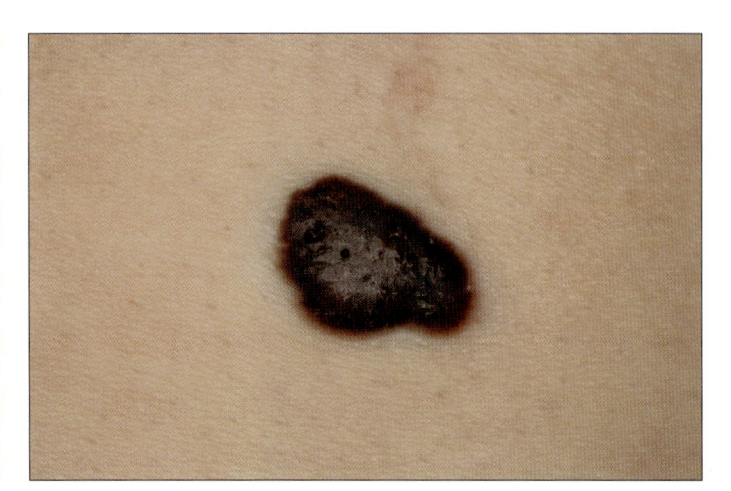

4.42 Benign seborrhoeic keratosis.

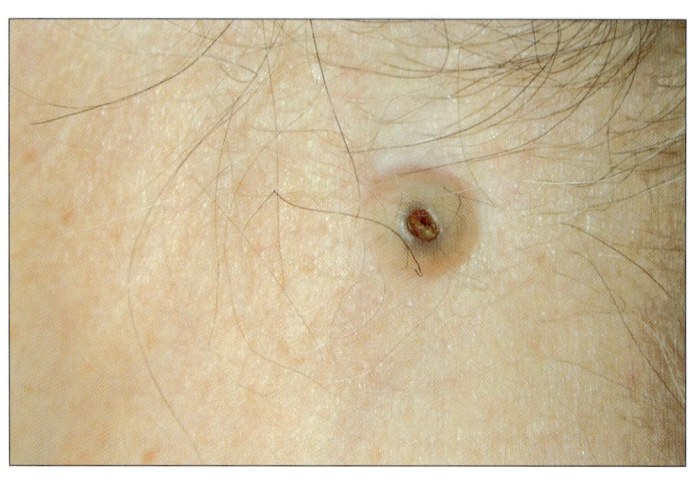

4.43 Senile comedone.

References

1. Glogau RG (2000). The risk of progression to invasive disease. *J Am Acad Dermatol* **42**:23–24.
2. Lebwohl M (2003). Actinic keratosis: epidemiology and progression to squamous cell carcinoma. *Br J Dermatol* **149** (Suppl 66):31–33.
3. Lee PK, Harwell WB, Loven KH, et al. (2005). Long-term clinical outcomes following treatment of actinic keratosis with imiquimod 5% cream. *Dermatol Surg* **6**: 659–664.
4. Tseng WP, Chu HM, How SW, et al. (1968). Prevalence of skin cancer in an endemic area of chronic arsenicism in Taiwan. *J Natl Cancer Inst* **40**:453–463.
5. Copcu E, Sivrioglu N, Culhaci N (2004). Cutaneous horns: are these lesions as innocent as they seem to be? *World J Surg Oncol* **2**:18.
6. Karagas MR, Greenberg ER (1995). Unresolved issues in the epidemiology of basal cell and squamous cell skin cancer. In: *Skin Cancer: Mechanisms and Human Relevance*. H Mukhtar (ed). CRC Press, Boca Raton, Florida, pp. 79–86.
7. Kricker A, Armstrong BK, English DR, Heenan PJ (1995). Does intermittent sun exposure cause basal cell carcinoma? A case-control study in Western Australia. *Int J Cancer* **60**:489–494.
8. Lear JT, Heagerty AH, Smith A, et al. (1996). Multiple cutaneous basal cell carcinomas: glutathione S-transferase (GSTM1, GSTT1) and cytochrome P450 (CYP2D6, CYP1A1) polymorphisms influence tumour numbers and accrual. *Carcinogenesis* **17**:1891–1896.
9. Lear JT, Smith AG, Heagerty AH, et al. (1997). Truncal site and detoxifying enzyme polymorphisms significantly reduce time to presentation of further primary cutaneous basal cell carcinoma. *Carcinogenesis* **18**:1499–1503.
10. Stevenson O, Ahmed I (2005). Lentigo maligna: prognosis and treatment options. *Am J Clin Dermatol* **6**:151–164.
11. Blessing K, Evans AT, al-Nafussi A (1993). Verrucous naevoid and keratotic malignant melanoma: a clinico-pathological study of 20 cases. *Histopathology* **23**:453–458.
12. Roberts DL, Anstey AV, Barlow RJ, et al. (2002). British Association of Dermatologists; Melanoma Study Group. UK guidelines for the management of cutaneous melanoma. *Br J Dermatol* **146**:7–17.

Chapter 5

Hand and foot dermatoses

John SC English, MRCP

Introduction

The commonest dermatosis of the hands and feet is dermatitis or eczema (the two terms are synonymous), but other inflammatory conditions must be differentiated (*Table 5.1*). As with all other parts of the skin the distribution, configuration, and morphology of the rash are helpful pointers in making a diagnosis. Is the rash all over the hands or feet, or just on one? Are the lesions confluent or discrete and what is the morphology of the lesions? Are there vesicles, dryness, cracking, and hyperkeratosis? Looking for signs of skin disease elsewhere is useful especially in establishing a diagnosis of psoriasis. It could be that the patient has a chronic fungal infection of the hands and then they are likely to have fungal infection of their feet. The feet should always be examined in conjunction with the hands.

Hand and foot dermatitis

Introduction
The patterns of hand dermatitis can be divided into four groups (*Table 5.2*). Dermatitis predominantly affects the backs of the hands, the fingers, the palms, or the whole hand. Hand eczema can be divided into either allergic, irritant, or endogenous, or a mixture of all three (**5.1**).

Table 5.1 Conditions affecting the hands and feet

- Dermatitis
- Psoriasis
- Pustular psoriasis
- Fungal infections
- Infestation
- Other inflammatory dermatoses

Table 5.2 Patterns of hand eczema

Dorsa of hands	Fingers	Palms	Whole hand
ICD	ICD	ACD	ACD
ACD	ACD	ICD	ICD
	Endogenous eczema	Endogenous eczema	Endogenous eczema

ACD, allergic contact dermatitis; ICD, irritant contact dermatitis

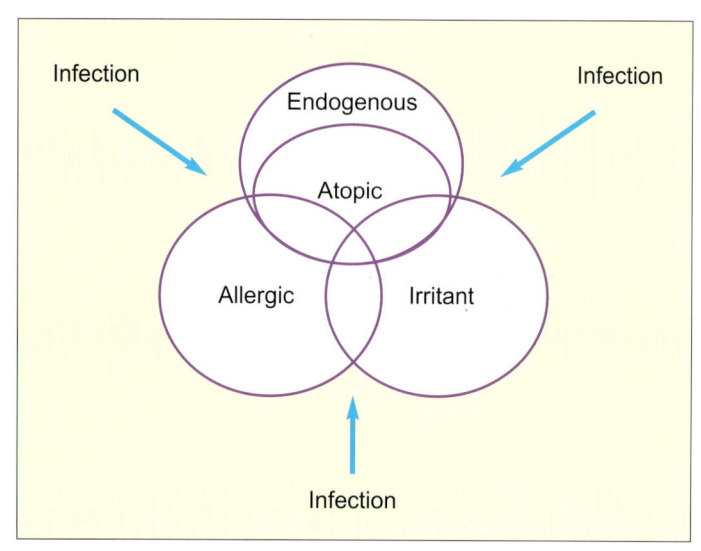

66 Hand and foot dermatoses

5.1 The various causes of hand eczema.

Clinical presentation
Irritant contact dermatitis (ICD)
Irritant dermatitis of the hands tends to affect the finger webs and the backs of the hands, but can affect the palmar surface (5.2–5.4). It is due to a direct toxic effect of exposure to irritant substances. The commonest causes are soaps, detergents, solvents, and occlusive effect of rubber gloves. Almost any chemical given enough exposure can be irritant, even water. Friction can also play a role in causing dermatitis. It is much more common than allergic contact dermatitis (ACD). ICD is not so common on the feet, as shoes are worn and this tends to cause occlusion and sweating. Juvenile plantar dermatosis of the feet is probably an irritant effect of drying out of sweaty feet after wearing occlusive trainers (5.5).

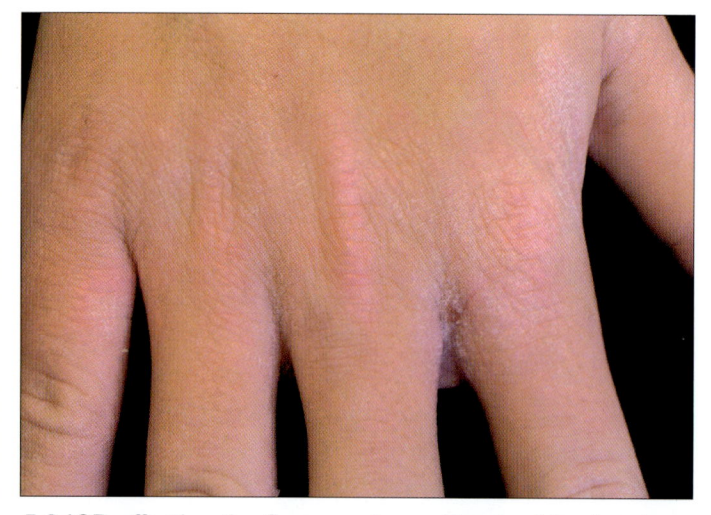

5.2 ICD affecting the finger webs and back of the hand.

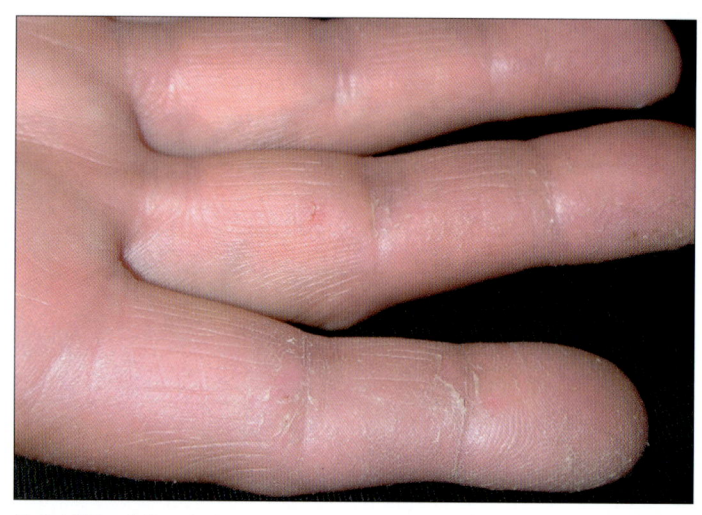

5.3 ICD of the palmar aspect of the fingers.

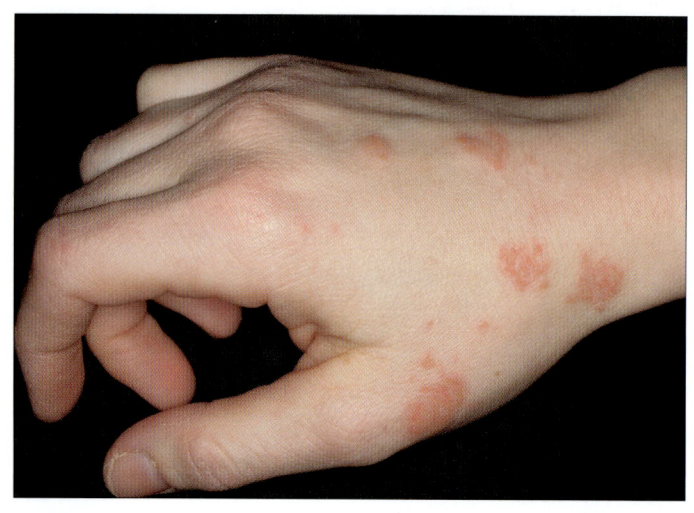

5.4 ICD discoid pattern affecting the back of the hand.

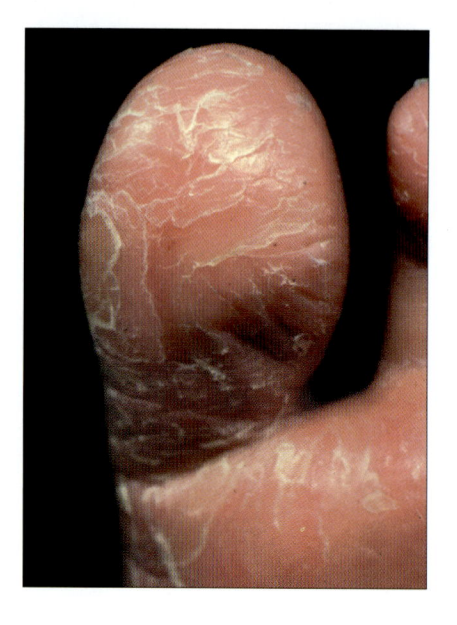

5.5 Juvenile plantar dermatoses.

Hand and foot dermatoses

Allergic contact dermatitis

The pattern of ACD is variable; predominantly vesicles will usually be present, especially on the palmar surface, and any part of the hand can be affected (**5.6–5.10**). ACD of the feet can affect the dorsal or plantar surface. The dorsal surfaces are often associated with leather allergy and the plantar surface with rubber allergy, due to the fact that leather on the insoles of shoes tends to be vegetable tanned and not chromium tanned, and the soles usually tend to be made of rubber (**5.11–5.13**). However, patients can be allergic to the glues, which often can contain rubber and therefore may get a pattern that can affect any part of the foot (**5.12**). However, even with careful examination of the hands and feet it is frequently not possible to tell whether sensitization has occurred (**5.14**) and therefore patch testing is strongly recommended (see Chapter 1).

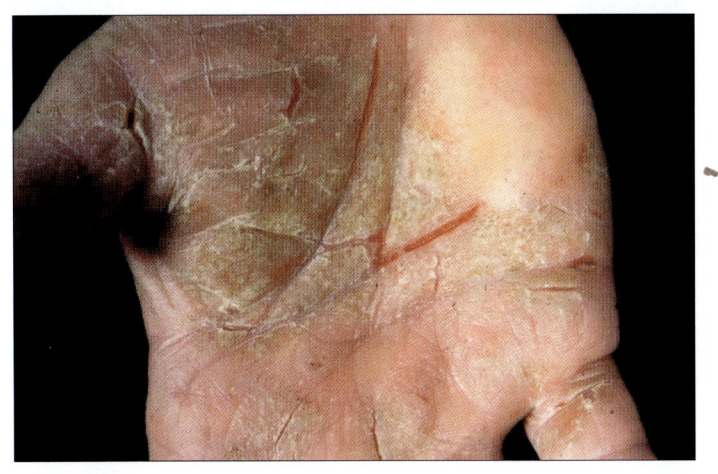

5.6 ACD from isopropyl phenyl phenylenediamine in bicycle tyres.

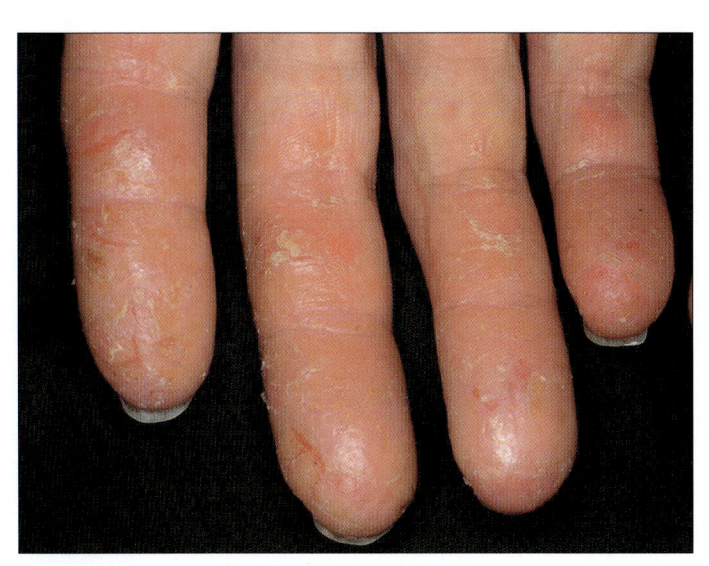

5.7 ACD from epoxy resin paint.

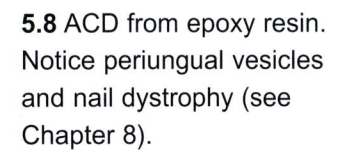

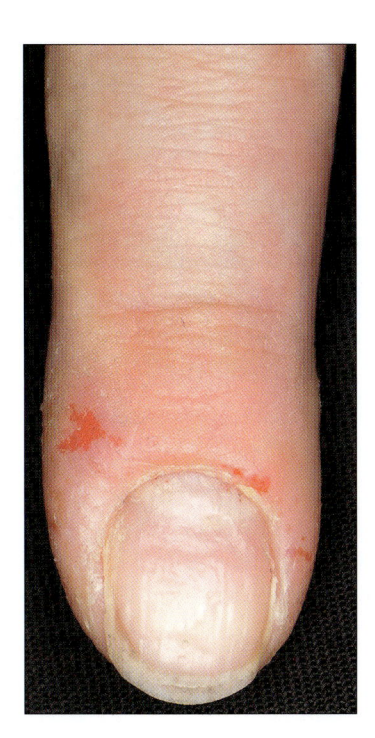

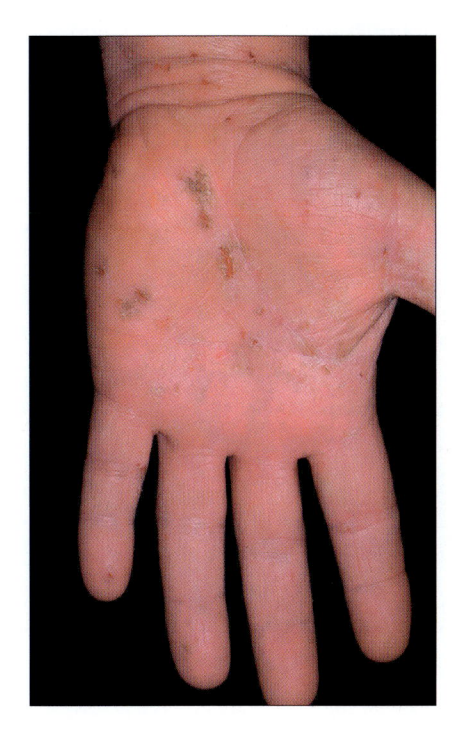

5.8 ACD from epoxy resin. Notice periungual vesicles and nail dystrophy (see Chapter 8).

5.9 ACD from methylchloroisothizolinone in a liquid soap.

68 Hand and foot dermatoses

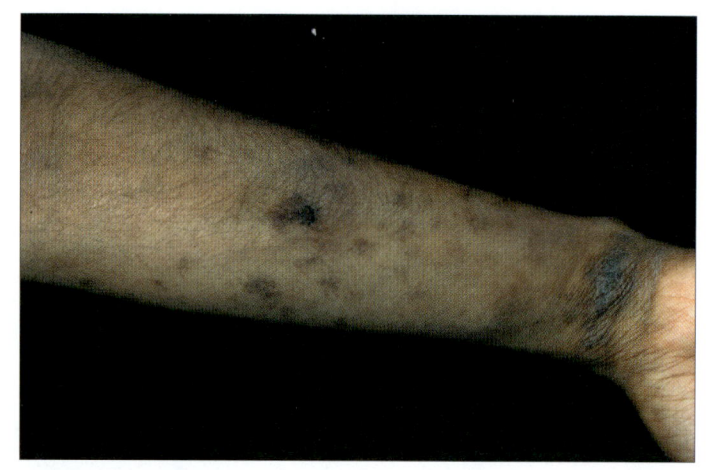

5.10 ACD from thiurams in rubber gloves mimicking ICD pattern of dermatitis.

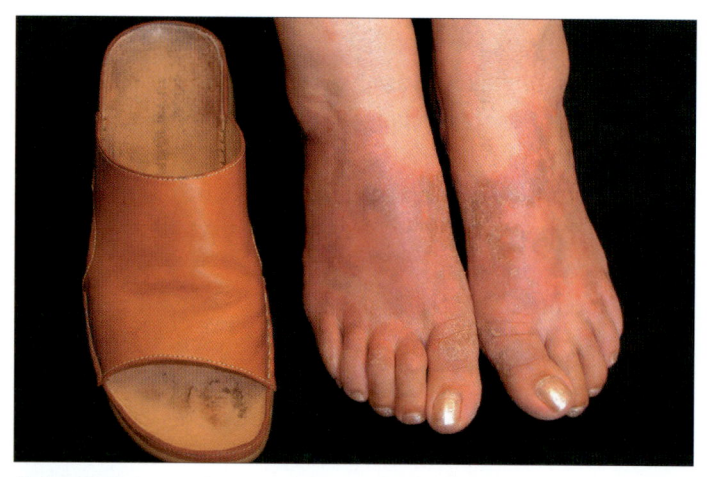

5.11 ACD from chromium-tanned leather.

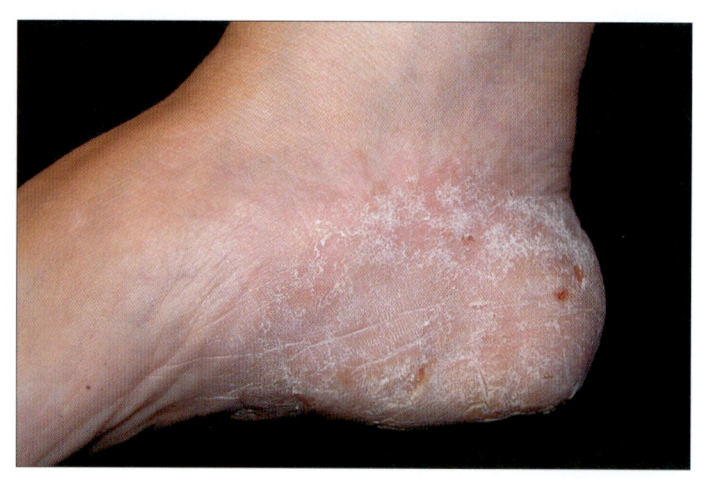

5.12 ACD from mercaptobenzothiazole in a shoe lining.

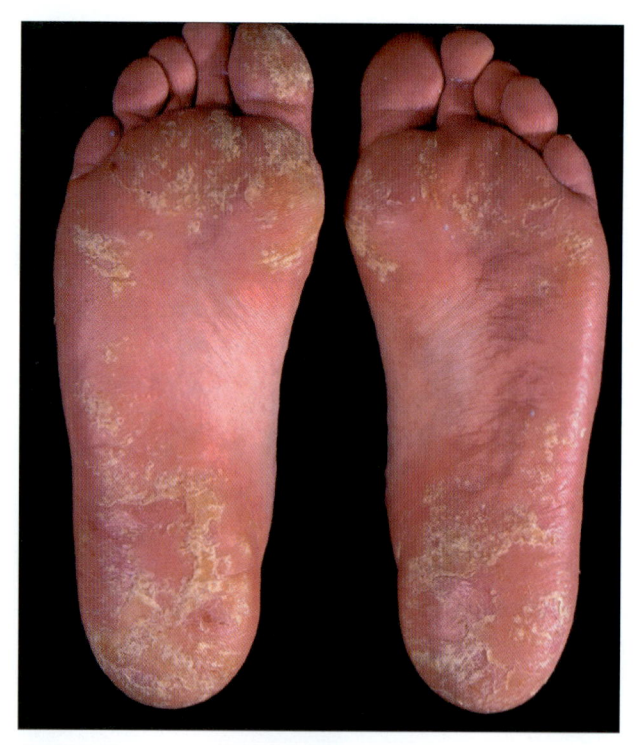

5.13 ACD from mercaptobenzothiazole in rubber soles. Notice the weight-bearing area of the foot is affected.

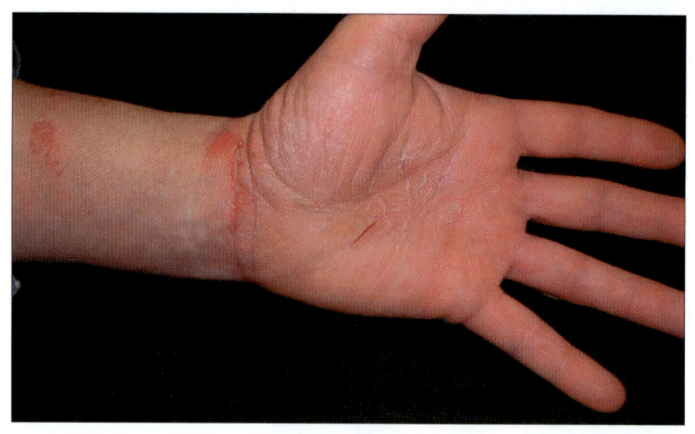

5.14 ACD from imidazolidinyl urea mimicking endogenous hyperkeratotic hand eczema.

Endogenous eczema
Endogenous eczema can have any pattern and affect any part of the hands or feet. It is a diagnosis made on exclusion, with negative patch tests and no history of irritant exposure.

One variety of endogenous eczema is that of recurrent pompholyx of the palms and soles, which may well be associated with bacterial infection (**5.15–5.17**).

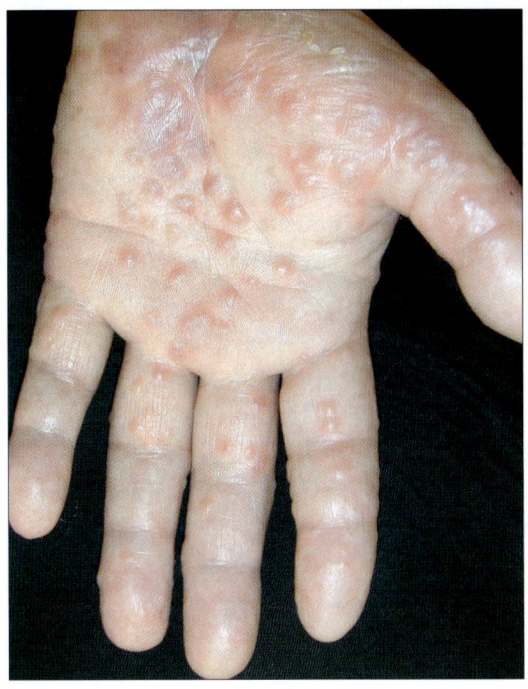

5.15 Vesiculo-bullous hand eczema reaction (id reaction) from infected foot eczema.

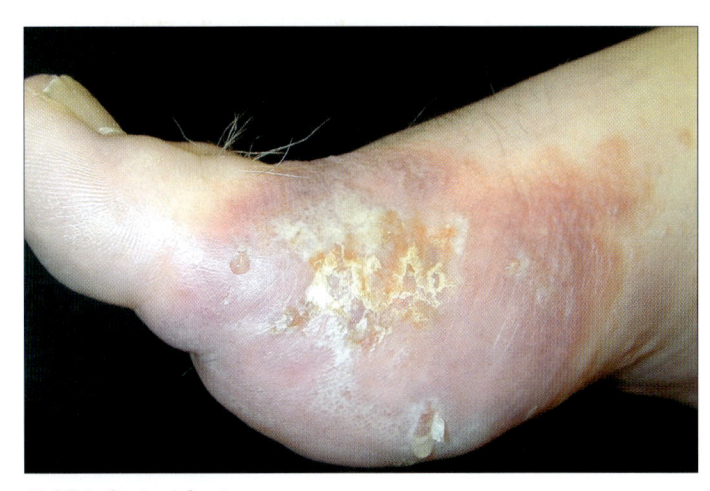

5.16 Infected foot eczema.

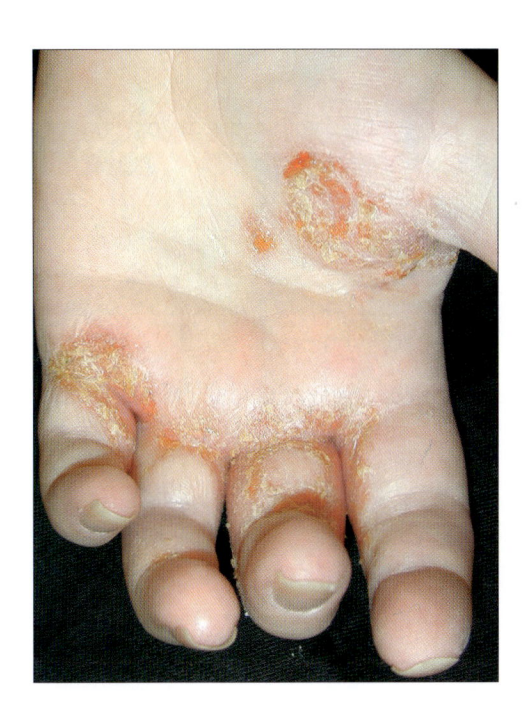

5.17 Chronic infected endogenous hand eczema.

Differential diagnosis

Table 5.3 highlights the features that help to distinguish between ICD and ACD. Elicitation of the aetiology of hand dermatitis rests more on a detailed history and the results of patch tests than on the clinical distribution or the pattern of the hand eczema.

Management

Allergen avoidance is advised if allergens have been identified through patch testing. If ICD has been diagnosed, then exposure reduction to the irritants is key to the management of ICD. With endogenous eczema topical steroids and emollients would be the treatment of choice, possibly with antibiotics if infection was thought to be playing a part. Emollients and topical steroids would also be used for ACD and ICD.

Prognosis

The prognosis is not always good with allergen avoidance in ACD patients. Some allergens, especially potassium dichromate through cement or *Compositae* plant allergens (chrysanthemums and dandelions), can cause a chronic dermatitis leading to suffering for many years. Otherwise exposure elimination will usually 'cure' a patient of hand eczema, especially if the allergen is easily avoidable such as epoxy resin (**5.7**, **5.8**). The prognosis for irritant dermatitis can also be bad if exposure reduction cannot be achieved. Often patients will have continued exposure to irritants in the home, rather than workplace. Once the dermatitis has broken out it is difficult to get it healed. Endogenous eczema can run a protracted course, and sensitization to medicament allergens or other allergens can, of course, occur. Treatments other than topical steroids would be hand and foot PUVA for resistant cases and even systemic immunosuppressants such as azathioprine and cyclosporin. Topical immunomodulators (calcineurin inhibitors) are not particularly effective as it is difficult for the large active molecules to penetrate the stratum corneum of the palms and soles.

Table 5.3 Characteristics of irritant and allergic contact hand dermatitis

	ICD	ACD
Lesions	Oligomorphic with redness, scaling, chapping	Polymorphic with redness, papules, vesicles, crusts, exudation, erosions, lichenification
Demarcation	Patchy, relatively clear	Diffuse, tendency to spread (face, wrist, axillae, genitals)
Localization	Fingertips, fingerwebs, dorsum of the hand, ball of the thumb	Interdigital, fingers, palmar and dorsal side
Course	Chronic, aggravation by climate changes, wet work, detergents, gloves	Relapsing, healing in weekends and holidays
Epidemiology	More persons affected in same work environment	One person affected in same work environment
Patch testing	Negative, positive – nonrelevant	Relevant positive, negative – allergen missed

Psoriasis

Introduction

Unfortunately patients sometimes develop a hyperkeratotic condition of the hands (**5.18**, **5.19**), often without signs of psoriasis elsewhere. There is usually no vesiculation and it is mainly a painful cracking of the skin that they complain of. Friction plays an important part in this. Psoriasis can affect just the palms and soles; however, if one carefully looks elsewhere, one sometimes finds evidence of psoriasis.

Clinical presentation

Psoriasis of the palms or soles (**5.20**, **5.21**) tends to present with painful cracking rather than itching or bleeding. Friction is an important cause of koebnerization of psoriasis of the palms and soles.

5.18 Palmar psoriasis.

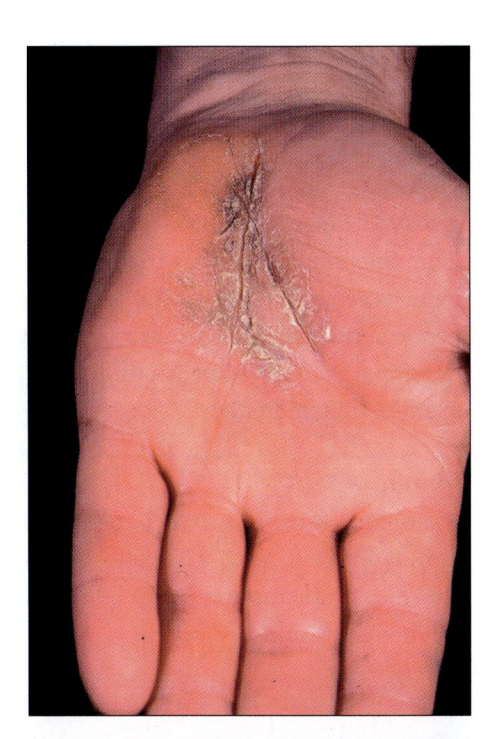

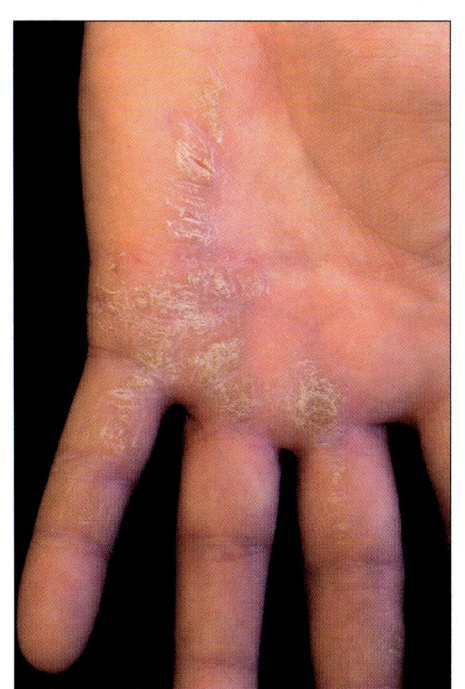

5.19 Palmar psoriasis.

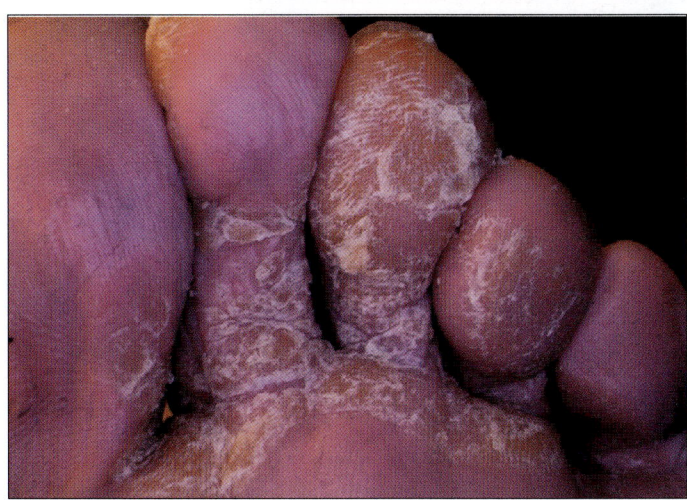

5.20 Psoriasis of the toes.

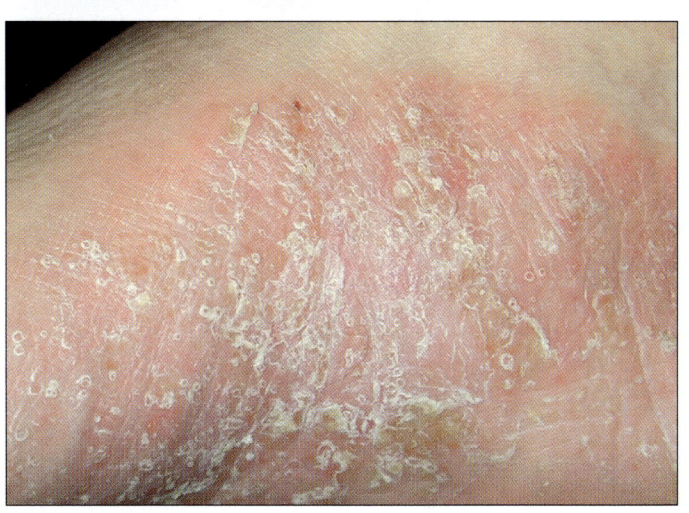

5.21 Psoriasis of the instep of the foot.

72 Hand and foot dermatoses

Differential diagnosis
Hyperkeratotic hand dermatitis or tylotic eczema shows hyperkeratotic plaques, centrally located in both palms, with a tendency to painful fissures (5.22). The histopathology reveals a slight focal parakeratosis and hyperkeratosis, with a spongiotic dermatitis rather than acanthosis and extended rete ridges. It is a separate entity, which has to be differentiated from psoriasis. It is usually far itchier than palmar psoriasis. Familial palmar keratodermas can present in adulthood and are differentiated by the family history (5.23).

Management
Topical steroids, including potent topical steroids, often under polythene occlusion, are necessary to help palmar psoriasis and plantar psoriasis. Use of emollients helps to prevent fissuring.

Prognosis
Psoriasis of the palms and soles does not respond as well as dermatitis to topical steroids and the prognosis is usually worse. Second-line treatment such as oral retinoids or topical PUVA are often necessary.

Fungus infection

Introduction
Fungus infection of the feet is extremely common; up to 5–10% of the population have fungus infection of the toe webs, spreading on to their plantar surface and the dorsal aspect of the feet. Fungus infection of the hands is less common and tends to be more asymmetrical.

Clinical presentation
Fungal infection of the hands presents with dryness and scaling, usually unilateral (see Chapter 9, 5.24, 5.25). With fungus infection of the feet the nails will often be involved. A spreading ringworm-like infection to the dorsum of the foot (5.26), or dry moccasin-form of fungal infection affecting the soles can be seen.

Differential diagnosis
The differential diagnosis includes psoriasis, hyperkeratotic hand eczema, or even ICD. *Table 5.4* lists the differences between psoriasis, fungus infection, and eczema of the hand. Scrapings of the skin should be sent for mycological examination and culture.

Management
If fungus infection has been diagnosed, then topical terbinafine will usually be effective. If it has been a very chronic problem and also affects the nails, then oral terbinafine would be needed.

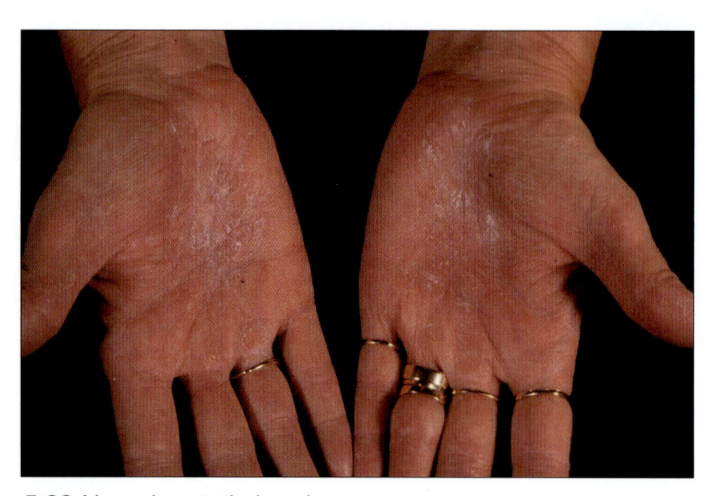

5.22 Hyperkeratotic hand eczema.

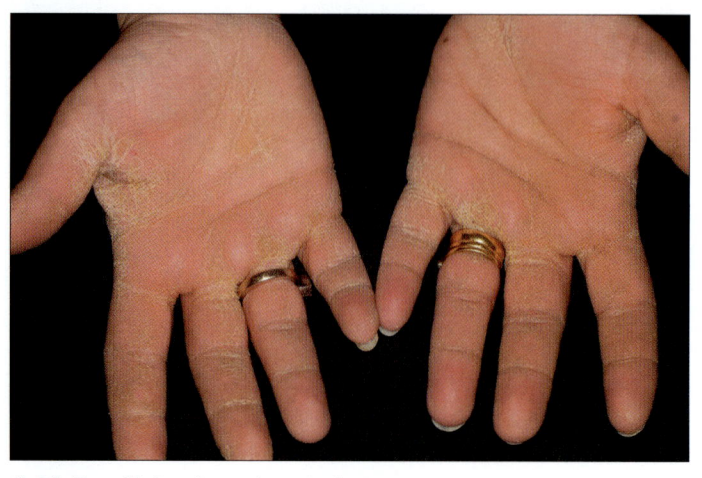

5.23 Familial palmar keratoderma.

Hand and foot dermatoses

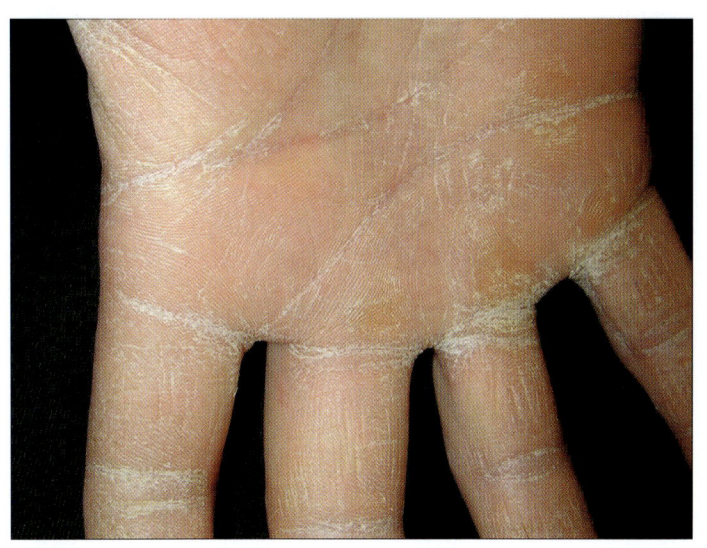

5.24 Fungal infection of the palm.

Prognosis
It is easy to be caught out by fungus infections of the hands; if there is asymmetrical scaling then a fungus infection must be thought of and scrapings for mycology taken.

Providing the fungus responds to terbinafine then the prognosis is good and clearance will occur. However, if it is a resistant case then further courses of terbinafine will be needed.

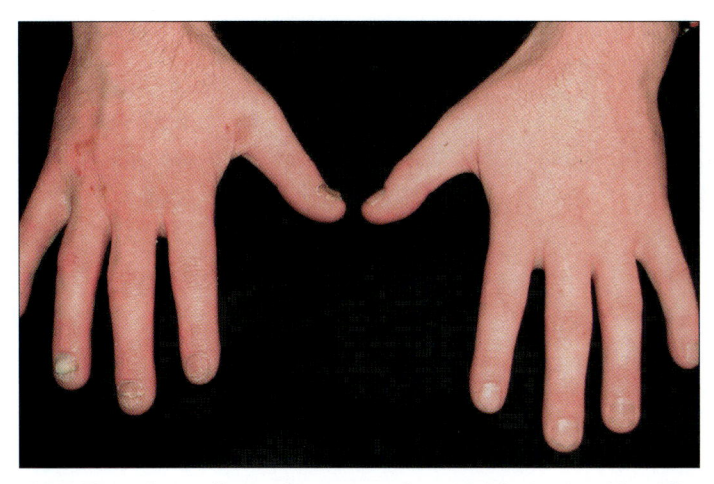

5.25 Note the unilateral presentation of this rash with nail involvement. Tinea manum.

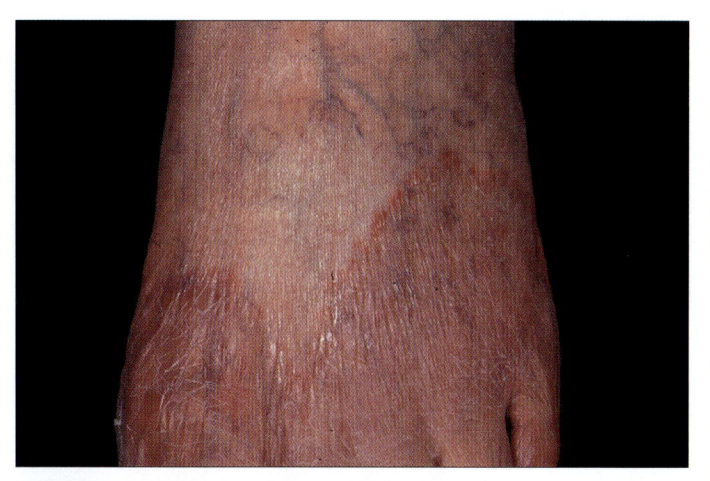

5.26 An active edge of fungal infection of the skin of the back of the foot.

Table 5.4 The differences between hand psoriasis, tinea manum and hand eczema

Psoriasis	Tinea manum	Hyperkeratotic hand eczema
Not usually itchy	Can be itchy	Itchy
Painful fissuring	Sometimes fissuring	Painful fissuring
Dry silvery scale	Usually dry, scaly	Vesicular, scaly
Well-defined lesions	Active edge on back of hand	More diffuse lesions
Nail and knuckle involvement	Nails often involved	Nails not involved
Koebner phenomena		

74 Hand and foot dermatoses

Palmo-plantar pustulosis

Introduction
This is a variant of psoriasis, a localized form of pustular psoriasis affecting the palms and soles. Probably less than 10% of patients with palmo-plantar pustular psoriasis will have signs of psoriasis elsewhere.

Clinical presentation
It presents with localized vesicles and pustules on the palms and soles which can be very painful; patients often liken it to walking on broken glass (**5.27–5.29**). In the early phase sometimes the pustules are not so obvious, but they usually fade to leave brown spots.

Differential diagnosis
Vesicular hand eczema and fungus infection are the differential diagnosis. It is sometimes difficult to make the diagnosis of palmo-plantar pustulosis if there is predominantly a vesicular component to it.

Management
Potent, or very potent topical steroids under polythene occlusion are usually necessary to gain some control.

Prognosis
Prognosis is often poor, with palmo-plantar pustulosis running a prolonged course; however, if control can be achieved then hopefully, it will remain clear for a long period of time. Further treatment options include oral retinoids and local hand/foot PUVA.

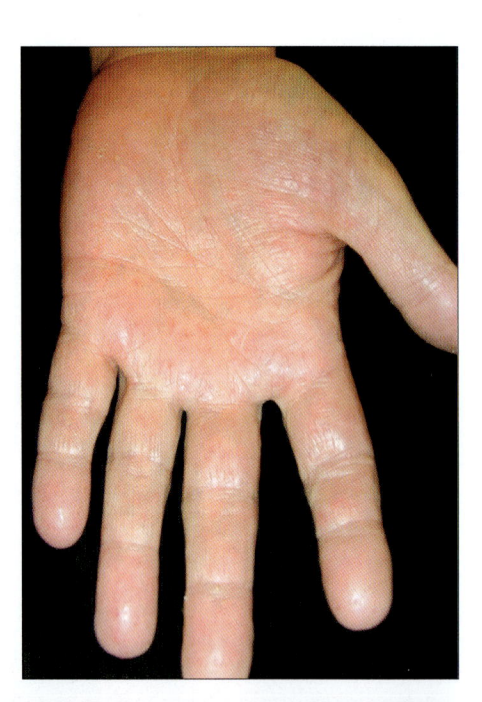

5.27 Palmar pustular psoriasis – not vesicular hand eczema!

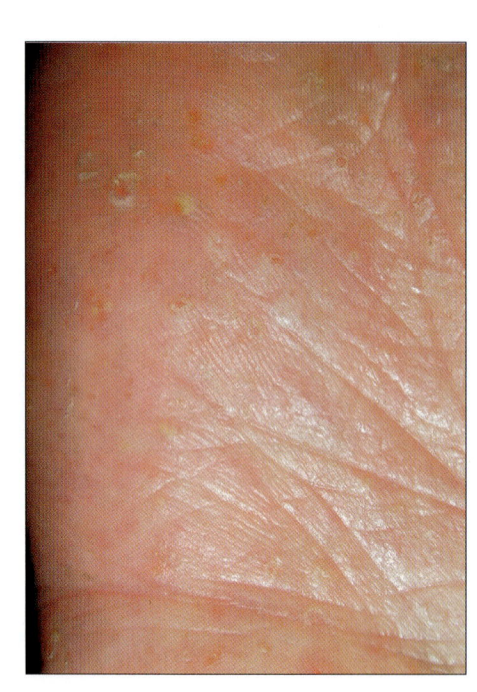

5.28 Close-up of **5.27** showing there are pustules.

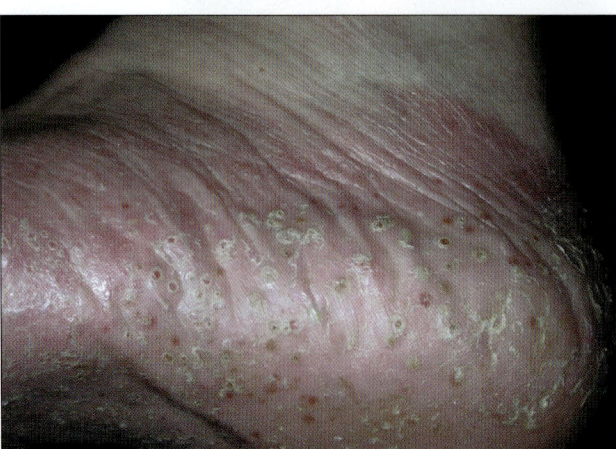

5.29 More obvious plantar pustular psoriasis.

Miscellaneous conditions affecting the hands and feet

A variety of inflammatory dermatoses can affect the hands. The commonest include lichen planus, granuloma annulare (see Chapter 2) and bullous pemphigoid (see Chapter 3) (**5.30–5.32**). Rarer dermatoses such as dermatomyositis and vasculitis are also seen (**5.33, 5.34**). Scabies commonly affects the finger webs and hands and feet, and this is often the first place to look when one suspects scabies, as the burrows are more visible here than elsewhere (see Chapter 3). Crusted scabies can cause a diagnostic problem on occasion, especially when it is very severe (**5.35**). Scabies infestation is very easily caught from these patients.

5.30 Lichen planus of the wrist spreading to the palm. Wickam striae can be seen on the wrist lesions.

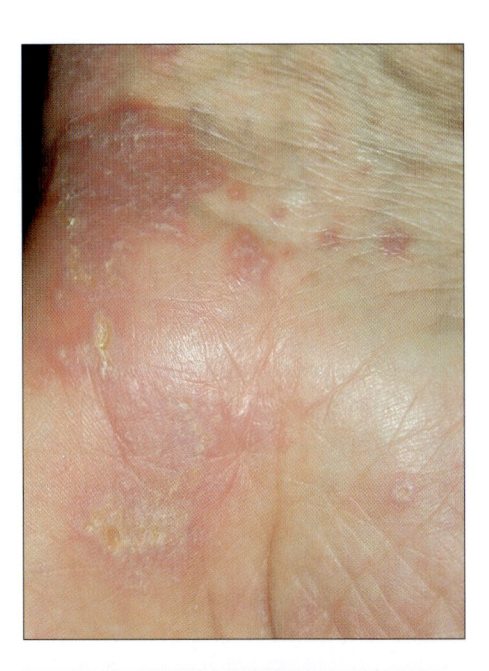

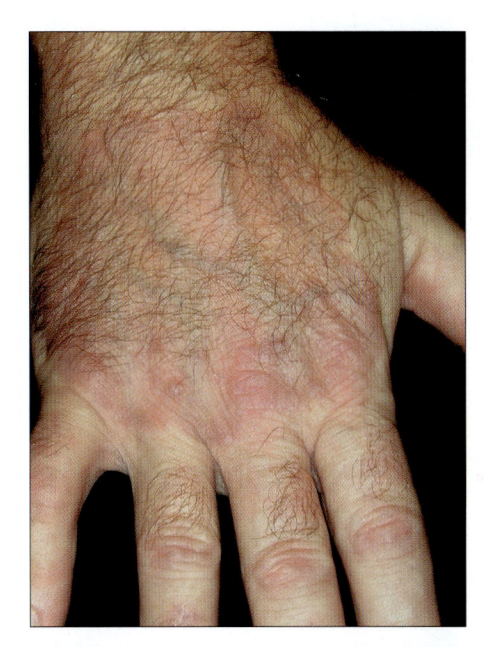

5.31 Granuloma annulare on the back of the hand mimicking a fungal infection or ICD.

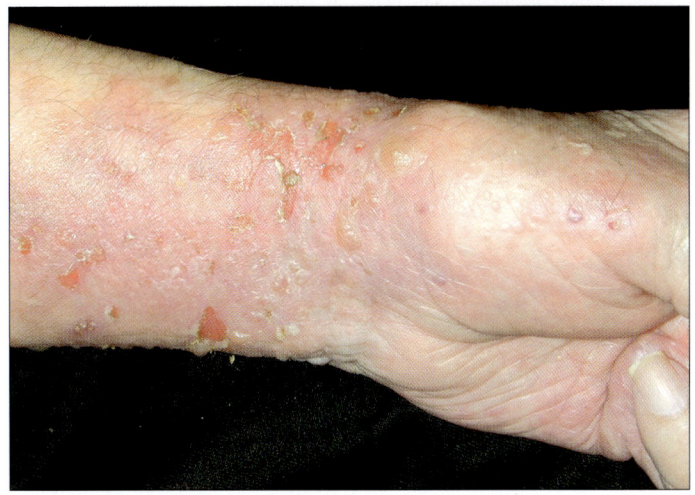

5.32 Vesiculobullous eruption of bullous pemphigoid.

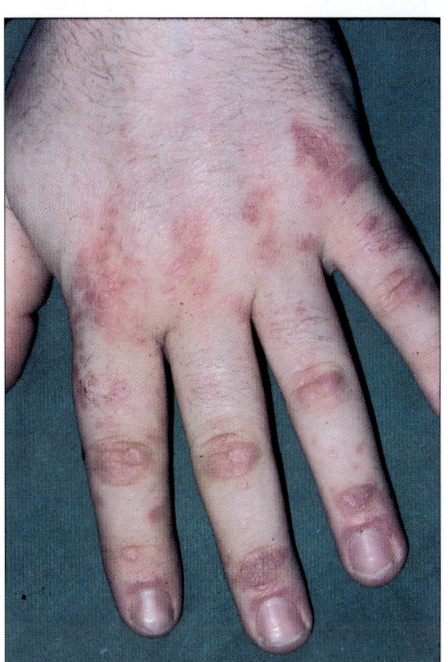

5.33 Dermatomyositis (Gottron's papules) on the knuckles and over the interphalangeal joints.

76 Hand and foot dermatoses

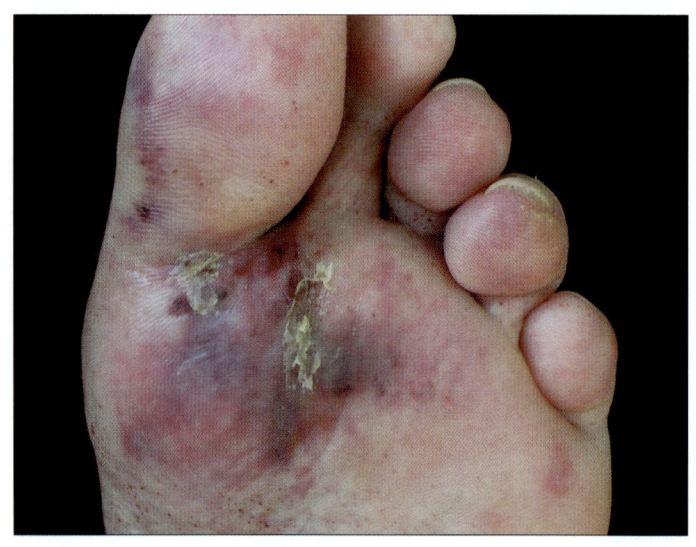

5.34 An area of necrosis and haemorrhagic vesicles on the sole of a foot due to small vessel thrombosis in a patient with phospholipid syndrome.

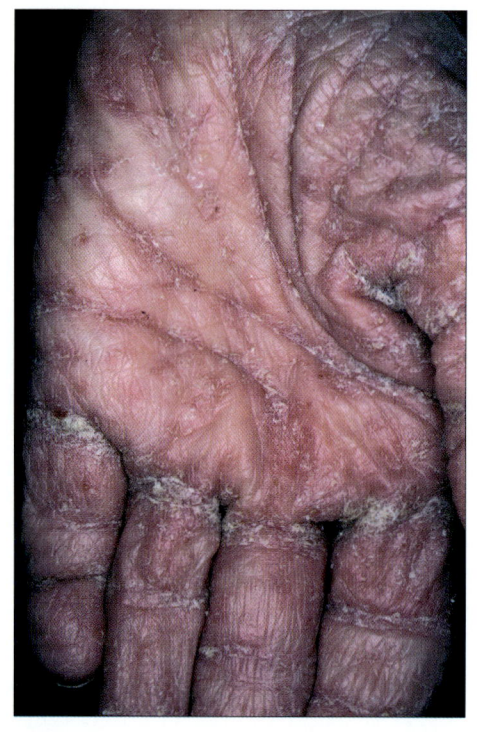

5.35 Norwegian scabies in an elderly patient from a nursing home.

Further reading

Menne T, Maibach H (eds) (2001). *Hand Eczema* (2nd edn). CRC Press, Boca Raton, Florida.

English JSC (ed) (1999). *A Colour Handbook of Occupational Dermatology*. Manson Publishing, London.

Chapter 6

Facial rashes

*Paul Farrant, MRCP and
Russell Emerson, MD, MRCP*

Introduction

Facial rashes cause cosmetic embarrassment to patients and are an important source of anxiety. The face is involved in many different diseases because it contains numerous sebaceous glands and is constantly exposed to the environment. This chapter describes the common dermatological diseases and an approach to differentiating them from each other.

History

It is important to take a thorough history of the presenting skin complaint and exposure to external factors including ultraviolet light (UV), cosmetic products, prescribed topical creams, and systemic therapies. This should include a medical history and enquiry about other medical symptoms including muscle weakness, joint pains, and past history of skin problems. *Table 6.1* lists the clinical features of common facial rashes.

- Scale: rashes with associated scale suggest psoriasis (silvery-white), seborrhoeic dermatitis (greasy, yellow), eczema, contact dermatitis, or possibly a fungal infection.
- Pustules and papules: acne, rosacea, perioral dermatitis, folliculitis and pseudo folliculitis barbae. Multiple small papules on the cheeks are seen in tuberous sclerosis and polymorphic light eruption following UV exposure.
- Vesicles/milia/cysts: vesicles are seen with herpetic infections. Milia are common but may be a feature of porphyria. Cysts are common on the face and can occur in isolation (epidermoid, pilar) or as part of an acneiform eruption.
- Swelling: periorbital swelling is seen with angio-oedema (urticaria), dermatomyositis, and rosacea. Swelling and redness of one cheek are seen with erysipelas. Acute contact dermatitis often causes localized itching and swelling which becomes dry or scaly, whereas urticaria/angio-oedema does not.
- Pigmentation: macular pigmentation on the cheeks is suggestive of melasma. The face is also a common site for simple lentigo, lentigo maligna, and seborrhoeic keratoses.
- Atrophy/scarring: discoid lupus is associated with scarring. Atrophoderma vermiculatum, a facial variant of keratosis pilaris, causes atrophy over the cheeks.

A stepwise approach to the management of patients with erythema/scaling and papules/pustules is seen in **6.1** and **6.2**, respectively.

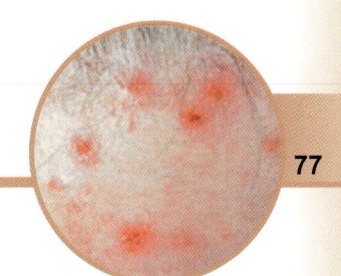

Facial rashes

Table 6.1 Clinical features of facial rashes

Skin erythema and scaling
- Seborrhoeic dermatitis
- Atopic eczema
- Tinea
- Psoriasis
- Keratosis pilaris

Papulo-pustular
- Rosacea
- Acne
- Adenoma sebaceum
- Polymorphic light eruption
- Rare: sarcoidosis, granuloma faciale

Vesicles/bullae
- Herpes simplex/zoster
- Erysipelas
- Erythema multiforme
- Pemphigus

Pigmentation
- Melasma/chloasma
- Solar lentigines
- Drug-induced
- Lentigo maligna
- Poikiloderma of Civatte

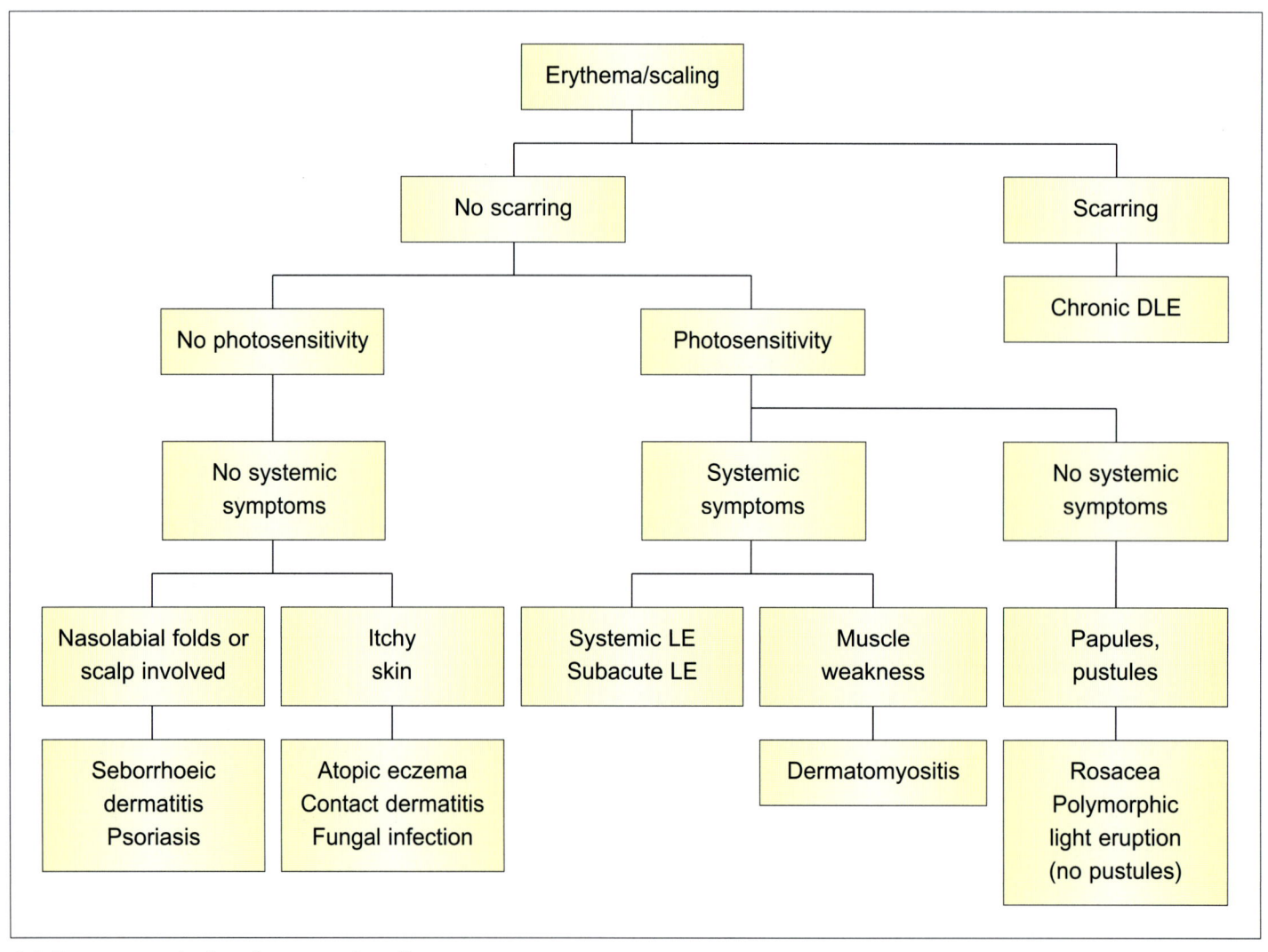

6.1 Management of erythema and scaling.

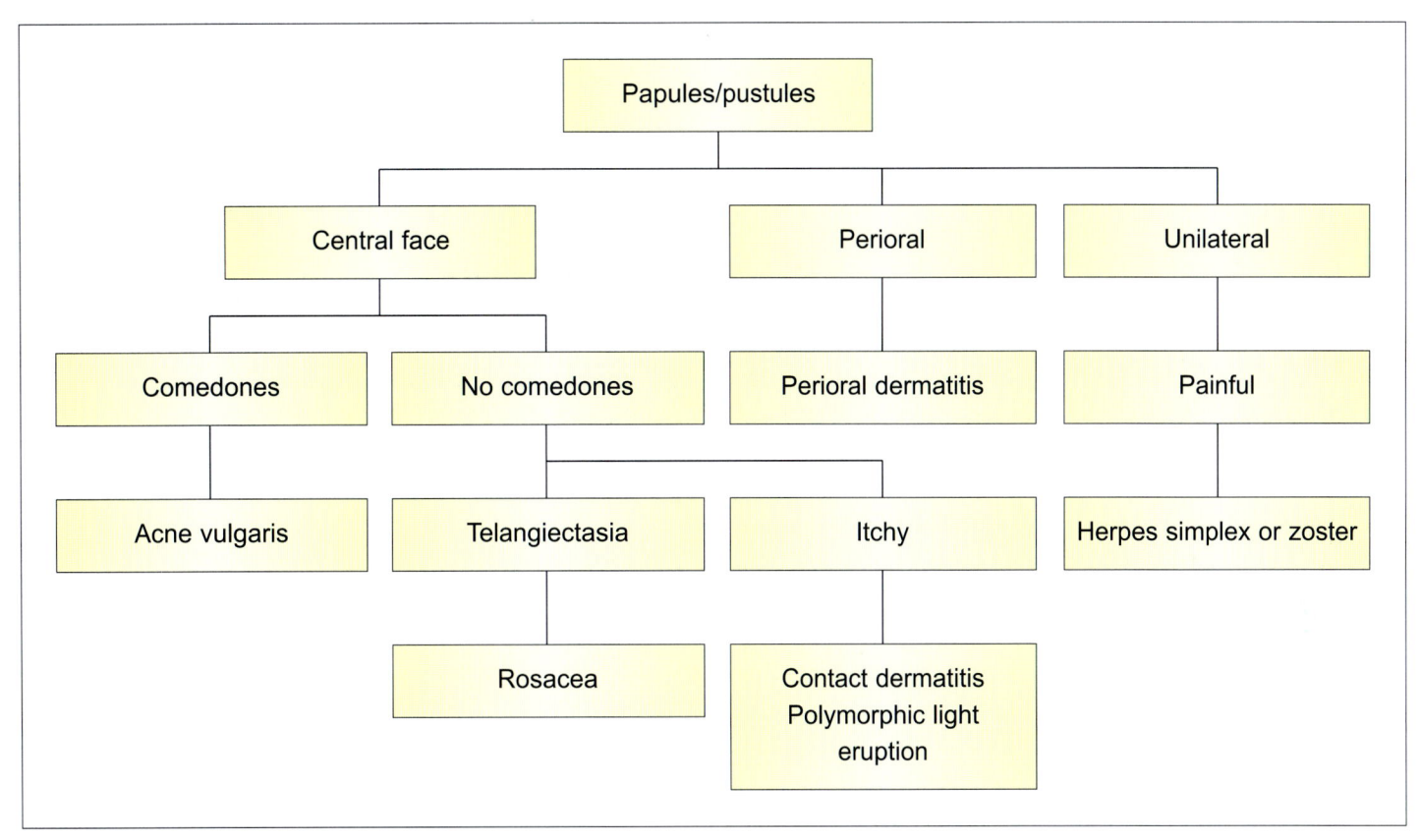

Facial rashes 79

```
                        Papules/pustules
         ┌──────────────────┼──────────────────┐
    Central face          Perioral          Unilateral
     ┌────┴────┐             │                  │
 Comedones  No comedones  Perioral dermatitis  Painful
     │       ┌─┴──────┐       │                  │
Acne vulgaris Telangiectasia  Itchy    Herpes simplex or zoster
              │                │
           Rosacea      Contact dermatitis
                        Polymorphic light
                            eruption
```

6.2 Management of papules and pustules.

Acne

Introduction
Acne is a disorder affecting the pilosebaceous unit associated with excess grease production of the skin, keratinization of the opening of the hair follicle, and inflammation due to bacterial infection with *Propionibacterium acnes* that may result in scarring.

Clinical presentation
Acne typically presents with open comedones (black heads), closed comedones (white heads), papules, pustules, and cystic lesions (**6.3**). The face, upper chest, and upper back are most commonly affected. Macrocomedones and scarring (both pitted and hypertrophic) are also features. A particular variant, acne excoriée, is characterized by marked excoriations on the face and is typically seen in young women (**6.4**).

Histopathology
Perifollicular inflammation with a predominance of neutrophils is seen. The hair follicles are often dilated, and filled with keratin. Rupture of the follicles can result in a foreign body reaction.

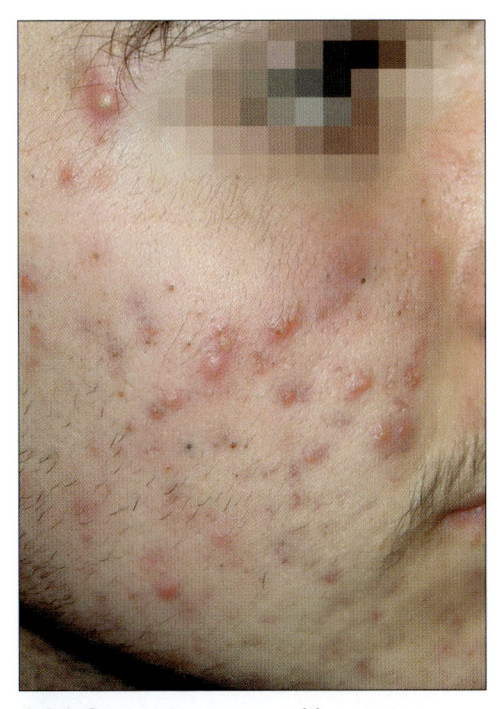

6.3 Inflammatory acne with numerous papules, pustules, and comedones.

Differential diagnosis

Folliculitis, rosacea, and perioral dermatitis can all mimic acne on the face. Acne-like conditions can also be precipitated by drugs (e.g. antiepileptics), topical and oral corticosteroids, oils applied to the hair line (pomade acne), and exposure to various chemicals (e.g. chloracne).

Management

Most acne will clear spontaneously by the mid twenties. Mild acne can be managed by topical agents, applied daily for 3–6 months. These include benzoyl peroxide (first line, good for noninflammatory acne), topical antibiotics (erythromycin, clindamycin), and topical retinoid related drugs (tretinoin and adapalene). Combinations of these agents can also be used, for example benzoyl peroxide in the morning and a retinoid in the evening.

Moderate acne is best managed with systemic antibiotics in addition to topical agents. These again require 3–6 months of treatment to achieve long-term clearance. These include oxytetracycline, lymecycline, erythromycin, and trimethoprim.

For unresponsive cases or severe acne associated with scarring, specialist referral is indicated. Such patients may require a 4–6 month course of oral isotretinoin. This achieves clearance in 85% of patients. Frequent side-effects include dryness of the lips, mucous membranes, and skin. It should be avoided in pregnancy and patients may require monitoring of their liver function and lipids. Any change in mood or tendency to depression during treatment should lead to cessation of therapy.

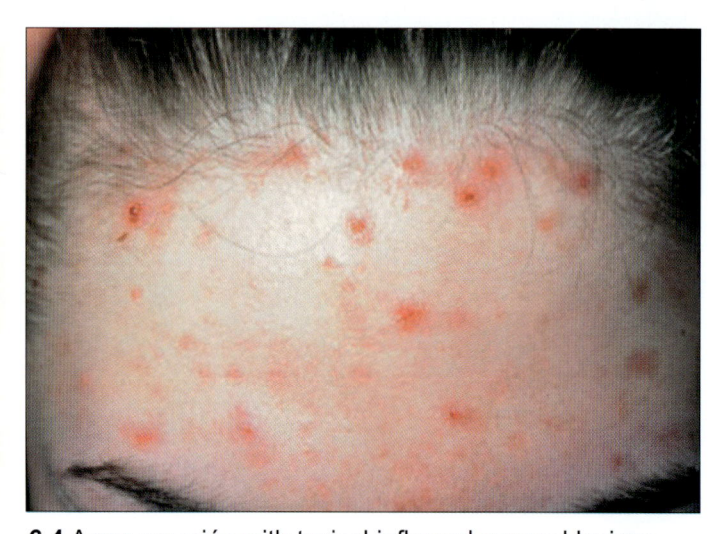

6.4 Acne excoriée with typical inflamed scarred lesions over the forehead.

Perioral dermatitis

Introduction

Perioral dermatitis typically affects young women in the 20–35-year-old age group. It is a variant of rosacea and may be precipitated by inappropriate use of moderate/potent topical corticosteroids.

Clinical presentation

It is characterized by small erythematous papules around the mouth and chin (**6.5A**). The area immediately adjacent to the vermillion border is usually spared. There may also be periorbital involvement. Comedones are not a feature.

Differential diagnosis

Acne vulgaris, steroid acne, rosacea, and seborrhoeic dermatitis are the main differentials.

Management

Patients should be advised to stop the application of topical corticosteroids and placed on a 2–4 month course of oral tetracycline antibiotics (**6.5B**). Topical tacrolimus and pimecrolimus may also be beneficial for flares.

Rosacea

Introduction

Rosacea is a common cause of facial redness in the 25–55-year-old age group, especially women.

Clinical presentation

Many patients have a history of flushing exacerbated by trigger factors including spicy foods, temperature changes, and alcohol. Facial redness typically occurs with small papules and occasional pustules (**6.6, 6.7**). The inflammatory changes typically affect the cheeks and nasolabial folds. Fixed redness may develop associated with superficial blood vessels (telangiectasia) and rarely sebaceous hyperplasia leads to an enlarged nose (rhinophyma) (**6.8**). Up to 15% of patients may have associated eye involvement presenting as conjunctivitis, keratitis, blepharitis, and cyst formation along the eyelid margin. Comedones are typically absent in rosacea.

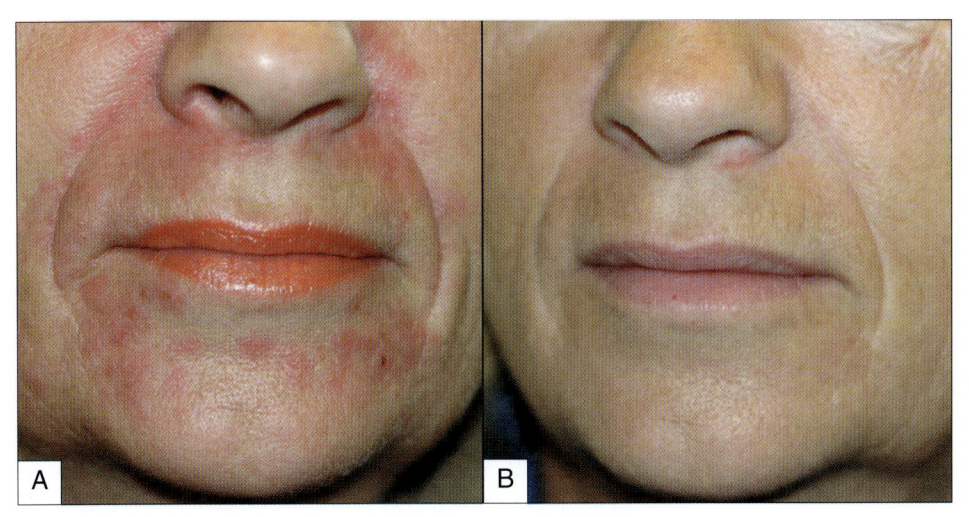

6.5 Perioral dermatitis before (**A**) and after (**B**) successful treatment with an oral tetracycline.

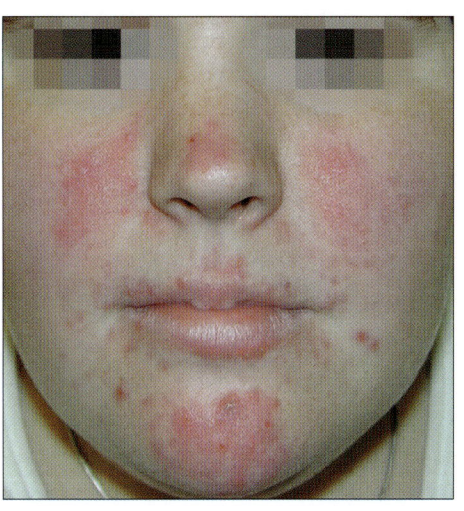

6.6 Papular lesions on the cheeks, nose, and chin with no evidence of comedones is typical of rosacea.

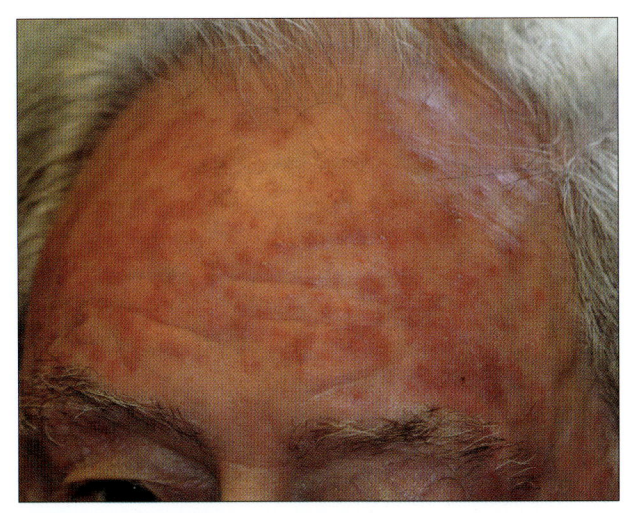

6.7 Severe rosacea of the forehead requires systemic treatment.

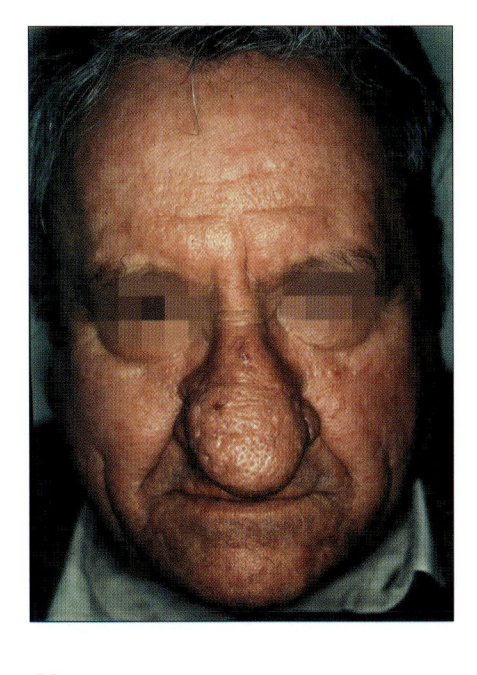

6.8 Rhinophyma is often associated with rosacea.

Histopathology

A mixed lympho-histiocytic perifollicular infiltrate may be present. In addition, there may be a perivascular infiltrate or granulomatous response. These changes are nonspecific. There may also be vascular dilatation, solar elastosis, and sebaceous gland hyperplasia indicating solar damage.

Differential diagnosis

Rosacea should always be suspected in patients with facial redness and papules. Other causes of flushing and erythema include eczema, seborrhoeic dermatitis, systemic lupus erythematosus, and the carcinoid syndrome.

Management

Patients should avoid trigger factors. Mild cases can be managed with topical metronidazole gel. More severe cases (**6.7**) require courses of systemic tetracyclines for 2–4 months. Many patients experience disease relapses and patients should be informed that it might be a chronic condition. Severe cases may need a specialist opinion and low-dose oral isotretinoin can be beneficial. Patients with rhinophyma and telangiectasia may benefit from skin surgery and laser therapy, respectively.

Atopic eczema

Introduction
Facial eczema commonly affects adults with severe eczema and can be a presenting feature of allergic contact dermatitis.

Clinical presentation
In infants the cheeks are a common site to be involved, with an ill-defined, red, scaling rash that is symmetrical. Episodes of infection are common and weeping and crusting are both common in this context. In adults, eczema can be either generalized (**6.9**, **6.10**), or more localized to specific areas such as the skin around the eyes and mouth. Lichenification of the skin may be present around the eyes (**6.11**).

Histopathology
See Chapter 3.

Differential diagnosis
The main differential diagnosis is contact dermatitis and all patients with facial eczema should be considered for patch testing to look for a contact allergen. Seborrhoeic dermatitis and psoriasis may also cause confusion.

Management
Soap and irritants should be avoided and emollients should be applied frequently. Treatment consists of topical steroids and/or topical calcineurin inhibitors. The skin on the face is particularly susceptible to the side-effects of topical steroids and treatment should be carefully monitored. Mild steroids (1% hydrocortisone) should be used initially and cream may be more cosmetically acceptable to patients. Moderate steroids may be necessary but used for limited periods of time (clobetasone butyrate, alclometasone dipropionate). Steroids should not be used continuously and there should be regular breaks from their use. They should not be used on the eyelids. The calcineurin inhibitors, tacrolimus ointment and pimecrolimus cream, are very useful on the face as they do not cause thinning of the skin.

Contact dermatitis

Introduction
Facial eczema can develop due to a number of external allergens including perfume, nail varnish, preservatives in cosmetic creams, nickel in jewellery, and plants. Typically, this occurs as a delayed type IV allergy and patients require referral to a dermatologist for specialist investigation with patch testing (see Chapter 1).

Clinical presentation
The sudden onset of facial eczema in a patient with no previous history of skin problems should raise suspicion of contact allergy. Contact dermatitis is more frequently seen in individuals with eyelid dermatitis (perfume/nail varnish) (**6.12**), localized ear involvement (topical medicaments used for otitis externa/nickel in ear rings), and scalp involvement (hair dyes). A detailed clinical history is useful in pinpointing the onset of the symptoms, exacerbating factors, and improvement following avoidance, but patch testing is usually necessary to identify the cause.

Histopathology
The pathological features are similar for other types of eczema. Eosinophils may be more conspicuous and Langerhans cells, when stained with S100, are more numerous.

Differential diagnosis
Atopic eczema, seborrhoeic dermatitis, and psoriasis should be considered.

Management
Patients with suspected contact allergy should be advised to stop all cosmetic products, use unperfumed soaps, and apply regular moisturizers. Topical corticosteroids may be necessary for disease flares. Specialist referral for patch testing is usually indicated to identify the culprit allergen or allergens.

Facial rashes 83

6.9 Ill-defined erythema with lichenification of the inner canthus is typical of chronic atopic eczema.

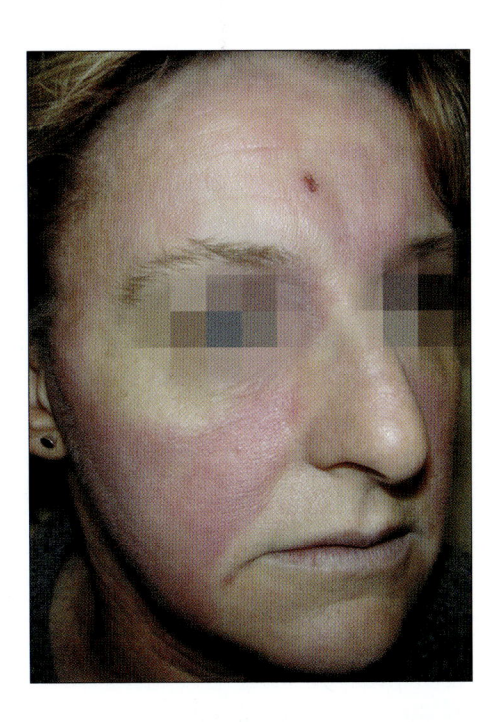

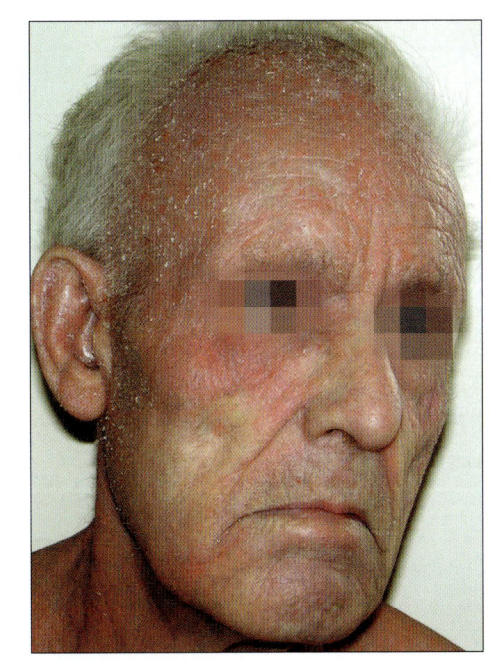

6.10 Sub-acute facial eczema.

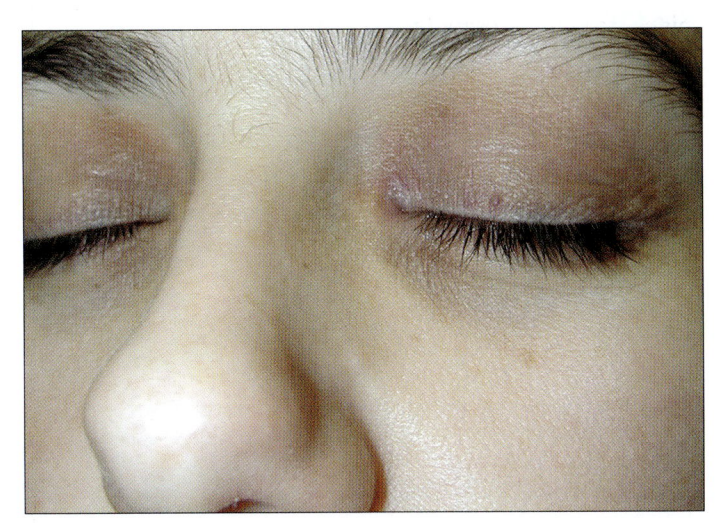

6.11 Localized atopic eczema causing lichenification of the eyelids.

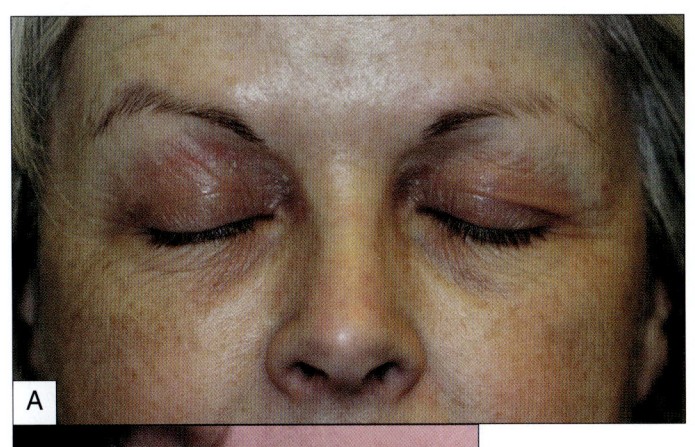

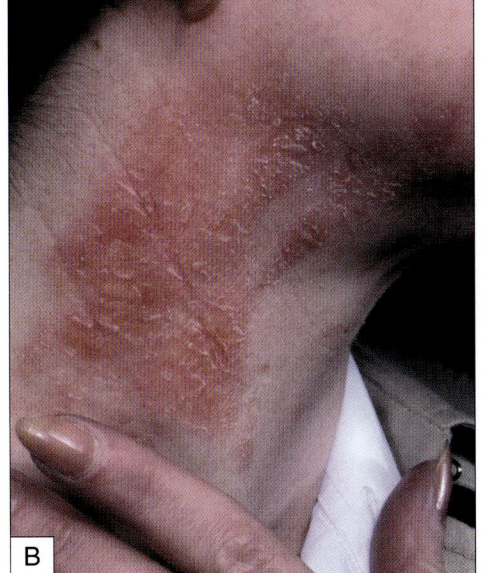

6.12 Contact dermatitis caused by nail varnish often causes a rash on the eyelids (**A**) and neck (**B**).

Seborrhoeic dermatitis

Introduction
Seborrhoeic dermatitis is a chronic condition that typically produces redness and pronounced scaling around the naso-labial folds and hair-bearing areas of the skin. There is an association with HIV infection, Parkinson's disease, and stress. The exact aetiology is unknown although *Pityrosporum ovale*, a skin commensal, is thought to play a role.

Clinical presentation
Infants present with thick yellow scales on the scalp – 'cradle cap'. In adults, there is an erythematous rash with thick scale (**6.13**) that has a predilection for the eyebrows, nasolabial folds, glabella, and scalp (dandruff and erythema). It can occur in the beard and moustache areas. There may also be involvement of the external auditory meatus, upper trunk, axillae, and groin.

Histopathology
The pathological findings are nonspecific but typically there is spongiosis, hyperkeratosis, parakeratosis associated with the hair follicles, and exocytosis of neutrophils.

Differential diagnosis
Psoriasis can mimic seborrhoeic dermatitis and may even coexist (sebo-psoriasis). Dermatophyte infection may also cause a red scaly rash, but tends to be asymmetrical and has an active scaly border. Skin scrapings may be necessary to rule out fungal infection if in doubt.

Management
Many patients experience a chronic disease with remission and relapses. Therapy is aimed at disease suppression and at reducing yeast overgrowth of the skin, thought to contribute to the disease process. Topical imidazoles may be used alone or in combination with mild topical steroids to treat associated inflammation (1% hydrocortisone). Ketoconazole/selenium sulphide shampoos may be used in dilute form to control scalp dandruff and washed gently into affected areas of the body. More potent steroids may be required in more resistant cases and pimecrolimus/tacrolimus are of benefit in persistent disease.

6.13 Localized scaling of the eyebrows and naso-labial fold with ill-defined erythema is suggestive of seborrhoeic dermatitis.

Psoriasis

Introduction
The face can be involved in patients who have psoriasis, but often this is limited to the hairline.

Clinical presentation
Psoriasis usually produces isolated red plaques on the forehead, outer cheeks, and naso-labial folds. It usually has a sharply marginated border with a silvery-white scale (**6.14A**). It rarely occurs in the absence of psoriasis at other body sites and careful examination should be made looking for fine scaling and redness at other sites including the hairline (**6.14B**), ears, and elbows. Sometimes patients present with a clinical picture of psoriasis and seborrhoeic dermatitis – sebo-psoriasis (**6.14C**).

Histopathology
See Chapter 3.

Differential diagnosis
Seborrhoeic dermatitis and contact dermatitis should be considered.

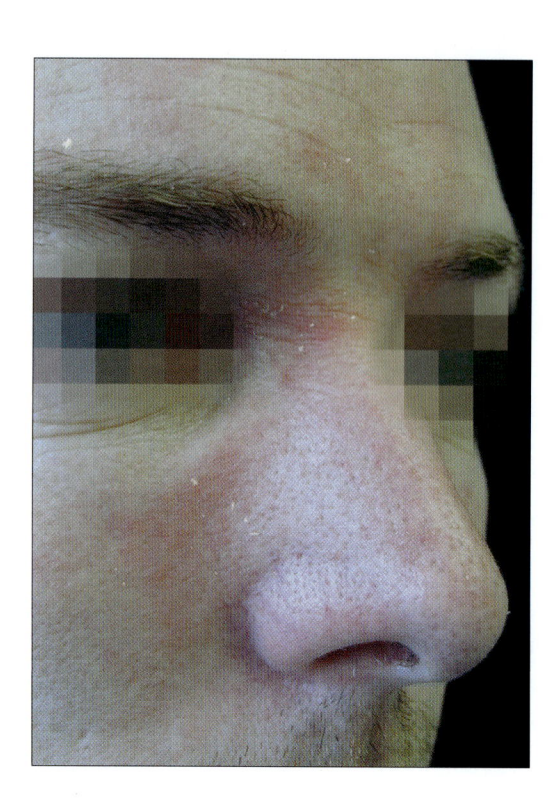

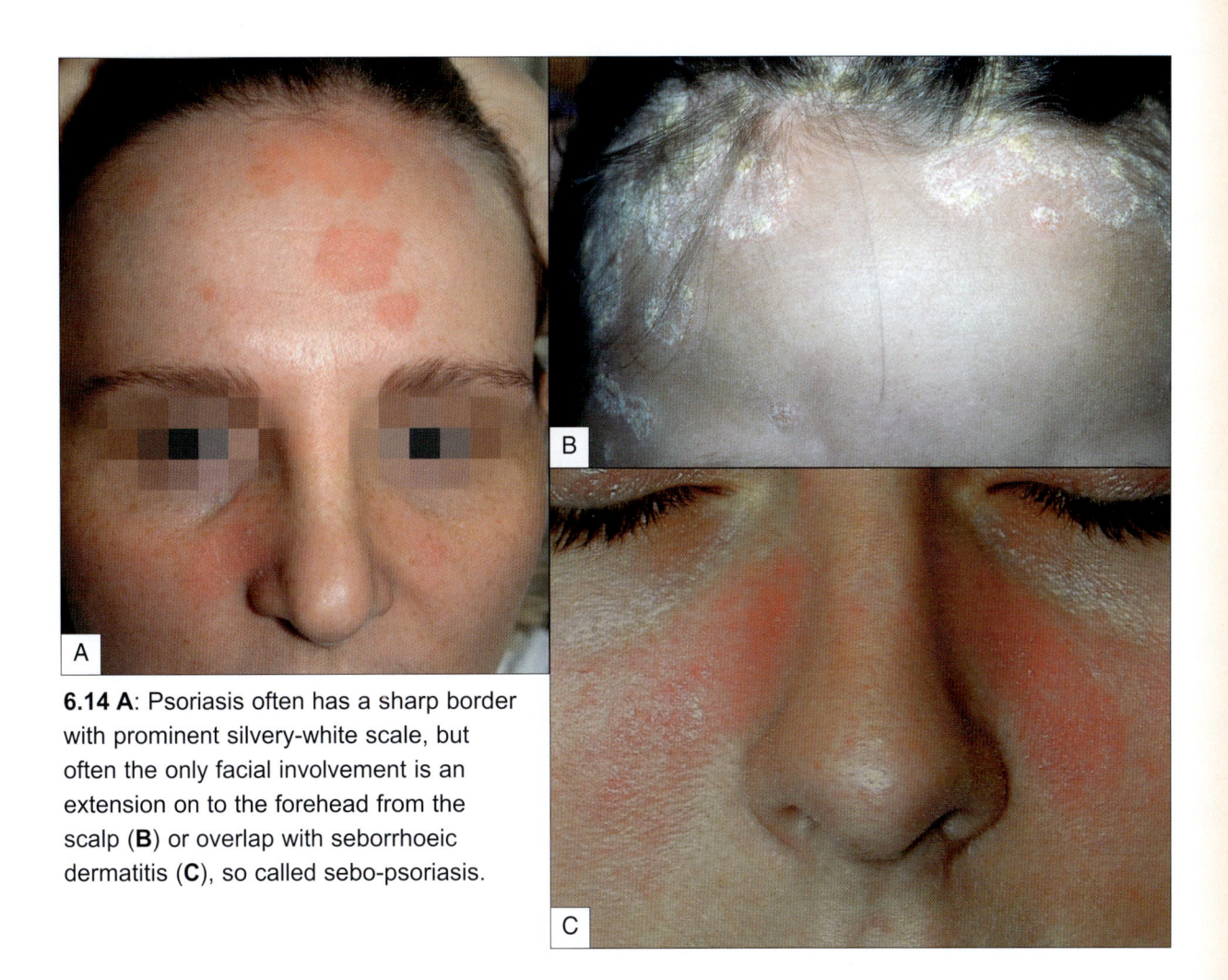

Facial rashes

6.14 A: Psoriasis often has a sharp border with prominent silvery-white scale, but often the only facial involvement is an extension on to the forehead from the scalp (**B**) or overlap with seborrhoeic dermatitis (**C**), so called sebo-psoriasis.

Management

Patients should be advised to apply regular emollients, avoid soaps, and apply topical steroids (1% hydrocortisone and clobetasone butyrate) on a once/twice daily basis when disease is active. Tacrolimus and pimecrolimus may be useful for more chronic persistent disease. Severe cases (**6.15**) may benefit from phototherapy or systemic therapy, particularly if there is more extensive involvement of other body sites.

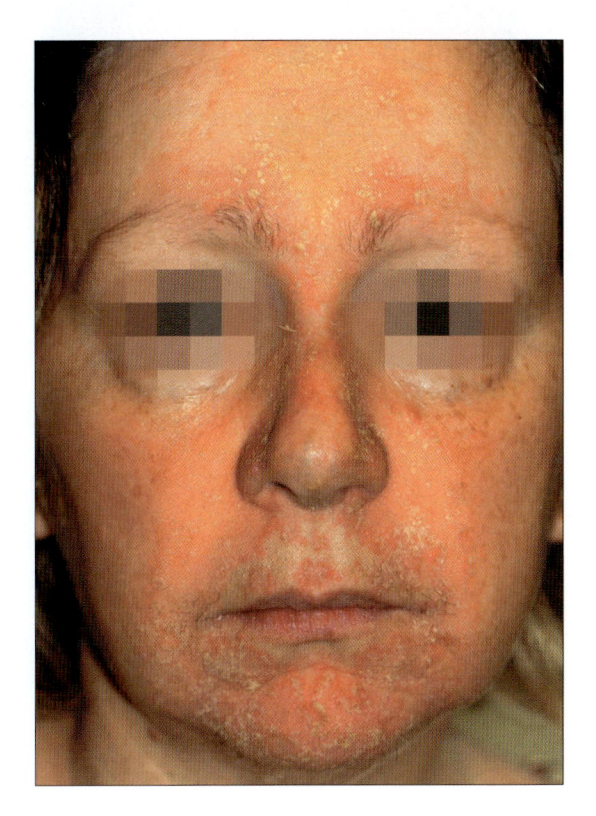

6.15 The face is often spared in psoriasis but disease flares may lead to a severe facial rash.

86 Facial rashes

Melasma

Introduction
Melasma is an acquired pigmentation that typically occurs on the cheeks and is associated with oral contraceptives and hormone replacement therapy. It can also occur during pregnancy. Extensive sun exposure is a common feature in the patient's history.

Clinical presentation
Melasma presents as a uniform brown macular area of increased pigmentation usually over the cheeks (**6.16**). It often affects both cheeks and is very well demarcated.

Histopathology
There is an increase in the amount of melanin in keratinocytes, as well as an increase in epidermal melanocytes and dermal melanophages. Solar elastosis is usually present in the papillary dermis.

Differential diagnosis
Postinflammatory hyperpigmentation should be considered.

Management
High-factor sunscreens are necessary for all patients complaining of melasma and should be applied on a daily basis all year round. Spontaneous resolution may be seen in melasma induced by pregnancy/hormonal therapy. Depigmentating creams (containing hydroquinone 2–4%) may be prescribed for more resistant cases on a twice-daily basis for 4–6 months (**6.16B**).

Lupus erythematosus

Introduction
Lupus erythematosus is an autoimmune disorder with frequent involvement of the skin and photosensitivity. There is a spectrum of disease, which includes discoid lupus (DLE), subacute cutaneous lupus (SCLE), and systemic lupus erythematosus (SLE).

Clinical presentation
Patients with cutaneous DLE usually present with well-defined patches of redness, atrophy, pigmentary disturbance,

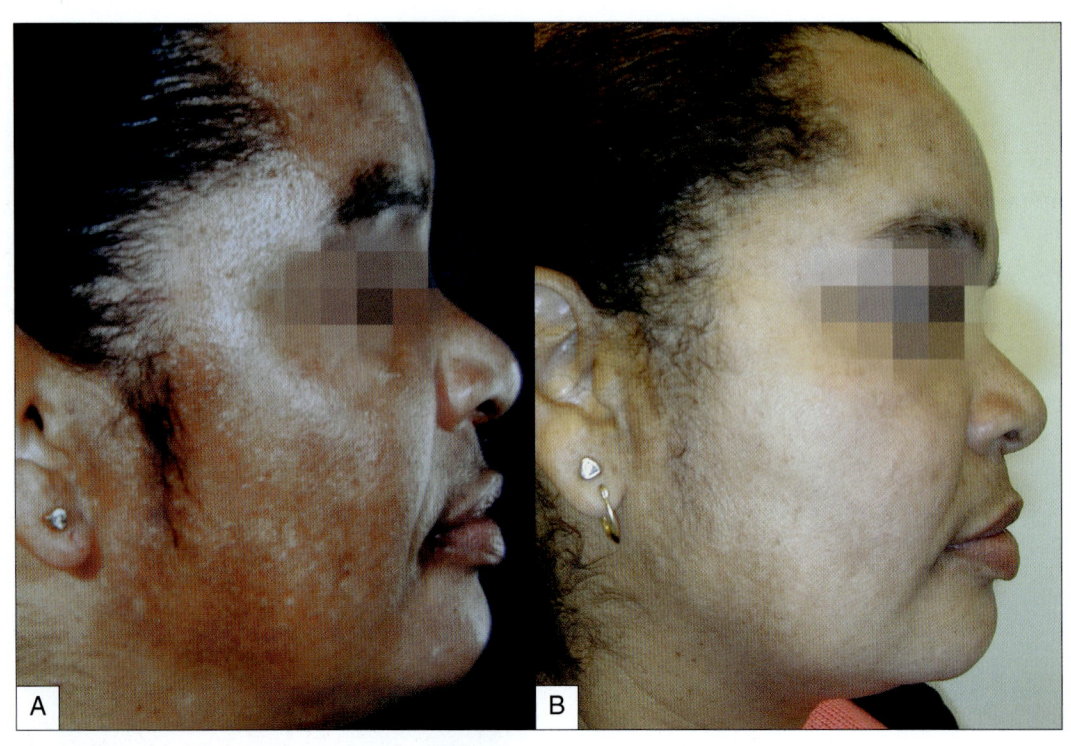

6.16 Melasma before (**A**) and after (**B**) treatment with hydroquinone.

and follicular plugging of hair follicles (**6.17**, **6.18**). The most common sites include the cheeks, bridge of the nose, ears, neck, and scalp. Scalp involvement is frequently observed and a scarring alopecia may develop (see Chapter 8). In other forms of lupus, the patient typically has systemic symptoms including tiredness and joint pains. In systemic lupus, the erythema tends to be more widespread on the face with a typical malar 'butterfly' flush (**6.19**). In subacute cutaneous lupus, there are multiple erythematous plaque-like lesions, which may be annular and resemble psoriasis (**6.20**). All forms of cutaneous lupus are aggravated by UV light exposure.

Histopathology

In cutaneous lupus there is intense inflammation of the basal layer of the skin associated with a dermal perivascular and perifollicular lymphocytic infiltrate. Basement membrane thickening may occur along with pigmentary incontinence. In DLE there may be marked hyperkeratosis, dilated hair follicles, keratin plugging, and epidermal atrophy.

Differential diagnosis

Isolated plaques of DLE may resemble psoriasis, seborrhoeic dermatitis, contact dermatitis, tinea (**6.21**), Jessner's (**6.22**), and lupus vulgaris. The facial butterfly rash of SLE is rare and may be confused with rosacea, which is common. The majority of patients with systemic or subacute lupus feel systemically unwell.

Management

Patients with cutaneous lupus require specialist referral and management. All patients with lupus should be advised to avoid direct sun exposure and use high factor (>SPF30) UVA/UVB sunscreens. DLE lesions usually respond to potent topical corticosteroids, which control inflammation and reduce the incidence of permanent scarring. More severe cases need oral antimalarial therapy with hydroxychloroquine. In SLE and more resistant cases, immunosuppressive drugs may be required.

6.17 Erythematous scarring of the ear with follicular plugging and atrophy.

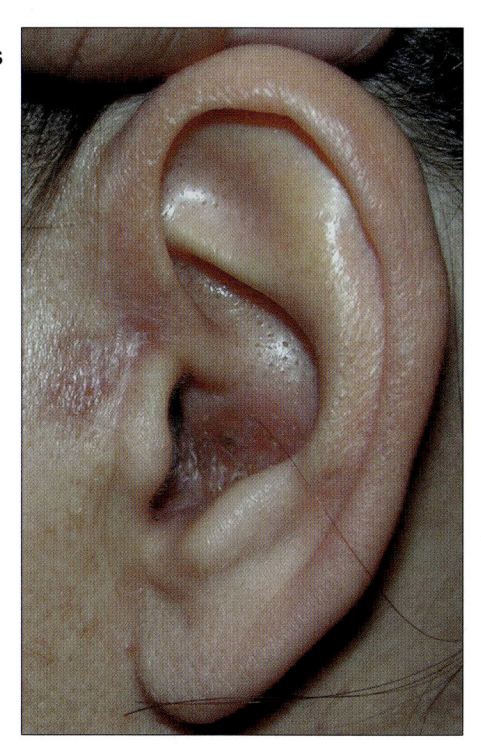

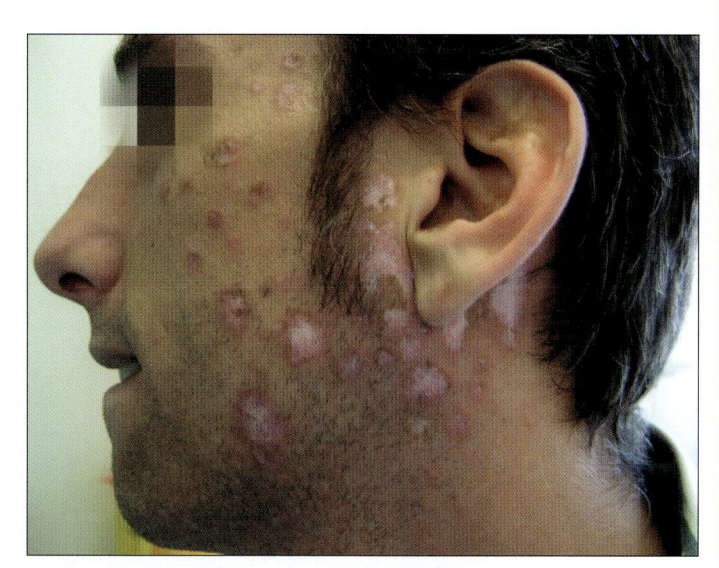

6.18 Chronic scarring DLE of the face.

88 Facial rashes

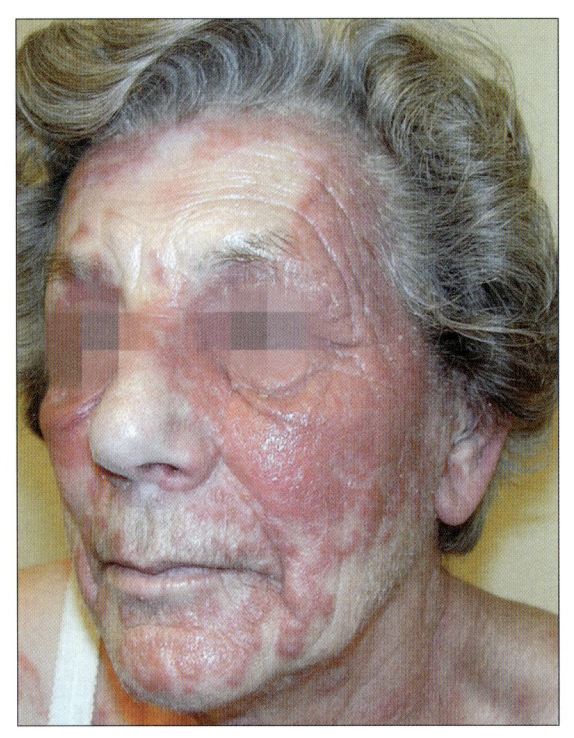

6.19 Severe facial rash of SCLE.

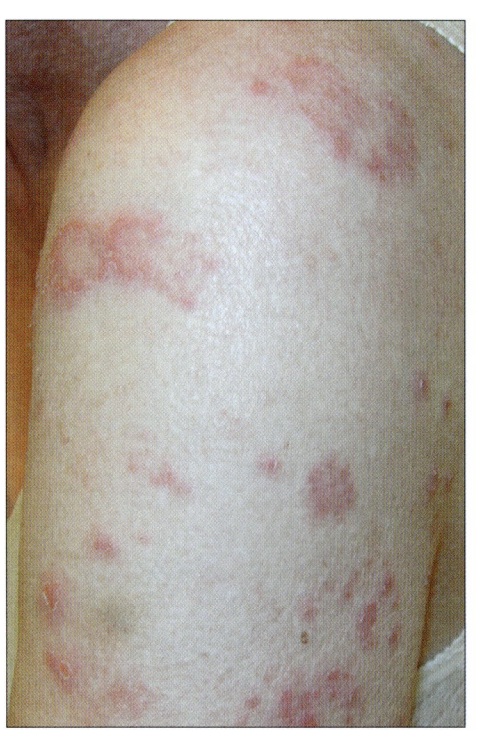

6.20 Annular scaly erythematous plaques in SCLE.

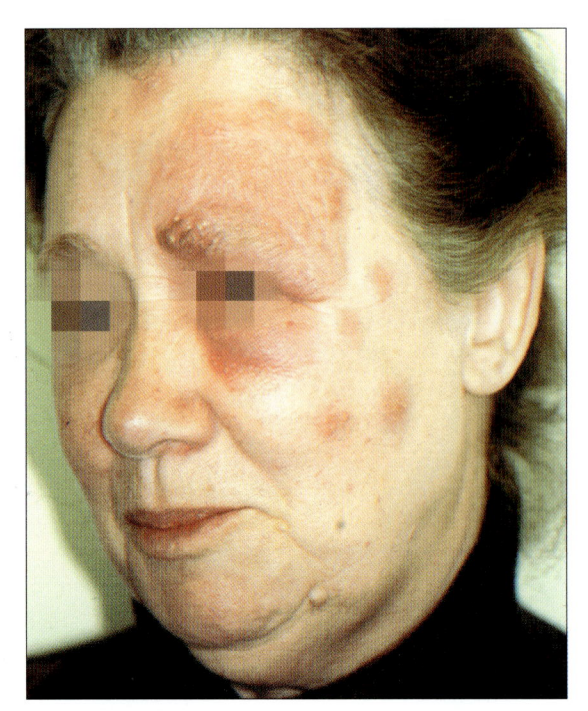

6.21 Tinea facei. This should be included in the differential for lupus and psoriasis on the face.

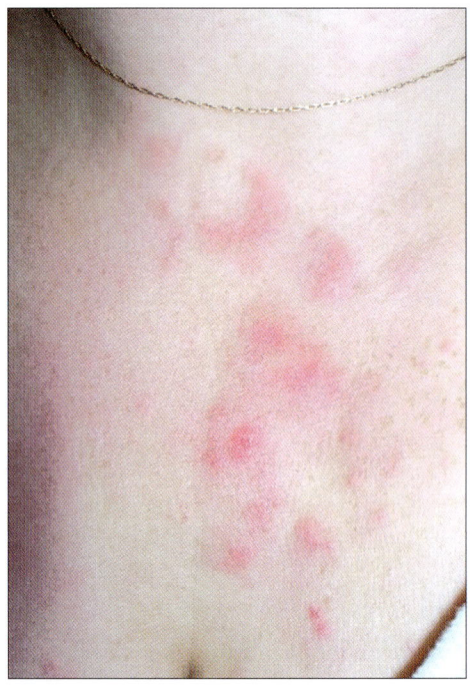

6.22 Jessner's benign lymphocytic infiltrate affecting the chest. There is no scaling and the lesions tend to disappear after a few weeks.

Dermatomyositis

Introduction
This rare autoimmune disorder can cause a facial rash, together with papules over the knuckles (Gottron's papules), and proximal myopathy. A third of adult cases are associated with underlying internal malignancy. There is no association with malignancy in the childhood variant.

Clinical presentation
The classical appearance on the face is a purple, periorbital, oedematous rash, known as the heliotrope rash (**6.23**). The forehead, cheeks, and neck may also be involved, together with Gottron's papules, erythema on the extensor surface of the arms, nail fold telangiectasia (**6.24**), and muscle weakness (proximal myopathy).

Management
Patients with suspected dermatomyositis should be referred for a specialist opinion and further investigation. Systemic therapy with oral prednisolone and other systemic immunosuppressive agents is usually required for several months.

Tuberous sclerosis

Introduction
This autosomal dominant condition is associated with a number of cutaneous features, one of which occurs on the face – adenoma sebaceum. In addition to this, patients may have periungual fibromas (see Chapter 8), ash leaf macules, and a connective tissue naevus known as a 'shagreen patch'. Eye and neurological features are also common.

Clinical presentation
Multiple, small, skin-coloured papular lesions that coalesce to form a cobbled appearance (**6.25**) occur on the cheeks, naso-labial folds, and chin from early childhood. 50% will have some angiofibromas by 3 years of age.

Management
Other clinical features of tuberous sclerosis should be sought and the diagnosis confirmed. Genetic counselling should be offered to parents planning a family. The facial lesions can be removed by a number of surgical means for cosmetic purposes.

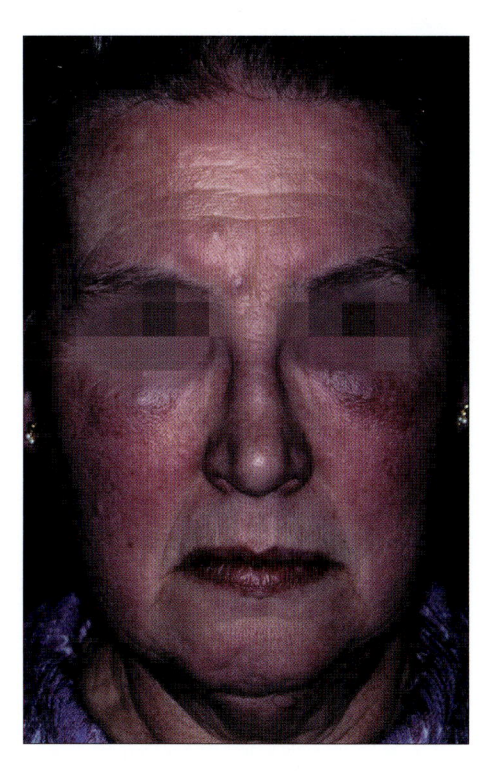

6.23 Periorbital oedematous rash of dermatomyositis (heliotrope rash).

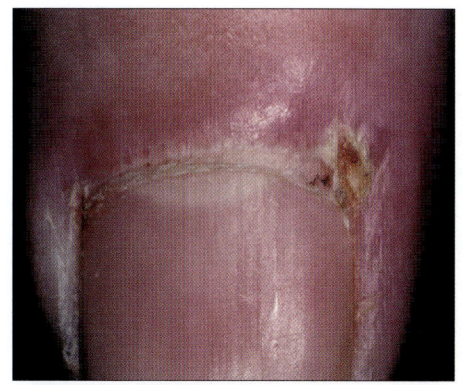

6.24 Prominent vessels of nail folds in dermatomyositis.

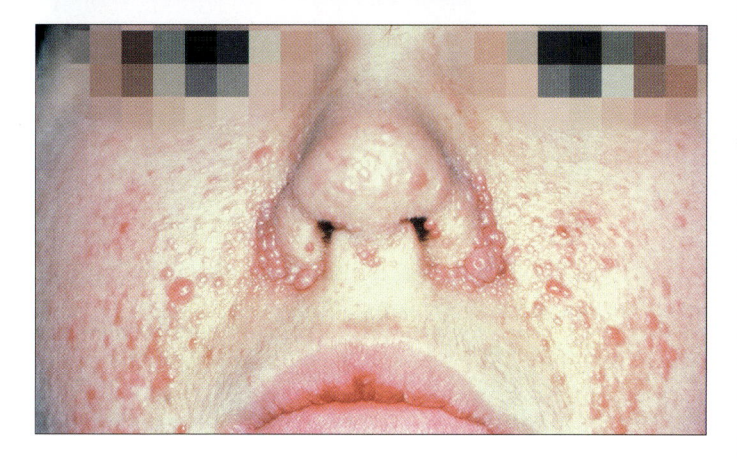

6.25 Erythematous papules associated with adenoma sebaceum.

Keratosis pilaris

Introduction
Keratosis pilaris is a common disorder of keratinization affecting the hair follicles of Caucasian children and young adults. It most commonly affects the outer aspect of the arms (**6.26**) but has two forms that can affect the face, ulerythema ophryogenes and atrophoderma vermiculatum.

Clinical presentation
In ulerythema ophryogenes there is involvement of the eyebrows, with redness, hairloss and prominent keratin at the site of hair follicles.

Atrophoderma vermiculatum is a rare variant of keratosis pilaris, affecting the cheeks (**6.27**), causing a honeycomb, atrophic appearance, with prominent keratotic papules and a background erythema.

Further reading

Ashton R, Leppard B (2004). *Differential Diagnosis in Dermatology*. Radcliffe Publishing, Oxford.

Cunliffe WJ, Strauss J, Gollnick H, Lucky AW (2001). *Acne: Diagnosis and Management*. Taylor & Francis, London.

Du Vivier A (2002). *Atlas of Clinical Dermatology*. Churchill Livingstone, Oxford.

Lowe NJ (2003). *Psoriasis: A Patient's Guide*. Taylor & Francis, London.

Mckee PH, Calonje E, Granter SR (2005). *Pathology of the Skin*. Mosby, Philadelphia.

Wolff K, Johnson R, Suurmond R (2005). *Fitzpatrick's Colour Atlas and Clinical Synopsis of Dermatology*. McGraw-Hill, New York.

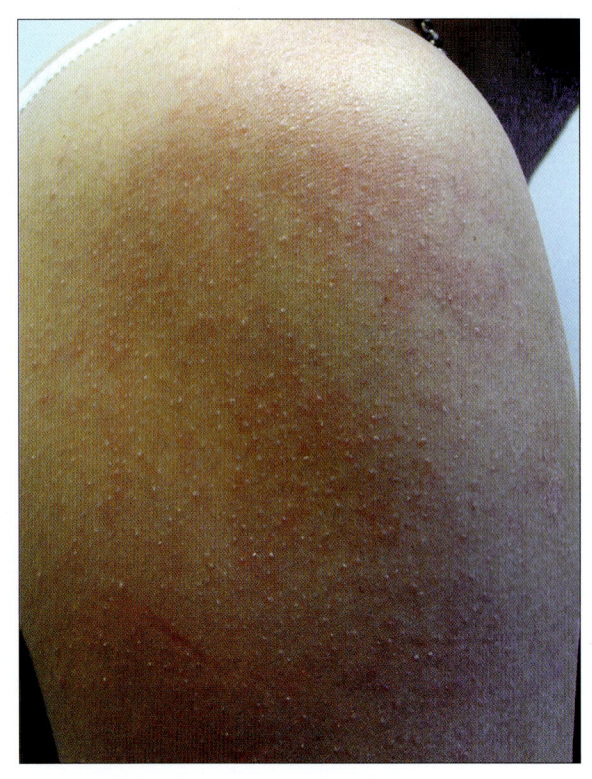

6.26 Keratosis pilaris typically affects the outer aspects of the arms.

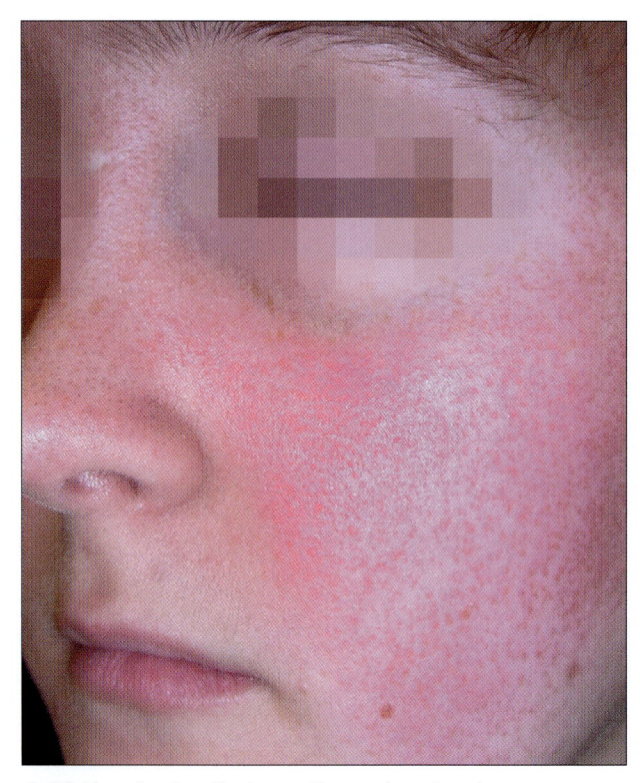

6.27 Keratosis pilaris on the outer cheeks.

Chapter 7

Genital and oral problems

Sheelagh M Littlewood, MBChB, FRCP

Introduction

Genital and oral disease is often regarded as a difficult subspeciality. There are several reasons for this. Firstly, the appearance of dermatoses on genital skin may be very 'nonspecific' and the characteristics of disease seen elsewhere may be absent in this area. It is important, therefore, to search for clues to diagnoses of diseases of oral and genital skin on nonmucosal surfaces.

Many diseases of the genital area result in scarring that would not be expected to occur in nongenital disease. This results in a 'common end-stage' appearance of shiny, smooth, featureless scarred tissue with little evidence of the original underlying disease, but could equally represent, for example, lichen sclerosus or lichen planus.

As the area is moist, occluded and subjected to friction and chronic irritation from urine and faeces, it is an excellent environment for infection and this often complicates other disease processes. It is important to remember that patients often attribute disease in the genital area to poor hygiene and as a result overwash the area, adding an irritant dimension to an already complex picture.

Many doctors and most patients are not familiar with the normal variation in the anatomy of this area and have little, or no, experience of normal appearances in an asymptomatic patient. This can result in misdiagnosis and unwarranted anxiety.

Lichen sclerosus

Introduction

Lichen sclerosus (LS) is a chronic inflammatory condition which tends to produce scarring that preferentially affects the genital area. It is 6–10-fold more prevalent in women. The aetiology is unknown, but a strong association with autoimmune disease is recognized. Occasionally, the disease can be asymptomatic and found purely by chance. However, the vast majority of patients complain of pruritis and soreness. In men, the condition only affects the uncircumcised. It can be asymptomatic but tends to produce not only itching and burning, but also bleeding, blistering, sexual dysfunction, and difficulties with urination when the urethral meatus is involved.

Clinical presentation

In either situation the classical features are pallor and atrophy as demonstrated by a wrinkling of the skin and textural change, plus an element of purpura, erosions, fissuring, telangiectasia, hyperkeratosis, bullae, or hyperpigmentation. Atrophy results in loss of the labia minora and burying of the clitoris, and pseudocysts of the clitoral hood from adhesions can occur.

The introitus can be significantly reduced and perineal involvement produces a classic figure-of-8 shape, extending around the anus (7.1–7.4). The histopathology can be very distinctive and can be useful in differentiating the condition from lichen planus, lichen simplex, and cicatricial pemphigoid. Typical findings are epidermal atrophy, hydropic degeneration of the basal layer, hyperkeratosis with follicular plugging, oedema, and homogenization of collagen in the upper dermis with an inflammatory infiltrate below. The dermis shows sparse elastic fibres with swollen collagen

92 Genital and oral problems

fibres, dilatation of blood vessels, and extravasation of red blood cells. There is often localized or diffuse squamous hyperplasia which may be the result of chronic scratching, but equally can indicate malignant transformation. There should be a low threshold for biopsy, sometimes repeatedly, of hyperkeratotic suspicious areas to exclude squamous cell carcinoma (SCC).

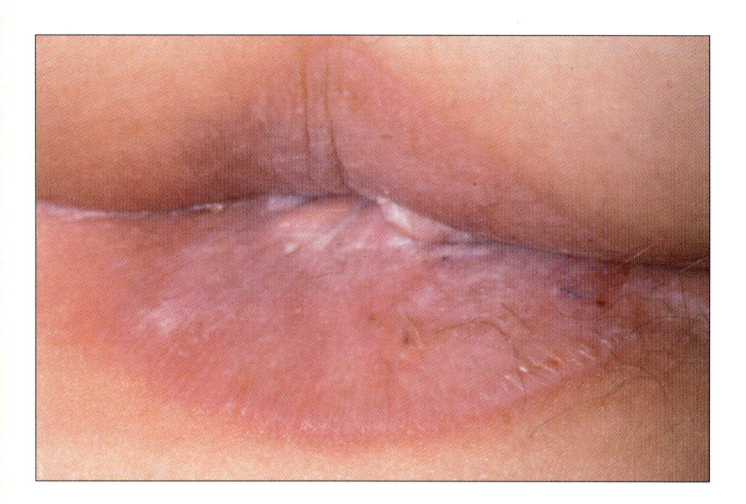

Management

First-line treatment is now recognized as ultra-potent topical steroids, 0.05% clobetasol propionate, for 3 months initially. It is important to advise on avoiding irritants, and the use of bland emollients and soap substitutes. Previous treatments such as topical testosterone have been shown to be ineffective. Surgery is not indicated for uncomplicated disease but is useful for complications such as introital narrowing and removal of pseudocysts. The disease runs a chronic course and the development of SCC is well recognized, with an incidence of 4–5%. Topical tacrolimus has also been used but its place has yet to be fully determined.

7.1 Perianal LS.

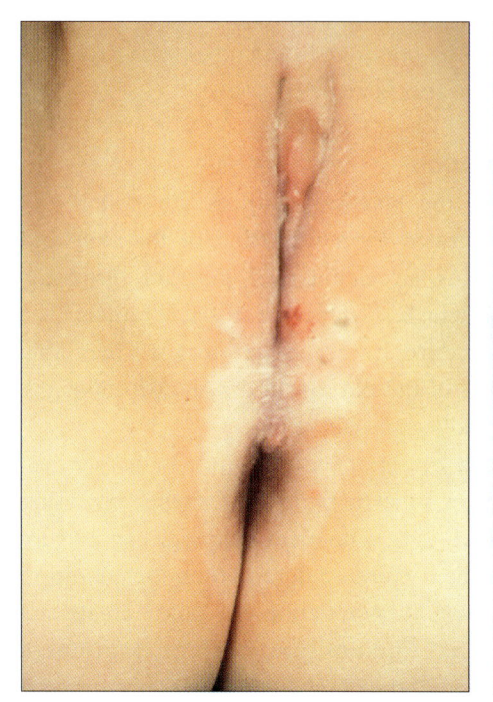

7.2 Juvenile LS.

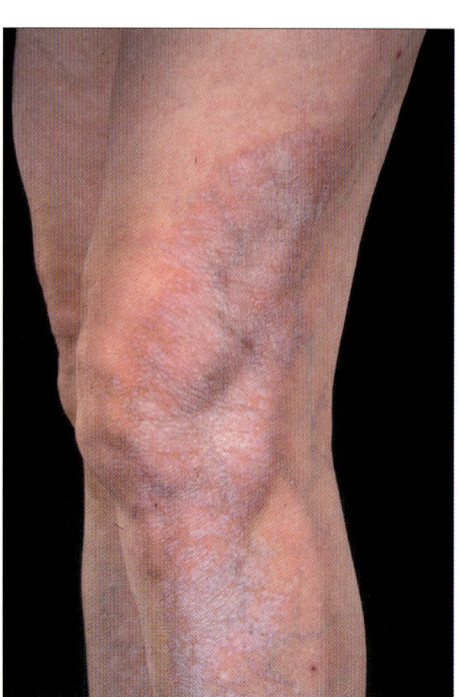

7.3 Nongenital LS on the leg.

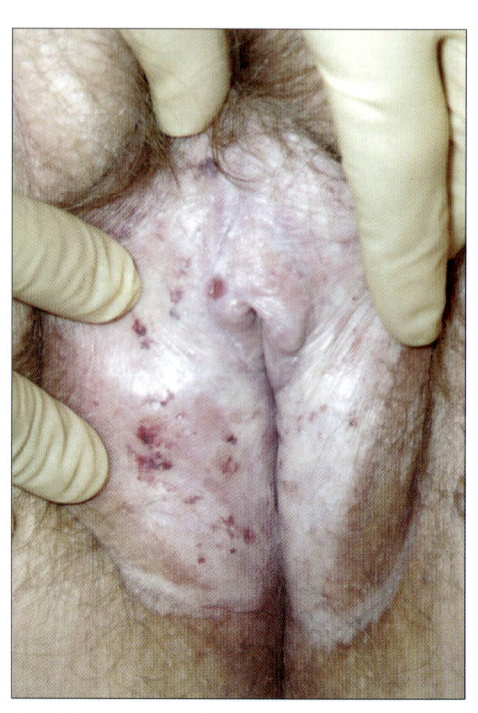

7.4 Extensive LS with petechiae and marked scarring.

Lichen planus

Introduction
Lichen planus (LP) is an inflammatory dermatosis that is believed to account for 1% of new cases seen in dermatology outpatients. Typical skin lesions are violaceous, itchy, flat-topped papules (7.5). The aetiology of LP is unknown, but it is believed to be an autoimmune disease. It can affect the skin or mucous membranes or both simultaneously.

Clinical presentation
Oral LP
Oral LP is one of the commoner conditions seen in oral medicine clinics. The prevalence ranges from 0.5% to 2.2% with a slightly higher prevalence in women.

There are three classes of clinical disease:
- Reticular, which is a net or plaque-like area which is often painless and is seen in about 20% of patients with typical cutaneous lichen planus (7.6).
- Erosive/atrophic, in which erythematous areas of thinned but unbroken epithelium occur. This includes the gingival condition of desquamative gingivitis.
- Ulcerative lesions, in which the epithelium is broken.

The latter two are typically very painful and run a chronic relapsing course. More than one type can exist at any time and can affect the buccal mucosa, lateral border of the tongue, and gingiva.

Genital LP
LP can affect the perigenital skin with a classic presentation of violaceous flat-topped papules (7.7). It can also affect the mucosal side of the labia, where it typically produces a glazed erythema, which bleeds easily on touch and tends to erode, hence the term 'erosive LP'. The early glazed erythema is very nonspecific and is difficult to diagnose correctly as it can resemble a number of other inflammatory diseases. However, LS tends to affect the outer aspect of the labia minora, as opposed to LP, which affects the inner. In a typical case of mucosal LP, the erythema is bordered by a white, occasionally violaceous border, which can be an important diagnostic clue. If present then this is the ideal place to biopsy. However, it is often absent resulting in diagnostic difficulty. One should always examine the mouth and other cutaneous sites, and look for evidence of vaginal disease, as this can be very helpful in making the diagnosis.

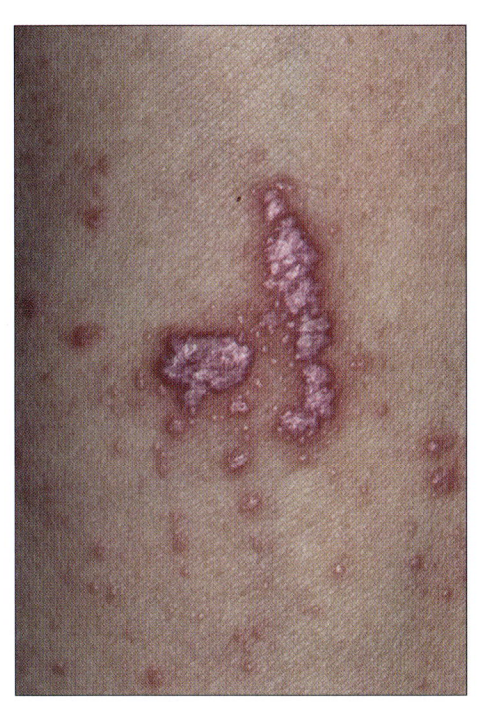

7.5 Polygonal flat-topped papules of LP on the wrist. Wickham striae are easily seen.

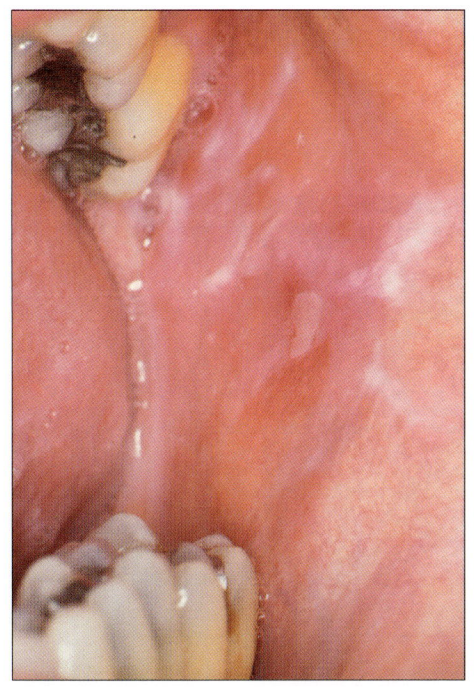

7.6 Lace-like Wickham striae of the buccal mucosa.

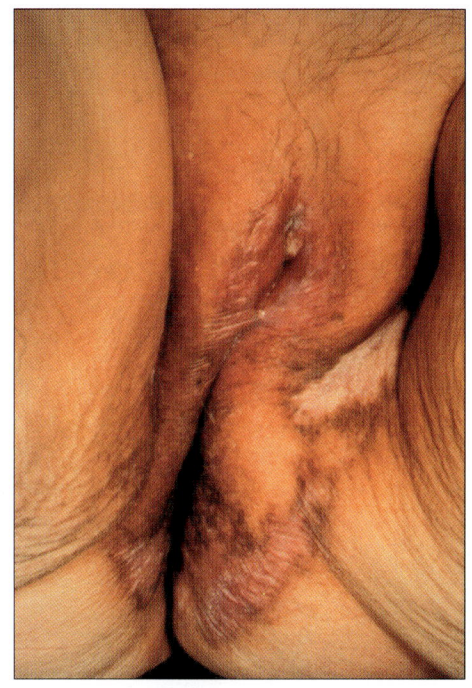

7.7 Chronic LP of the anogenital area with hyperpigmentation and gross scarring.

94 Genital and oral problems

The erosive form of genital LP can be associated with a similar condition in the mouth, the vulvo-vaginal-oral syndrome.

In males, LP tends to present with classical itchy, violaceous papules, but has a particular tendency to produce annular lesions (**7.8**). Occasionally an erosive form is seen in males, with mucosal lesions and red erosive changes on the glans and shaft. This can result in a scarring process similar to that in the vulva, resulting in a phimosis. The differential diagnosis would include psoriasis, Zoon's balanitis, LS, and erythroplasia of Queyrat.

The classical histology consists of basal epidermal damage, colloid bodies, pigmentary incontinence, epidermal acanthosis, hypergranulosis, and a dense band-like lymphocytic infiltrate below a saw toothing of the rete ridges. However, the mucosal erosive form loses many of these characteristics and in contrast tends just to show an attenuated thinned epidermis, parakeratosis, and large numbers of plasma cells.

Management
Treatment is with an ultra-potent topical steroid. Erosive disease tends to run a chronic course, although occasional patients go into remission. Other treatment options include systemic steroids, methotrexate, hydroxychloroquine, and oral retinoids, particularly in hypertrophic cases. There does seem to be an increased risk of malignancy although the degree of this is uncertain.

Zoon's balanitis

Introduction
Zoon's balanitis is a condition affecting middle-aged and older uncircumcised men. It is believed to be an irritant mucinitis produced by the particular environment associated with the presence of a 'dysfunctional foreskin'.

Clinical presentation
It presents as an indolent, asymptomatic, well-demarcated, glistening, shiny red or orangey patch on the glans or mucosal prepuce (**7.9**). There is no involvement of the penile shaft or foreskin. There is often purpura and haemosiderin resulting in so-called cayenne pepper spots. The lesions can be solitary or multiple. Histology is that of epidermal attenuation, diamond- or lozenge-shaped basal cell keratinocytes, and spongiosis. There may be ulceration or erosion and a band of plasma cells in the dermis. It is sometimes called plasma cell balanitis, but the presence of plasma cells is not diagnostic as they can be present in many mucosal conditions. The differential diagnosis includes LP, psoriasis, fixed drug eruption, secondary syphilis, erythroplasia of Queyrat, and a Kaposi sarcoma.

Management
Attention to hygiene, topical steroids, with or without antibiotics, should be the first line of treatment. However, if the condition persists or relapses then circumcision is the treatment of choice.

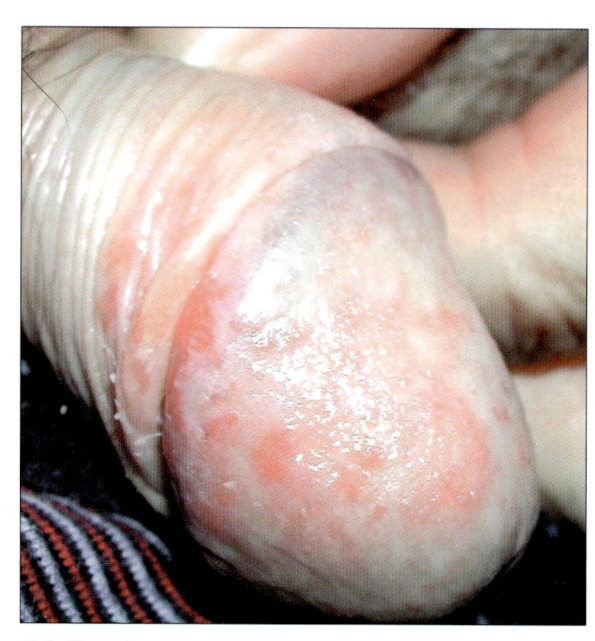

7.8 Annular LP of penis.

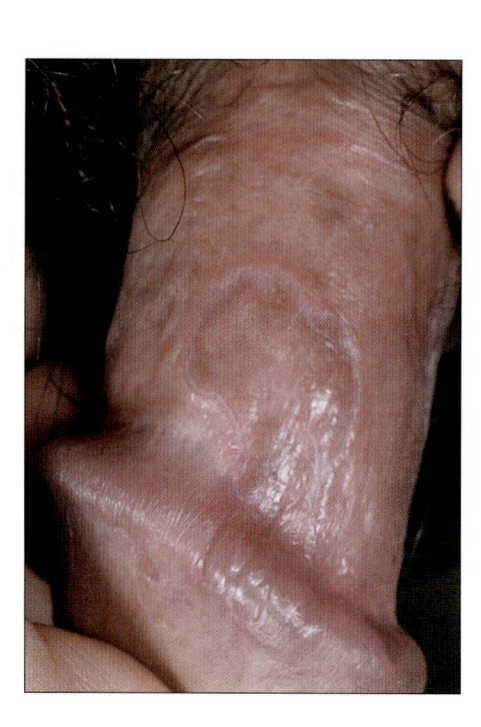

7.9 Zoon's balanitis.

Zoon's vulvitis

Introduction
A similar condition affecting the vulva has been described, but is a much rarer entity in women and there is doubt as to its existence. Typically, the lesions resemble those in males with well-circumscribed, glistening, orangey erythema, sometimes with cayenne pepper spots, which can affect any area of the vulva (7.10). The symptoms vary and the histology is similar to that in the male. Many cases are thought to represent LP.

7.10 Zoon's vulvitis.

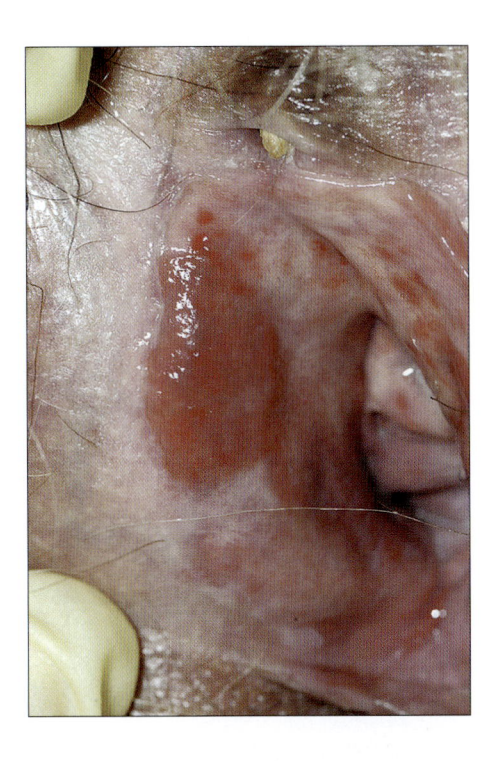

Autoimmune bullous diseases

Introduction
Pemphigoid, cicatricial pemphigoid, and pemphigus can affect the oral and genital areas (7.11, 7.12).

Clinical presentation
Bullous pemphigoid mainly affects the elderly; occasionally children have genital involvement. Typically, it presents with tense bullae which can arise from normal or erythematous skin. Histology shows subepidermal bullae and direct immunofluorescence IgG at the basement membrane.

In cicatricial pemphigoid the changes on histology and immunofluorescence are identical to pemphigoid, but the clinical presentation varies, in that it tends to affect mucous membranes more frequently with resultant scarring.

Pemphigus shows an intraepidermal blister on histology with IgG in the intracellular spaces. It affects younger patients and pemphigus vulgaris often presents with oral lesions in the form of extensive ulceration.

In the mucosal areas, intact blisters are seldom seen. In the absence of blisters elsewhere, or a history of blistering, the diagnosis can be difficult to make. The clinical presentation tends to be painful erosions and scarring, and in the mouth erythema and erosion of the gingiva. The differential diagnosis lies between all the bullous diseases as well as LP and LS and requires biopsy for histology as well as normal skin for immunofluorescence.

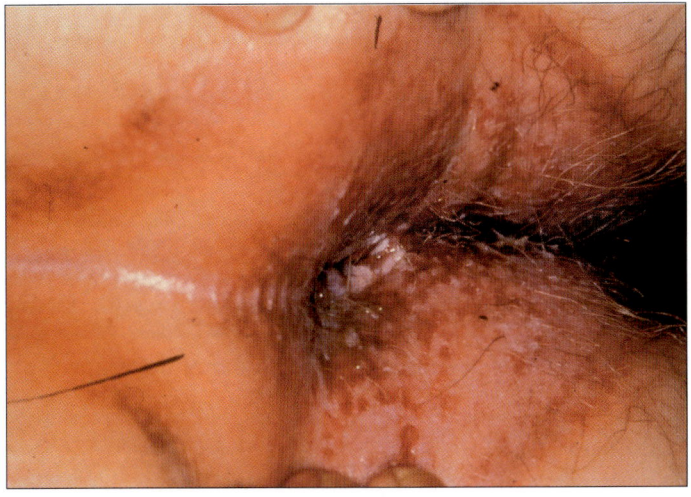

7.11 Perianal cicatricial pemphigoid.

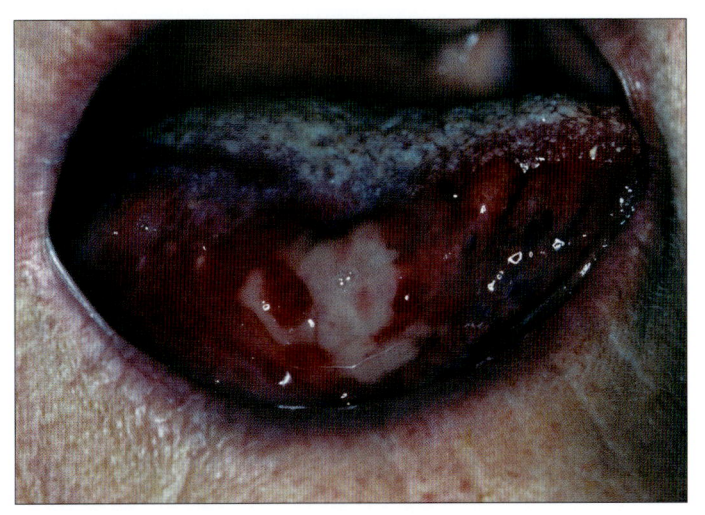

7.12 Oral ulceration due to cicatricial pemphigoid.

Genital and oral problems

Malignant lesions

Introduction
Dysplasia affecting the vulva is referred to as vulval intraepithelial neoplasia (VIN), and on the penis, penile intraepithelial neoplasia (PIN). VIN is further divided into categories I–III, depending on the degree of involvement of the epidermis. However, most of the information and work refer to full thickness dysplasia, or VIN III.

In the past, there have been many terms used to describe varying clinical appearances for what is now all regarded as VIN III. Other than as a clinical description there is no justification for this. The incidence of VIN has increased markedly in the last 25 years, mainly in younger women and it is strongly associated with sexually transmitted disease, smoking, and the presence of cervical intraepithelial neoplasia (CIN). There is a clear association between VIN and human papilloma virus (HPV), type 16 in particular. There is a subset of patients with VIN in whom HPV testing is negative. The HPV type tend to be younger patients and the disease multicentric and multifocal. The non-HPV type is found in older women and is more commonly unifocal and unicentric. The risk of progression to invasive carcinoma is low and has been estimated to be 3–4%. However, the risk for the older group of patients with solitary disease is almost certainly much higher, and in elderly women it is frequently associated with LS.

Clinical presentation
VIN lesions can vary from skin coloured, red or white papules and plaques to hyperpigmented lesions which are commonly multiple and multifocal (7.13). The larger single plaques can be pink, scaly, or eroded. Any nonhealing persistently eroded lesion on the genitalia should be biopsied.

In men, there can be a similar pink or reddish plaque, or eroded patches. A rarer form developing on the glans has a slow-growing, skin-coloured plaque which is scaly and may eventually involve the entire glans penis, becoming thick and crusted. This has been termed pseudoepitheliomatous keratotic and micaceous balanitis. Over time this may develop into a frank low-grade SCC (7.14).

Management
Treatment of PIN and VIN may involve local destruction or excision of solitary lesions, but for multifocal extensive lesions treatment is much more difficult. In many patients observation is often appropriate. Extensive surgery for multifocal disease is mutilating and unlikely to be curative. Laser, cryotherapy, topical 5-fluorouracil, or immiquimod for extensive areas have all been used but complete clearance is uncommon and recurrence frequent. Patients should be encouraged to stop smoking, as this is associated with progression to frank squamous carcinoma.

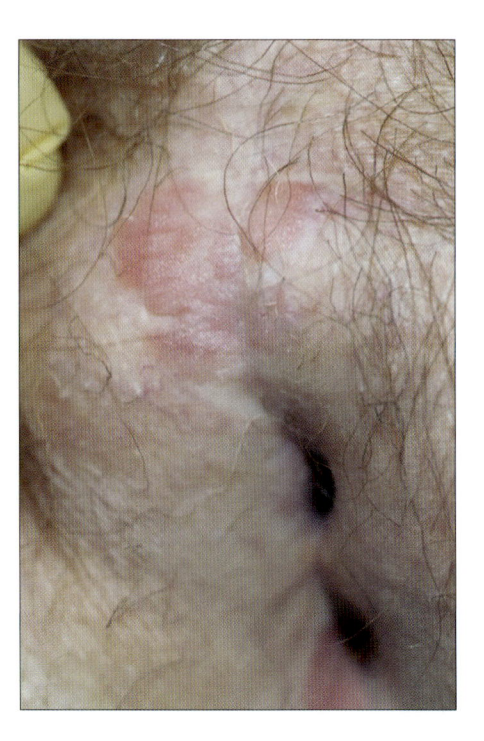

7.13 LS and VIN.

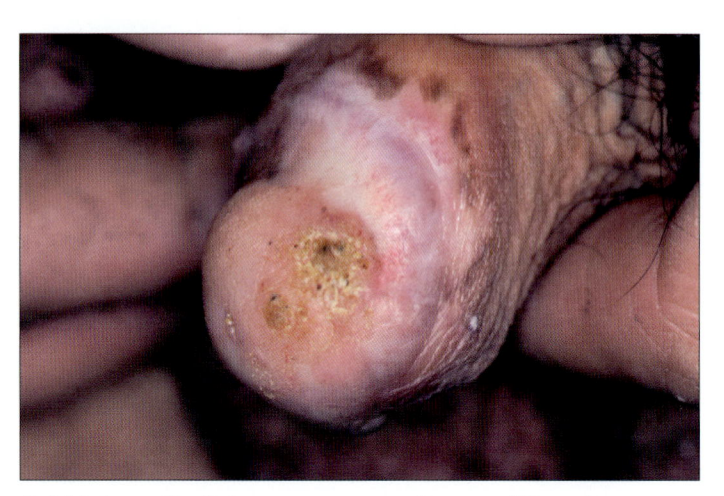

7.14 Intraepithelial squamous carcinoma of the glans.

Eczematous conditions

Introduction
Eczematous rashes in the vulva are common. Atopic eczema can affect the genital area either acutely or chronically when, as the result of chronic scratching and rubbing, thickened erythematous scaly plaques develop often with overlying excoriation and fissuring (7.15).

Clinical presentation
This appearance is termed 'lichen simplex'. It can be bilateral or unilateral and the labia majora are the most frequently affected sites, although the labia minora, vestibule, mons pubis, and inner thighs can all be affected. In both men and women, the perianal area is a site of predilection and, in men, the scrotum is a frequently involved site (7.16). The diagnosis is usually simple to make on the basis of lichenification and excoriation (7.17).

Management
The treatment involves breaking of the 'itch-scratch cycle', replacing irritants with bland emollients and soap substitutes, topical steroids of medium to high potency, occasionally systemic steroids, sedating antihistamines for night-time itch and, sometimes, selective serotonin reuptake inhibitors for daytime itching.

Contact dermatitis, both irritant and allergic, often complicates the picture. This is not surprising as many patients self-medicate and aggressively over-cleanse the area. Vulval skin reacts more readily to irritants than other areas, and the barrier function is often substantially weaker. Examination reveals varying degrees of redness, swelling, and scaling, sometimes with ulceration. In chronic cases, lichenification and excoriation, together with abnormalities of pigmentation, become prominent. Secondary infection is not uncommon.

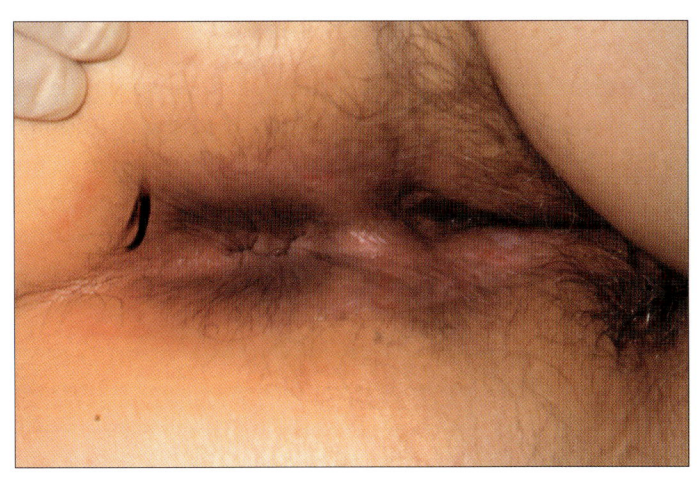

7.15 Perianal eczema.

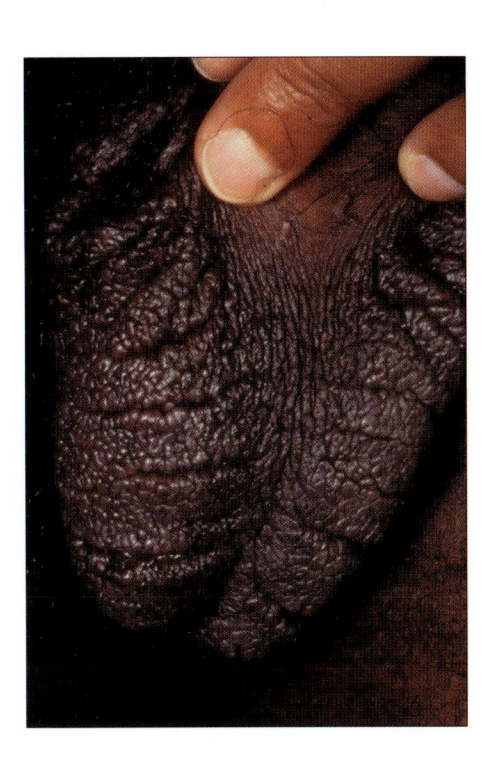

7.16 Lichen simplex of the scrotum.

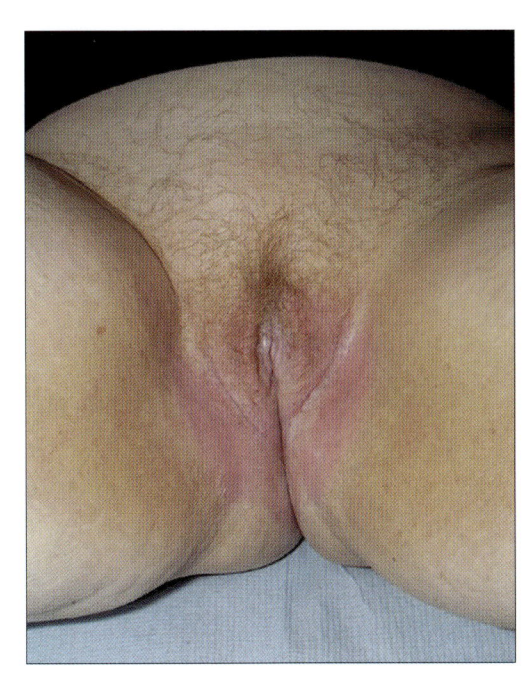

7.17 Vulval eczema.

Allergic contact dermatitis can be difficult to distinguish from irritant dermatitis and they do sometimes overlap. The most common allergens are fragrances, preservatives, topical medications, rubber products, nail polish, and nickel. The presentation can be acute, subacute, or chronic and, in the acute phase, vesiculation, swelling, and spread beyond the site of contact are seen. In more chronic cases, the changes can be indistinguishable from those seen in an irritant dermatitis. The diagnosis is made from history and patch testing, and one should have a low threshold for patch testing of patients with vulval disease.

Vulval ulceration

Introduction

Vulval ulcers can broadly be classified as infectious, noninfectious, and malignant (*Table 7.1*). Although acute ulcers tend to be infectious in origin, the natural history depends on many factors including immune status, secondary infection underlying dermatological disease, and previously administered therapy (**7.18**). One should not guess at the aetiology of an ulcer and initiate treatment before appropriate investigations have been done. For acute ulcers this includes bacterial, viral, and sometimes fungal cultures. Even if bacterial or candidal infection is demonstrated, these may not be the primary cause of the ulcer. Any chronic ulcer necessitates a biopsy to exclude malignancy.

Further reading

Black M, McKay M (2002). *Obstetric and Gynaecological Dermatology*, 2nd edn. Mosby, Philadelphia.

Bunker CB (2004). *Male Genital Skin Disease*. Saunders, Edinburgh.

Ridley CM, Neill S (eds) (2002). *The Vulva* (2nd edn). Blackwell Scientific, Oxford.

Table 7.1 Aetiology of vulval ulcers

Infectious ulcers
- Syphilis
- Herpes simplex
- Herpes zoster
- Candida
- Chancroid

Noninfectious ulcers
- Pyoderma gangrenosum
- Urethral caruncle
- Trauma
- Behçet's syndrome
- Apthae
- Epstein–Barr virus

Malignant ulcers
- BCC
- SCC
- Malignant melanoma
- Extramammary Paget's disease

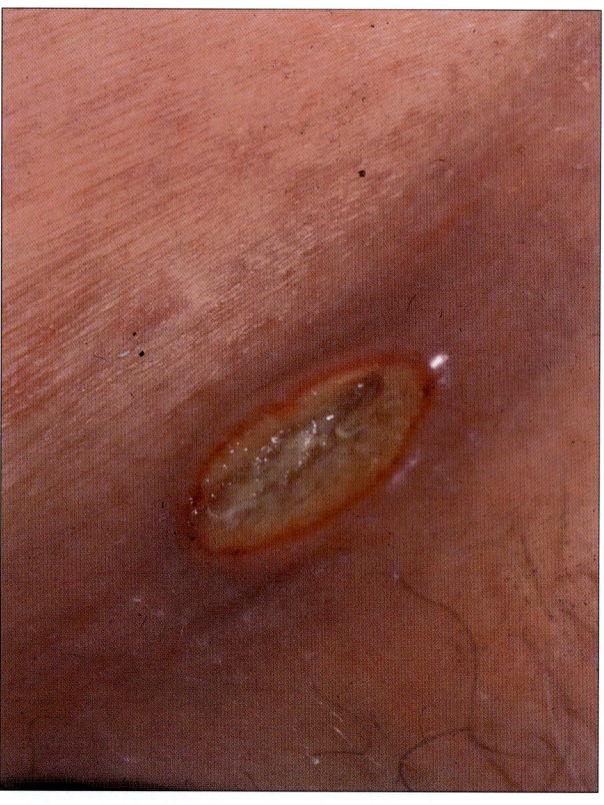

7.18 Perivulval ulcer.

Chapter 8

Scalp and nail disorders

Stuart N Cohen, BMedSci, MRCP

Introduction

Disorders of the scalp are common and may be intensely symptomatic. Hair loss, in particular, is frequently associated with a high degree of distress. Uncertainty regarding diagnosis makes counselling such patients even more difficult, so accurate diagnosis is especially important.

Although scalp involvement may be a feature of several of the most common inflammatory dermatoses, including psoriasis, atopic dermatitis, and seborrhoeic dermatitis, the focus of this section is on diseases with a predilection for the scalp, those that are scalp specific, and on disorders of hair. This latter group often leads to diagnostic difficulty. The value of simple blood tests should not be forgotten, as biochemical abnormalities such as iron deficiency commonly lead to hair loss and are easily correctable.

Many abnormalities of the nail unit result from general skin conditions, most typically psoriasis, but also atopic eczema, lichen planus, and others. In some cases, disease is restricted to the nails. Where the cause of a rash is unclear, specific nail changes may help to confirm the diagnosis. The nails may also give clues to systemic disease, with features of Beau's lines, leuconychia, yellow nail syndrome, and so on. Unfortunately, many conditions affecting the nail unit are difficult to manage, but care should be taken not to overlook a treatable problem such as onychomycosis.

DISORDERS OF THE SCALP AND HAIR

Alopecia areata

Introduction
This is a nonscarring alopecia with a prevalence of approximately 0.1%. It is associated with other organ-specific autoimmune diseases, such as thyroid disease and vitiligo. Atopy also appears to be linked. In monozygotic twins, a concordance rate of 55% has been found, suggesting that both genetic and environmental factors are relevant.

Clinical presentation
Alopecia areata usually presents with well-defined, circular patches of complete hair loss, with no evidence of scarring (**8.1**). Exclamation mark hairs (where the proximal shaft is narrower than the distal shaft) are often seen around the periphery of the patches. Other patterns include alopecia totalis (where the scalp is completely bald), alopecia universalis (where all body hair is lost), and ophiasis, in which there is hair loss over the temporo-parietal and occipital scalp. In diffuse alopecia areata, there is widespread thinning, rather than the usual well-defined patches (**8.2**). Several nail abnormalities may be associated.

Histopathology
A lymphocytic infiltrate is seen in the peribulbar and perivascular areas, the external root sheath, and invading the follicular streamers. Langerhans cells are also present.

Differential diagnosis
Localized hair loss is seen with trichotillomania, tinea capitis, traction alopecia, and pseudopelade of Brocque. History and clinical findings will differentiate the vast

majority of cases. Diffuse alopecia areata is more challenging, as telogen effluvium, iron deficiency-related hair loss, and androgenetic alopecia may look similar.

Management
If there is doubt about the diagnosis, hair microscopy and serum ferritin may exclude other possibilities. A biopsy is only rarely required. Treatment options include potent or very potent topical steroid applications, or intralesional steroid injection. For more extensive disease, contact sensitization with diphencyprone, PUVA, systemic corticosteroids, and ciclosporin have been used, but response rates are disappointing.

The disease may spontaneously remit, though some patients have regrowth in some areas at the same time as new hair loss in others. Regrowing hairs are often not pigmented. Ophiasis pattern, extensive disease, and associated atopy carry a worse prognosis.

Trichotillomania

Introduction
This is characterized by the plucking of hairs in a habitual manner. It does not necessarily reflect significant psychopathology, though it may be a sign of impulse control disorders, personality disorder, or psychosis.

Clinical presentation
Onset is most commonly in childhood. The scalp is the most common site, resulting in localized or patchy alopecia (**8.3**). The affected areas tend to have irregular borders and often contain broken hairs of varying lengths. Even in extensive cases, the occiput is usually spared.

Histopathology
Biopsy is rarely needed, though follicular plugging, melanin casts, trichomalacia, haemorrhage, and increased numbers of catagen follicles may be seen.

Differential diagnosis
Alopecia areata and tinea capitis are the main differentials. The former usually results in better defined areas of alopecia.

Management
Diagnosis is usually clinical, though mycological examination of plucked hairs and histology are helpful if there is doubt. Some cases, particularly in childhood, will spontaneously resolve. Treatments have included cognitive behavioural therapy and antidepressants.

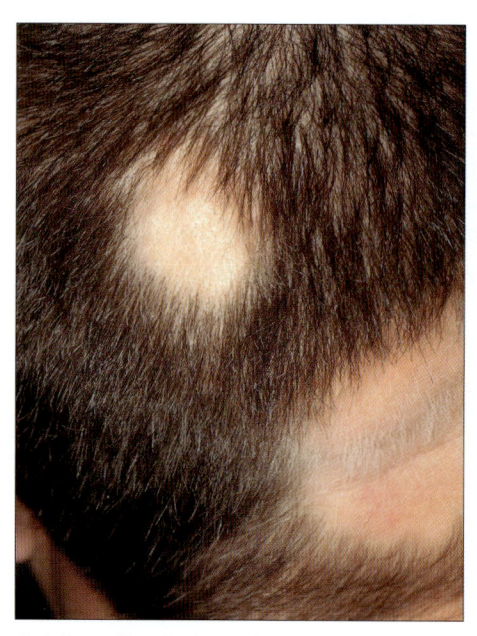

8.1 Localized alopecia areata with some fine downy regrowth, a good prognostic sign.

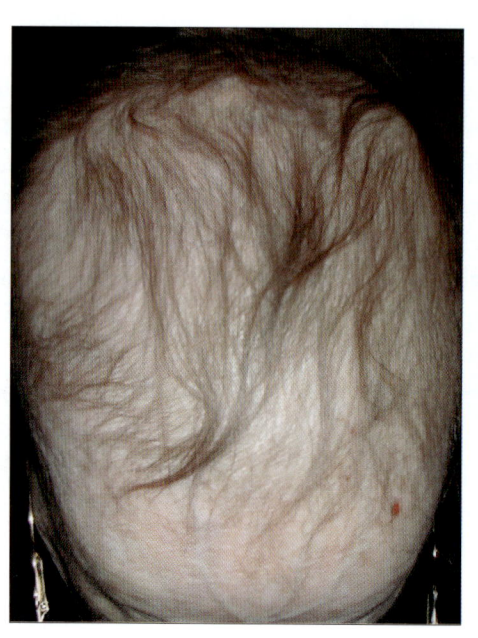

8.2 Diffuse alopecia areata.

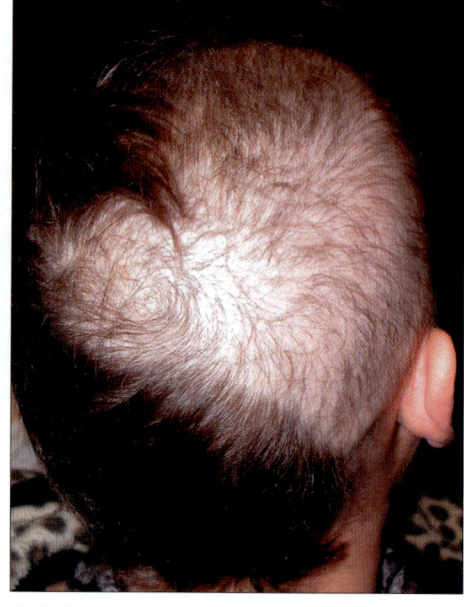

8.3 Trichotillomania. In this case, the majority of short hairs are the same length.

Tinea capitis

Introduction
Dermatophyte infection of the scalp occurs frequently in children, but rarely in adults. *Trichophyton tonsurans* and *Microsporum canis* are the commonest causative organisms.

Clinical presentation
Tinea capitis most commonly presents with discrete patches of alopecia, with or without scaling. Diffuse scaling may occur. Posterior cervical and posterior auricular lymphadenopathy is often present. Alopecia is usually reversed on treatment, but may be permanent after severe or long-standing infection.

An exaggerated host response may result in formation of a kerion (**8.4**). This is a boggy, purulent plaque with abscess formation and may give rise to systemic upset.

Differential diagnosis
Where scaling is prominent, the condition may mimic seborrhoeic dermatitis or psoriasis (such as in pityriasis amiantacea, **8.5**). The alopecia may be mistaken for alopecia areata or trichotillomania. Other causes of scarring alopecia may be considered if scarring is a feature. Kerion is frequently misdiagnosed as bacterial infection.

Management
The diagnosis should be confirmed by mycological studies. Samples may be obtained through skin scrapings and brushings, or from plucked hairs. Microscopy with potassium hydroxide will reveal the fungus, which may be cultured. If the diagnosis is suspected and these tests are negative, fungal staining of a biopsy specimen will identify hyphae or spores.

Tinea capitis always requires systemic therapy. Griseofulvin 10–20 mg/kg/day for 8–12 weeks or terbinafine 62.5 mg daily (10–20 kg), 125 mg daily (20–40 kg), 250 mg daily (>40 kg) may be used. For kerion, in addition to this, antibiotics for superadded infection may be necessary and topical steroids may be used to suppress inflammation.

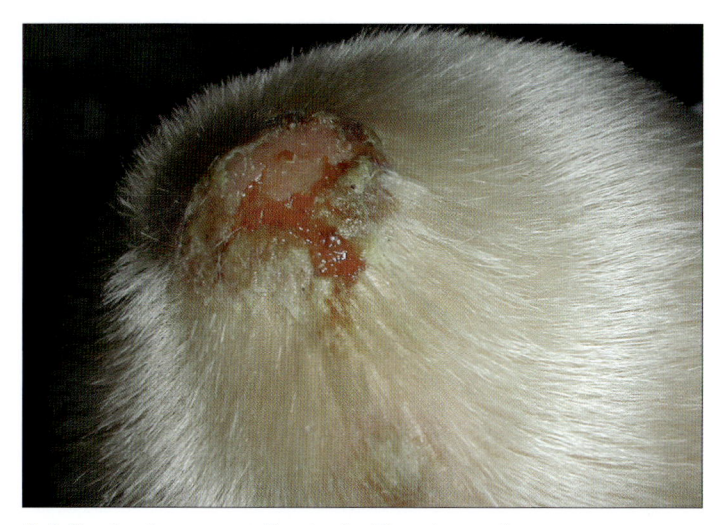

8.4 Scalp ring worm (kerion). (Courtesy of Dr Andrew Affleck.)

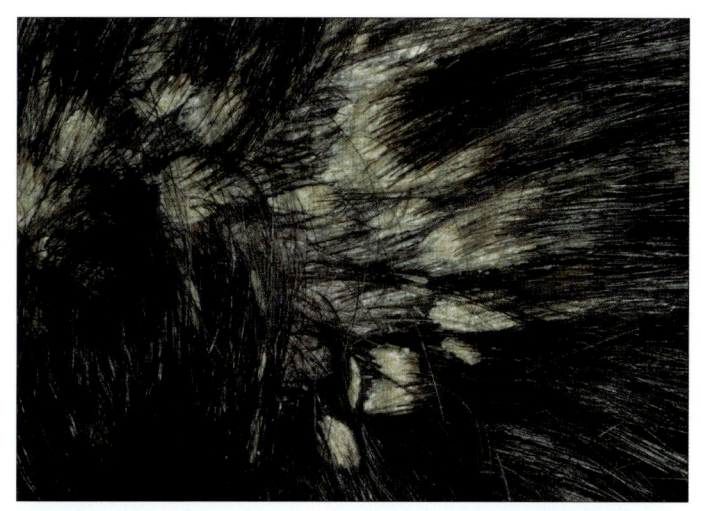

8.5 Pityriasis amiantacea describes build-up of thick, adherent scaling; it is usually in the context of psoriasis, but may also result from seborrhoeic dermatitis or tinea capitis.

Scalp and nail disorders

Folliculitis decalvans

Introduction
This is a form of painful, recurrent, patchy scalp folliculitis, which results in scarring and thus hair loss. It is thought to result from an abnormal response to *Staphylococcus aureus* toxins.

Clinical presentation
There is patchy, scarring alopecia, with crusting and pustules (**8.6**). There may be tufting of hairs (more than one hair erupting from a single follicle).

Histopathology
Histology shows hyperkeratosis, follicular plugging, and perifollicular inflammation.

Differential diagnosis
Other causes of scarring alopecia may look similar, including discoid lupus, lichen planopilaris, or pseudopelade of Brocque.

Management
Treatment options include topical or oral antibiotics, including combination treatment such as clindamycin and rifampicin, or oral isotretinoin. Small areas of scarring alopecia may be excised.

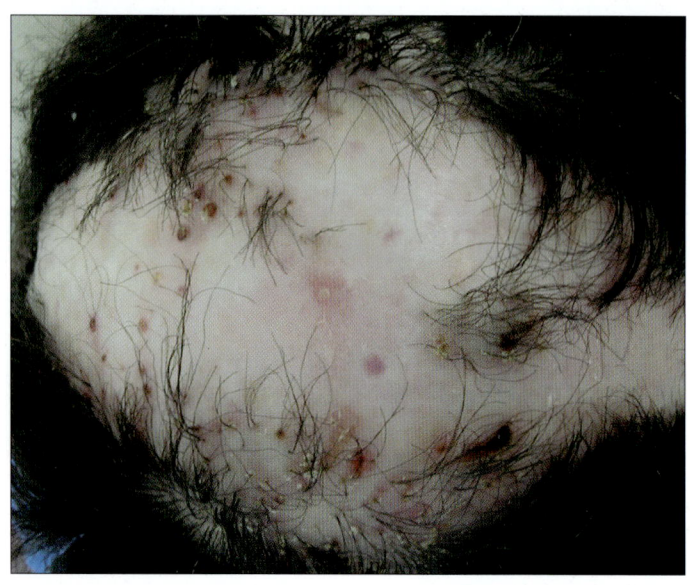

8.6 Scarring alopecia due to long-standing folliculitis decalvans. (Courtesy of Dr Andrew Affleck.)

Dissecting cellulitis of the scalp

Introduction
This condition is uncommon, usually affecting young, black men. Follicular hyperkeratosis is thought to represent the primary cause, though bacterial superinfection is frequent.

Clinical presentation
Multiple painful inflammatory nodules and fluctuant abscesses occur, giving a 'boggy' feel to the affected areas (**8.7**). It is most common over the occiput. As lesions settle with scarring, alopecia occurs.

Histopathology
Biopsy reveals neutrophilic folliculitis, granulomatous response to keratinous debris, and fibrosis.

Differential diagnosis
In advanced, or burnt-out disease, the boggy feeling may be lost, and the appearance may be similar to other causes of scarring alopecia such as folliculitis decalvans, discoid lupus, and pseudopelade.

Management
Oral antibiotics, intralesional steroid injection to inflammatory nodules, oral isotretinoin, incision and drainage, and local excision of discrete areas have been used.

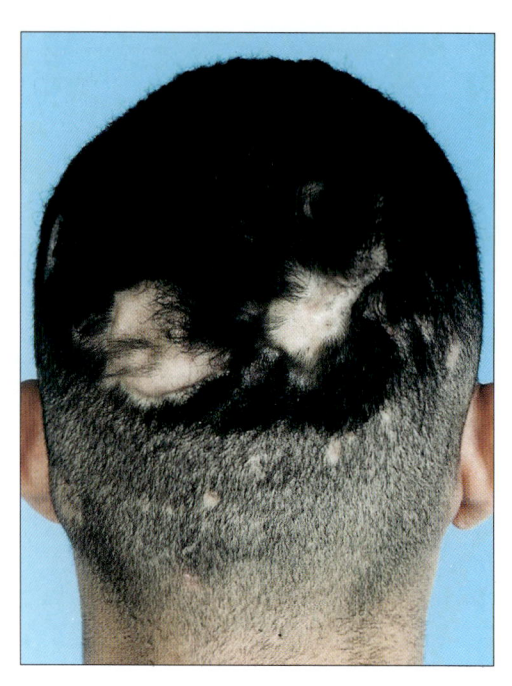

8.7 Scarring alopecia due to dissecting cellulitis of the scalp. (Courtesy of Dr Andrew Affleck.)

Acne keloidalis nuchae

Introduction
This occurs mainly in black men. The precise cause is unclear.

Clinical presentation
It usually begins on the nape of the neck with formation of small follicular papules (**8.8**). These then become firmer and more numerous, before coalescing into plaques. There is alopecia over the affected area and sometimes tufting of hairs, similar to that in folliculitis decalvans. Advanced disease may be associated with abscesses and sinuses.

Histopathology
Various types of inflammatory infiltrate may be seen, particularly in the upper third of the follicle. Hair fragments with surrounding granulomata may be seen, with scarring. True keloid changes are only seen later.

Differential diagnosis
Lesions may be similar to other types of folliculitis or acne. Advanced disease may mimic folliculitis decalvans, though the site is usually characteristic.

Management
Early disease may respond well to topical treatment with potent or very potent steroids, or retinoids. Antibiotics may be used to settle active folliculitis. More advanced disease may be improved with intralesional steroid or surgical intervention.

Lichen planopilaris

Introduction
This is lichen planus (LP) of the scalp. The cause of the condition is unknown.

Clinical presentation
There is patchy hair loss, perifollicular erythema, and scarring alopecia. There may also be evidence of LP at other sites, including nails and mucous membranes (**8.9**).

Histopathology
As in LP at other sites, biopsy shows hyperkeratosis, irregular acanthosis, basal layer liquefaction, Civatte bodies, and a band-like lymphocytic infiltrate at the dermo-epidermal junction; pigment incontinence may be marked.

Differential diagnosis
Appearances may be similar to other causes of scarring alopecia, but the violaceous rim around active areas is characteristic. Burnt-out lichen planopilaris may be indistinguishable from pseudopelade of Brocque.

Management
The diagnosis may be confirmed histologically. Treatment options start with topical steroids; intralesional or systemic steroids may be tried, or other agents such as oral retinoids and immunosuppressants. Some cases will resolve spontaneously.

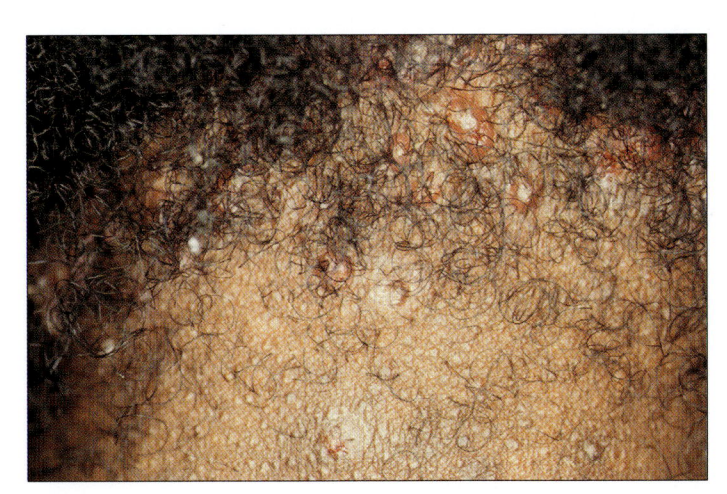

8.8 Acne keloidalis nuchae.

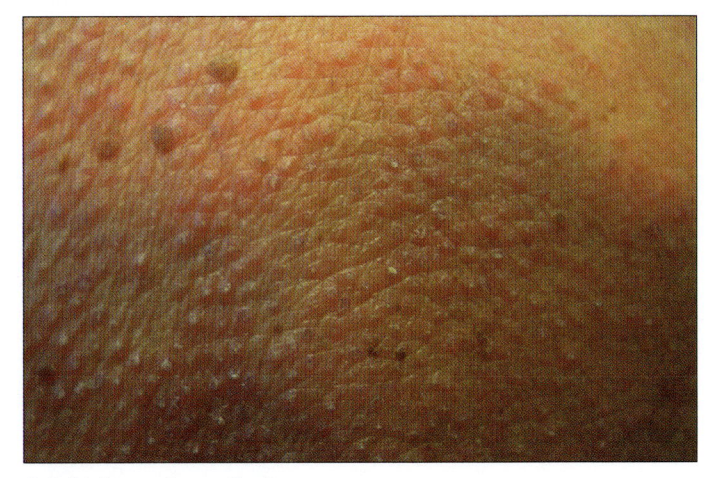

8.9 Lichen planopilaris.

Discoid lupus erythematosus

Introduction
Lupus is more common in blacks than whites. Discoid lupus is the commonest form seen in dermatology clinics. Lesions are most often seen on the face and scalp. Most patients have disease localized to the skin, with no detectable autoantibodies, but a small proportion (5–10%) may later develop systemic lupus erythematosus.

Clinical presentation
There is erythema, follicular plugging, sometimes induration, scarring alopecia, and commonly dyspigmentation, especially hypopigmentation (8.10). Disease is often photoaggravated.

Histopathology
Biopsy shows hyperkeratosis and damaged keratinocytes; there is often thickening of the dermo-epidermal and follicular basement membrane zones; in the dermis, there is often a pronounced lymphohistiocytic interface, and perivascular and periadnexal cellular infiltrate. Follicular plugging is seen, or follicular structures may be atrophic or absent.

Differential diagnosis
On the scalp, discoid lupus may appear similar to lichen planopilaris or tinea capitis. The scaling is different from that seen in psoriasis and, in established cases, alopecia is more prominent.

Management
Topical treatment consists of steroid applications; intralesional steroids may be used. Systemic options include hydroxychloroquine and methotrexate. High-factor sunscreen (SPF >30) should also be advised.

Pseudopelade of Brocque

Patchy scarring alopecia, with no active inflammation and no diagnosis evident on histology, is known as pseudopelade of Brocque (8.11). This may represent the end-stage of several other recognized conditions. Treatment is unsatisfactory, although excision of the affected areas is effective where practical.

Naevus sebaceus

This congenital lesion presents in early childhood as an oval or linear yellow-orange plaque, commonly on the head or neck (see Chapter 2). Alopecia is typical in scalp lesions. The lesion may become more verrucous with age and darker in colour. Not uncommonly, neoplasms develop within naevus sebaceus, many benign, but also basal cell carcinomata. Treatment consists merely of observation or excision.

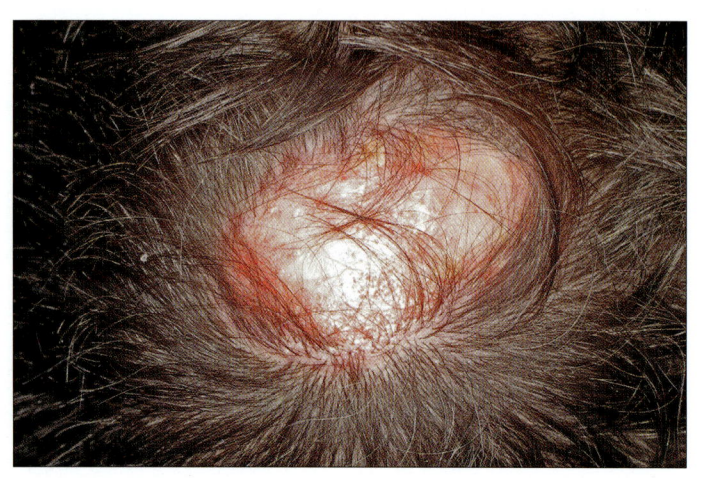

8.10 Chronic discoid lupus erythematosus of the scalp.

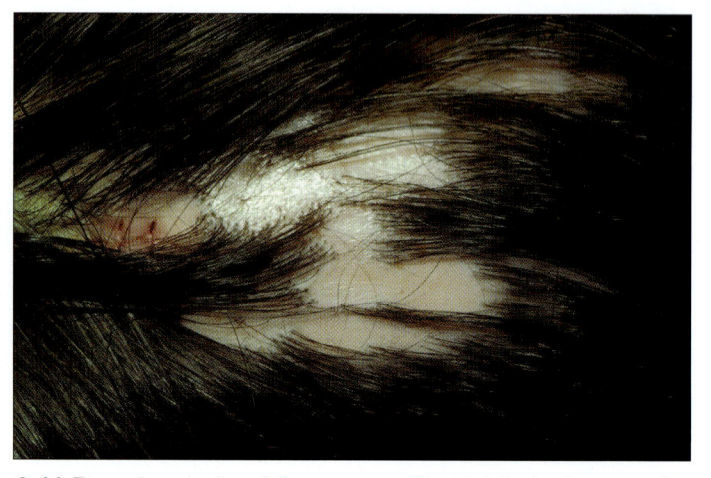

8.11 Pseudopelade of Brocque or 'footprints in the snow'.

Diffuse hair loss

Introduction
From the normal scalp, up to 150 hairs are shed per day. In telogen effluvium, a greater than normal proportion of hairs enter the telogen phase of the hair cycle, leading to increased shedding. Iron deficiency and thyroid dysfunction should be excluded in all cases of diffuse hair loss. Various chemotherapeutic agents and some other drugs also cause hair loss.

Clinical presentation
Telogen effluvium classically presents 2–4 months after a high fever, other severe illness, or pregnancy with increased shedding and diffuse hair loss. In other patients, particularly middle-aged women, it may be chronic. Here it is more difficult to distinguish from other causes of diffuse thinning.

Differential diagnosis
Diffuse thinning may result from androgenetic alopecia, although this is usually most marked over the crown. There may be a family history. Iron deficiency and thyroid disease should be excluded biochemically. Chronic telogen effluvium and diffuse alopecia areata should be considered. In the former, increased numbers of telogen hairs ('club hairs') are seen on hair microscopy; in the latter, exclamation mark hairs may be seen and histology is characteristic.

Management
Correction of biochemical abnormalities, such as iron deficiency, may lead to resolution. Telogen effluvium, especially where acute, usually resolves spontaneously after several months. Antiandrogens have been used in androgenetic alopecia, as has topical minoxidil. Stopping the latter may cause any benefits of treatment to be lost.

Traction alopecia

Introduction
Excessive tension put on hair may lead to hair loss. It tends to occur when a ponytail is aggressively pulled back, but also around tight braids (8.12). Regular hair straightening is another cause.

Clinical presentation
If caused by a ponytail, hair loss is seen in the temporal regions. The scalp appears normal.

Histopathology
Biopsy is not usually required and is nonspecific or normal.

Differential diagnosis
Diagnosis is usually clear from the distribution matching a history of putting hair under tension. Frontal fibrosing alopecia, which causes slowly progressive temporal and frontal recession, and loss of eyebrow hair, may appear similar. If this diagnosis is suspected, histology is helpful.

Management
Hair should be kept in a relaxed style, though hair loss may be permanent.

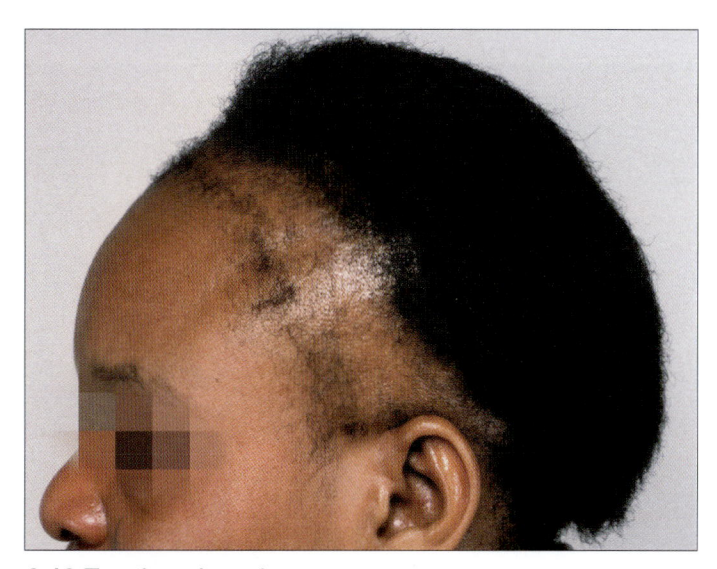

8.12 Traction alopecia.

Disorders of nails

Onychomycosis

Introduction
Fungal nail infection is common, with prevalence rates of 2–13%. Several factors predispose to onychomycosis, including local trauma, orthopaedic problems, affected close contacts, previous history, and tinea pedis. Infection may be due to dermatophytes or yeasts. Common organisms include *Trichophyton rubrum*, *T. interdigitale*, *Candida albicans*, and *Fusarium spp*.

Clinical presentation
Apart from abnormal appearance, there is sometimes associated pain. Toenails are far more commonly affected than fingernails (**8.13, 8.14**). In distal and lateral subungual onychomycosis (DLSO), the lateral nailfolds may be scaly and the nail is opaque or discoloured (**8.15**). There may be thickening and crumbling as well as nailbed hyperkeratosis. Superficial white onychomycosis produces chalky white patches on the surface of the nail, which may coalesce. Where there is loss of the cuticle due to proximal nailfold disease, fungi may enter, causing proximal subungual onychomycosis. Total dystrophic onychomycosis is usually a result of DLSO, but may occur with other subtypes. The entire nail is thickened, with a rough surface and mixed colours.

Histopathology
This is rarely necessary, though it may be helpful where there is diagnostic doubt, or suspected dual pathology. Fungal stains will confirm the presence of causative organisms.

Differential diagnosis
Psoriasis may look identical. Pitting and onycholysis may be diagnostic of this, though it should be remembered that psoriatic nails may be colonized by fungus. Yellow nail syndrome usually affects all nails, hyperkeratosis is lacking, and there is typically associated lymphoedema.

Management
Diagnosis should be confirmed by mycological study of nail clippings. Recurrent tinea pedis should be treated aggressively. Topical treatment of onychomycosis with amorolfine 5% lacquer as monotherapy is often ineffective, except in superficial nail plate infection. It may render systemic therapy more effective when used in combination. The systemic agent of choice is terbinafine 250 mg once daily, for 6 weeks in fingernail infections and 12 weeks in toenail infection. Alternatives include pulsed itraconazole 200 mg once daily for 1 week in 3 consecutive months or griseofulvin 500–2000 mg per day, continued until 1 month after clinical resolution. Griseofulvin has many interactions, as it induces hepatic enzymes.

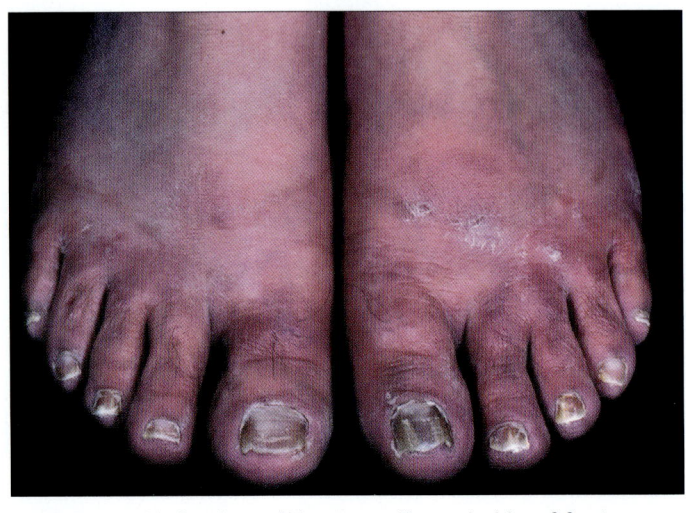

8.13 Fungal infection of the toenails and skin of feet.

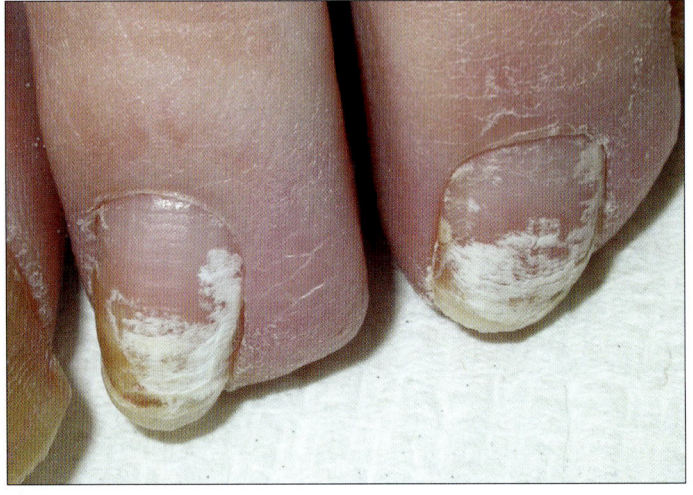

8.14 Superficial white onychomycosis of the toenails.

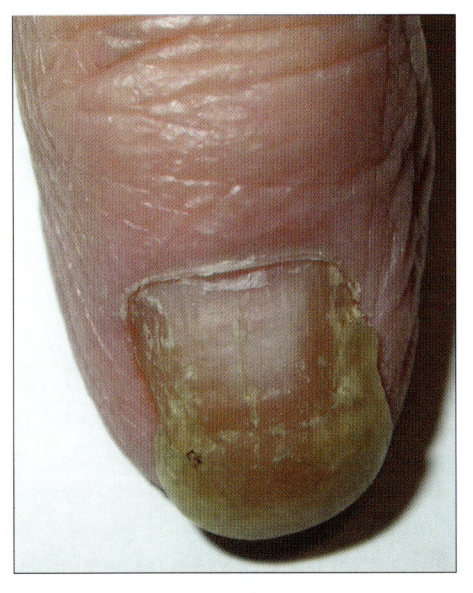

8.15 Distal and lateral subungual onychomycosis.

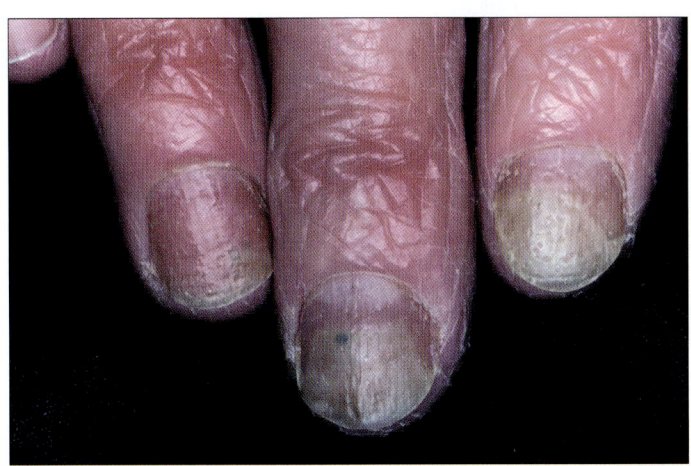

8.16 Psoriatic pitting and distal onycholysis of the fingernails.

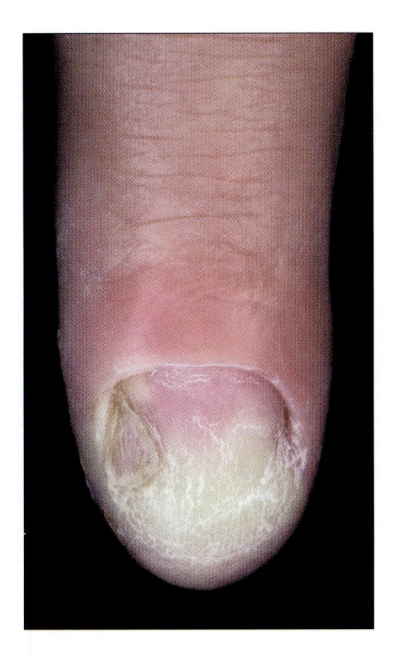

8.17 Acropustulosis of Hallopeau.

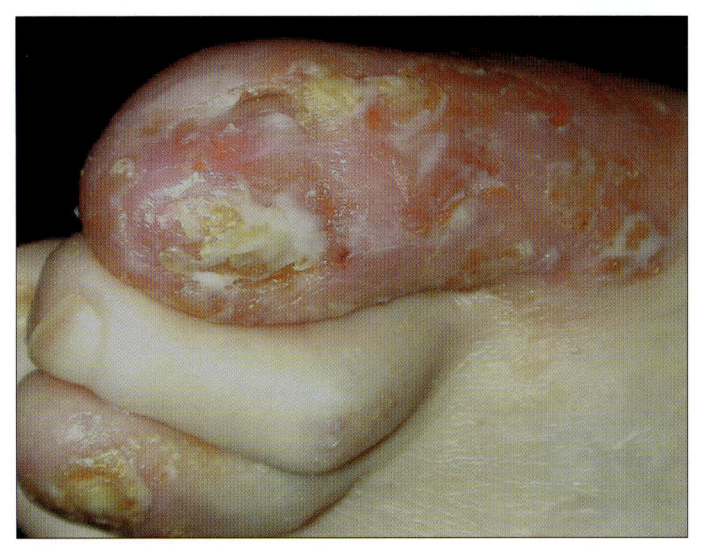

8.18 Acropustulosis of Hallopeau of the big toenail.

Psoriasis

Introduction
Psoriasis is common, with worldwide prevalence figures of 1–3%. Most patients with psoriasis will, at some point, have signs of nail involvement.

Clinical presentation
Pits are the most common change seen in psoriasis (**8.16**). These are punctate depressions, seen as a result of proximal matrix disease. They may be seen also in other dermatological conditions. Toenail disease often leads to discoloration, which may mimic onychomycosis. Subungual hyperkeratosis may lead to marked thickening of the nail plate. Focal parakeratosis produces an 'oil spot' or 'salmon patch'; if this extends to a free margin, onycholysis or separation of the nail plate from the nailbed results. Other abnormalities include splitting of the nail plate and paronychia. A variant of psoriasis, acropustulosis continua of Hallopeau, gives rise to sterile pustules around the nail unit (**8.17**). The nail may be completely lifted off (**8.18**).

Histopathology
Nail unit biopsy is often unnecessary, but shows acanthosis, neutrophil exocytosis, and parakeratosis; microabscesses or pustules may be seen and there may be a granular layer, usually absent from a healthy nail plate. Fungal hyphae may be seen indicating either infection or merely colonization.

108 Scalp and nail disorders

Differential diagnosis
Other features of psoriasis should be sought to confirm the diagnosis. The presence of an oil spot is highly suggestive of psoriasis. Differential diagnoses include onychomycosis; other causes of pitting include atopic disease, alopecia areata and LP; nail thickening may be seen in Darier's disease, pityriasis rubra pilaris, and pachyonychia congenita; Reiter's syndrome may be indistinguishable from psoriasis, though associated features of keratoderma blenorrhagica, urethritis, and uveitis should indicate the correct diagnosis.

Management
General hand care is important, including frequent use of emollients, keeping nails short, and protecting the hands from wet work and irritants. Very potent topical steroid application around the nail folds may help; injection of triamcinolone is possible, but requires ring block. The nails may improve with PUVA and oral treatment may be given in the form of the retinoid acitretin. Methotrexate or ciclosporin may also help.

Eczema

Introduction
Hand eczema commonly leads to disruption of the nail unit, though changes such as pitting may be a feature of a general atopic tendency. The nails may be exposed to a variety of allergens and irritants, and a combination of these may play a role in eczematous nail disease.

Clinical presentation
A wide variety of changes may be seen including thickening, pits, and transverse ridges (**8.19**). Nailbed disease gives rise to subungual hyperkeratosis and onycholysis. Often, but not always, there will be eczema around the nail units (**8.20**).

Histopathology
As with the skin, histology shows spongiosis and a predominately lymphocytic infiltrate. As in psoriasis of the nail, a granular layer is seen.

Differential diagnosis
The diagnosis is usually obvious from the cutaneous findings. Hand dermatitis may be difficult to distinguish from psoriasis and exogenous factors should be considered as possible causes or exacerbating factors.

Management
As with psoriasis, scrupulous hand care is advised, involving frequent use of emollients and soap substitute, and avoiding allergens, irritants, and wet work. Patch testing should be considered. Treatment involves emollients, and topical steroids may be applied to the nail folds. Infection should be treated with topical or systemic antibiotics. PUVA may be helpful.

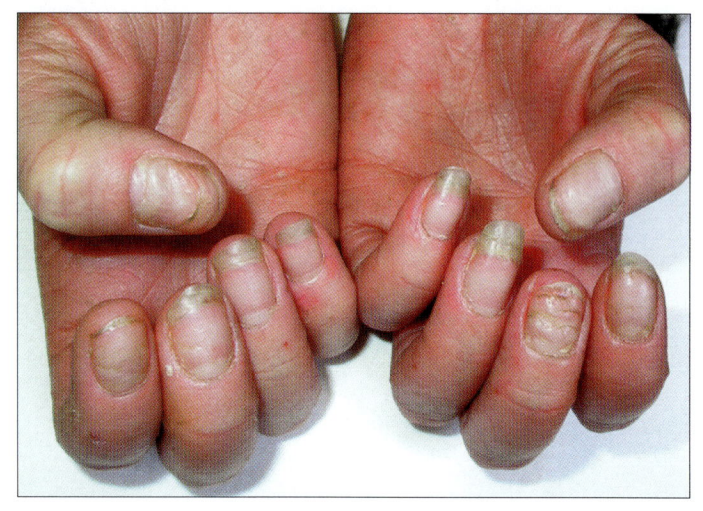

8.19 Nail dystrophy due to chronic periungual eczema showing thickening, pits, and transverse ridges.

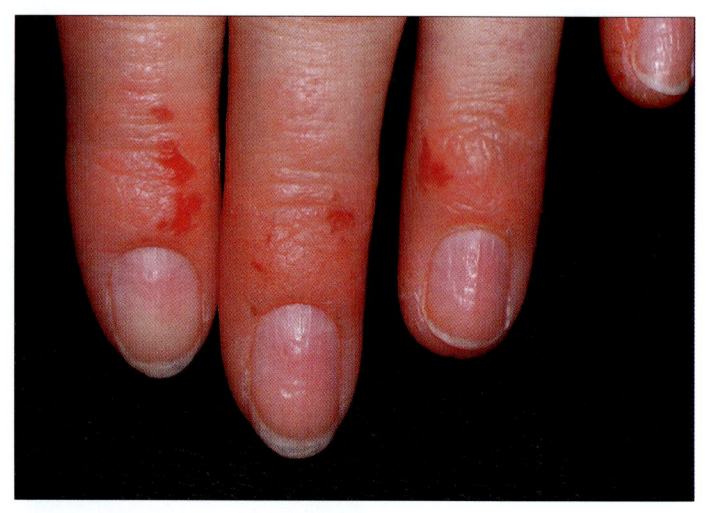

8.20 Eczematous nail dystrophy.

Lichen planus

Introduction
There are many different forms of LP. Typically, it manifests as a cutaneous, pruritic papular eruption, but may also affect the nails and mucosal surfaces. Nail disease is present in about 10% of cases. The cause is unknown.

Clinical presentation
LP nail disease may be the sole manifestation of the disease, or it may be accompanied by one of the other types. A variety of changes may be seen in the nail. These include superficial splitting of the nail (onychorrhexis), brittleness, subungual hyperkeratosis, and onycholysis (**8.21**, **8.22**). A sandpapered effect (trachyonychia) may result. Where all nails are affected, it is known as 'twenty nail dystrophy' (**8.23**).

Histopathology
The skin shows basal cell liquefaction with a band-like inflammatory infiltrate. In addition, there is marked spongiosis on nail histology.

Differential diagnosis
Examination of skin and mucous membranes may confirm the diagnosis. Isolated nail disease is more challenging. Onycholysis is commonly associated with psoriasis but may be due to various infectious, inflammatory or physical insults. Trachyonychia may also be seen associated with alopecia areata, psoriasis, ichthyosis, or ectodermal dysplasia. LP-like changes are also seen in graft-versus-host disease.

Management
Scarring nail changes will be permanent, but other effects may resolve spontaneously, especially in children. Potent or very potent topical steroids may be applied to the nail folds; triamcinolone may be injected into the nail unit under ring block anaesthesia.

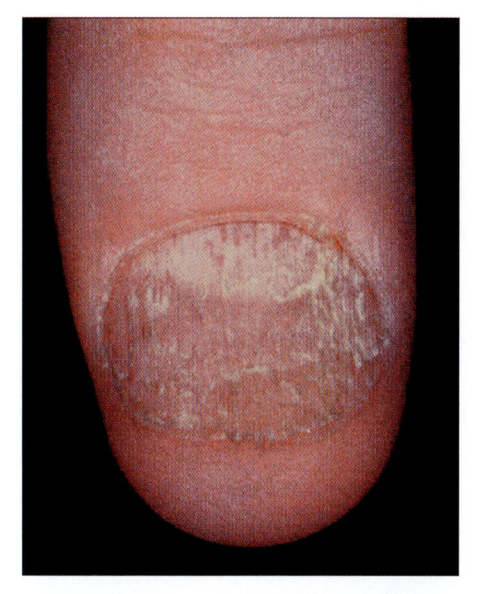

8.21 LP of the nail showing splitting of the nail and brittleness.

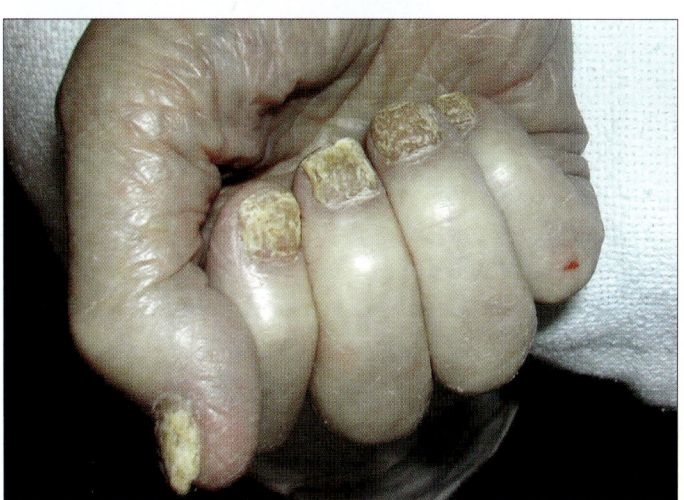

8.22 Subungual hyperkeratosis and onycholysis in LP nail dystrophy.

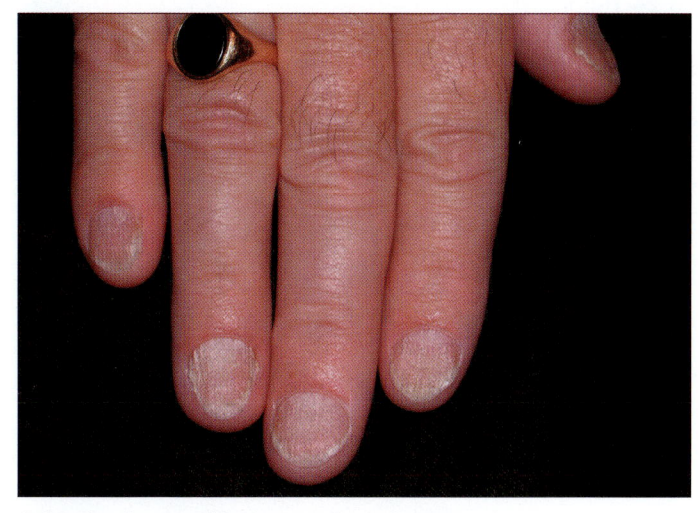

8.23 Trachyonychia in twenty nail dystrophy.

Alopecia areata

Introduction
This usually presents with patchy hair loss (see above), but nail changes are seen in a substantial proportion of those affected. These may occur synchronously with, or precede the hair loss.

Clinical presentation
One to twenty nails may be affected. There may be shallow pits; nails may be thickened and brown, appear sandpapered (trachyonychia, see above), or be thin, shiny, and fragile. Superficial splits, spoon-shaped nails (koilonychia), thinning, or thickening may be seen.

Histopathology
The nail matrix shows spongiosis. There may be a lymphocytic infiltrate; PAS-positive inclusions may be seen in the nail plate. The parakeratosis seen in psoriatic pits is lacking.

Differential diagnosis
The typical pattern of hair loss usually suggests the diagnosis. If this is lacking, appearances may be confused with psoriasis, LP, or onychomycosis.

Management
Potent or very potent topical steroids, or injected steroids may be effective. Systemic immunosuppressives may also reverse the nail changes.

Yellow nail syndrome

Classically associated with lymphoedema and respiratory disease, the nails show yellow-green discoloration, decreased growth rate, thickening and hardening of the nail plate, and loss of the cuticle (**8.24**). The cause is unknown and the condition may resolve spontaneously.

Onychogryphosis

This is characterized by overgrowth and increased curvature of the nail plate. It is most common in the elderly (**8.25**). Although mainly attributable to neglect, vascular and mechanical factors, and local skin disease may contribute. Treatment may include trimming, chemical destruction with 40% urea paste, or total ablation through phenol application.

Pincer nail

Pincer nail is usually an isolated familial abnormality of the big toe or thumb nails which develops in adulthood (**8.26**). The sides of the nail become ingrown and are very painful because of recurrent infections and associated swelling. Total ablation of the nail is often required to stop ingrowing of the sides of the nail and recurring infections.

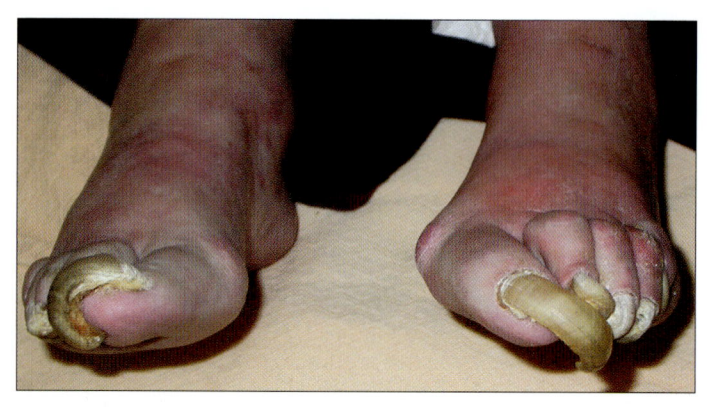

8.24 Yellow nail syndrome.

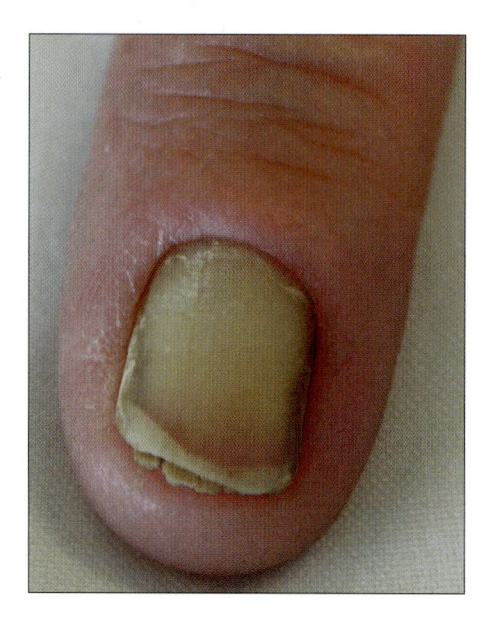

8.25 Onychogryphosis.

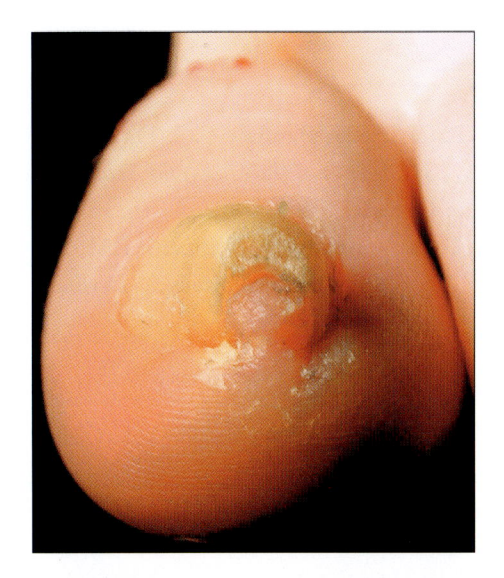

Scalp and nail disorders

8.26 Pincer nail.

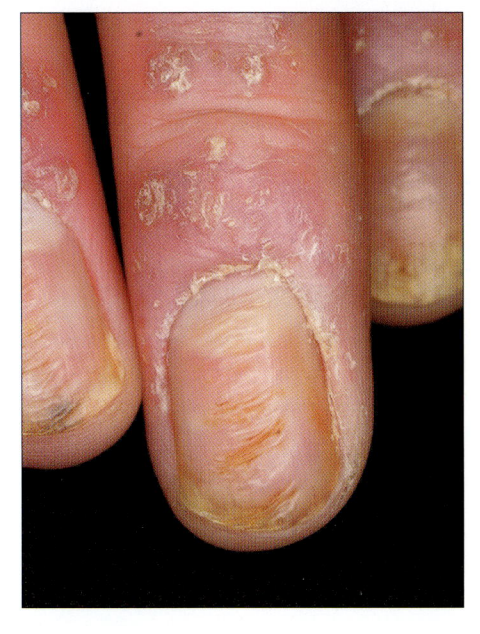

8.27 Median nail dystrophy in a patient with psoriasis.

Median nail dystrophy

Median nail dystrophy or washboard nail is due to repetitive disruption of the cuticle, often due to a nervous habit. There is a lower threshold for the development of this in patients with psoriasis (**8.27**, **8.28**).

Tumours of the nail unit

Any tumour of the nail unit, benign or malignant, may give rise to abnormalities of the nail plate. Such a diagnosis should be considered particularly where a single nail is affected. Differential diagnosis includes skin cancers (see Chapter 4), or benign lesions, such as glomus tumour, myxoid cyst (**8.29**), neurofibroma, periungual fibroma (**8.30**), and viral wart. Exostosis of the distal phalanx may also present similarly. Radiography and biopsy should be considered.

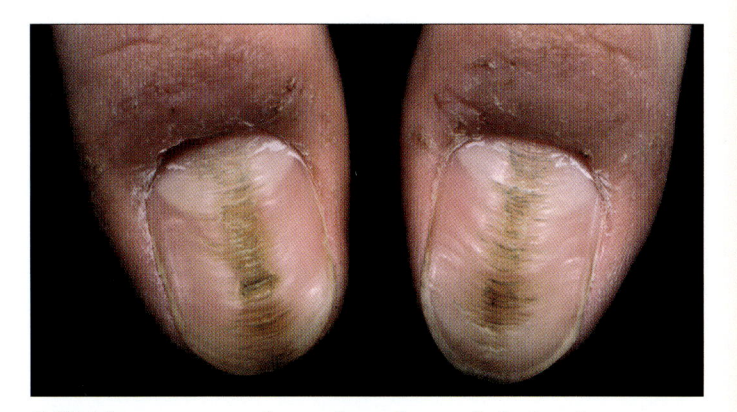

8.28 More common form of median nail dystrophy.

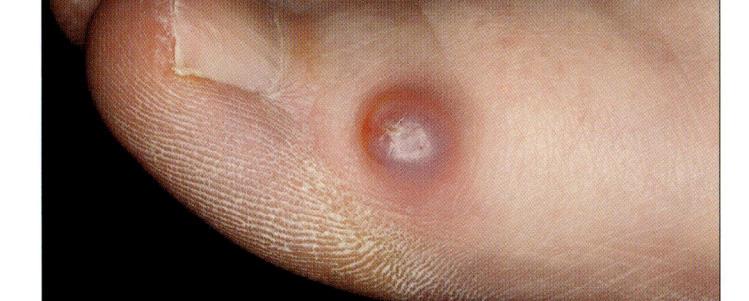

8.29 Myxoid cyst.

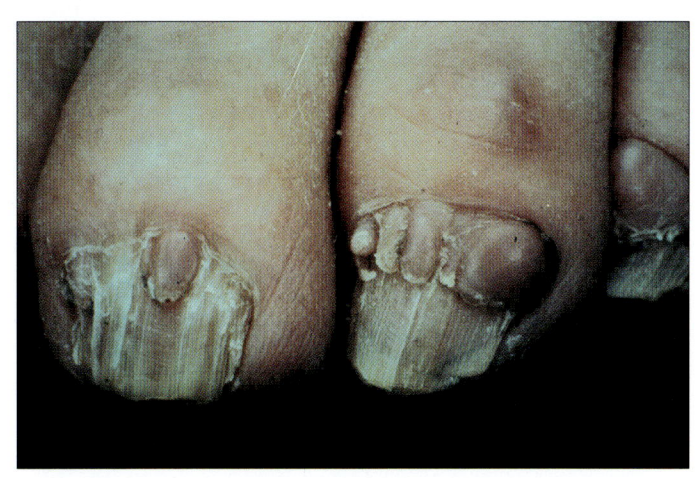

8.30 Periungual fibromas in a patient with tuberose sclerosis.

Further reading

Bolognia JL, Jorizzo JL, Rapini RP (eds) (2003). *Dermatology.* Mosby, London.

de Berker DAR, Baran R, Dawber RPR (1995). *Handbook of Diseases of the Nails and their Management.* Blackwell Sciences, Oxford.

Holzberg M (2006). Common nail disorders. *Dermatol Clin* **24**(3):349–354.

Sinclair RD, Banfield CC, Dawber RPR (1999). *Handbook of Diseases of the Hair and Scalp.* Blackwell Sciences, Oxford.

Tosti A, Iorizzo M, Piraccini BM, Starace M (2006). The Nail in Systemic Diseases. *Dermatol Clin* **24**(3):341–347.

Chapter 9

Skin infections and infestations

Neill C Hepburn, MD, FRCP

Introduction

Skin infections can be divided into bacterial, viral, or fungal whereas infestation will be with either an insect or a worm. The distribution, configuration, and morphology of the rash are important in helping to make the diagnosis but the history, including travel, will also be key. Often dermatitis becomes secondarily infected and can even at times be caused by infection (see Chapters 2 and 3). The use of swabs, tissue culture, histology, mycological studies, and serological tests will often be necessary to make or confirm the diagnosis.

BACTERIAL INFECTIONS

Impetigo

Introduction
A common, highly contagious, bacterial infection with streptococci and/or staphylococci.

Clinical presentation
Patients present with erythematous areas, which start in one area, but can rapidly spread and become numerous. They may form small bullae with breakdown (**9.1A**), or just moist crusty areas (**9.1B**). There is usually a peripheral collar of scale or crust but little surrounding erythema.

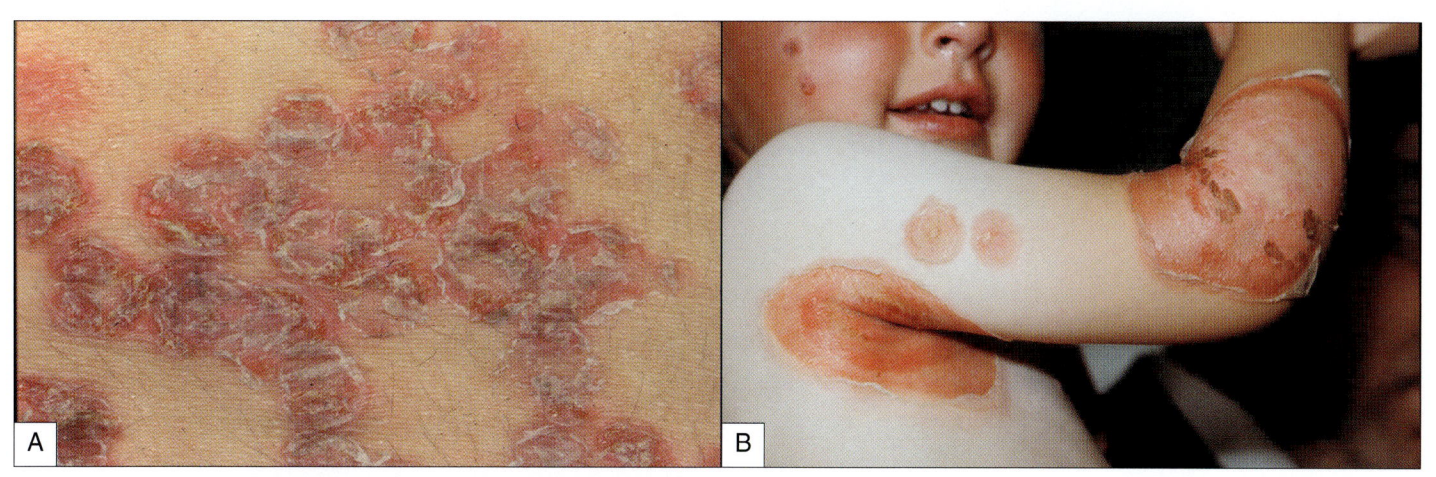

9.1 A, B: Impetigo. Note eroded areas with collarette of scale/crust.

Skin infections and infestations

Differential diagnosis
Infected eczema may look similar and, of course, those with eczema are predisposed to impetigo.

Management
The lesions should be swabbed to identify the infecting bacterium and its sensitivity. The area should be treated topically with fucidic acid or systemically with flucloxacillin or clarithromycin.

Prognosis
Recurrence is common. Swabs should be taken from the nares of the patient and family members.

Cellulitis

Introduction
Cellulitis and erysipelas are bacterial infections involving the dermis and subcutaneous tissues. Common pathogens are group A streptococci or *Staphylococcus aureus* in adults and *Haemophilus influenzae* type B in children. Breaks in the skin such as surgical wounds, abrasions, ulcers, or tinea pedis predispose to cellulitis by providing a portal of entry for the bacteria. Previous episodes of cellulitis, lymph node resections, and radiation therapy, which damage the lymphatics, also predispose to cellulitis.

Clinical presentation
Patients present with sudden onset of malaise and, within a few hours, the skin becomes erythematous, warm, oedematous, and painful. In cellulitis that involves the deeper layer, there is no clear distinction between involved and uninvolved skin. The skin may form bullae, which rupture (**9.2**). In erysipelas, which tends to involve the more superficial layers and cutaneous lymphatics, there is a clear line of demarcation between involved and uninvolved skin (**9.3**), and there is prominent streaking of the draining lymphatics.

Differential diagnosis
Secondarily infected eczema is common around leg ulcers but the skin is not warm to the touch. In necrotizing fasciitis, infection of the subcutaneous tissues results in destruction of fat and fascia with pain out of proportion to the clinical signs, and often only a mild fever but with diffuse swelling and pain (**9.4**). Urgent surgical debridement is needed.

Management
It is usually not possible to identify the infecting organism from blood cultures or skin swabs. Needle aspiration from the subcutaneous tissues and blood cultures can be helpful. Oral phenoxymethyl penicillin and flucloxacillin or erythromycin should be given. In patients who are allergic to penicillin, ciprofloxacin can be used. If the patient is toxic, antibiotics should be given intravenously initially.

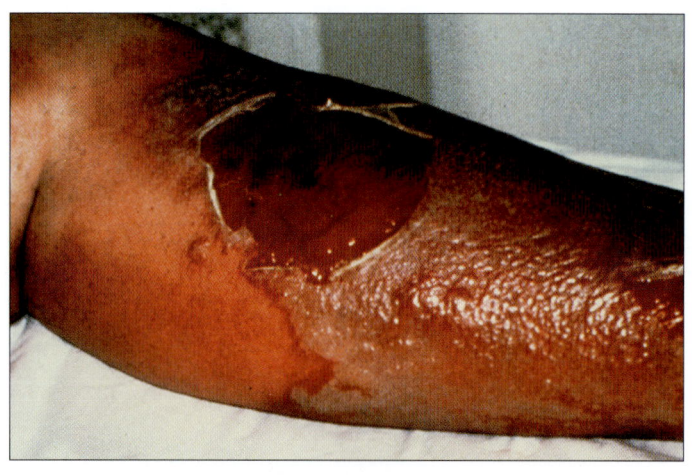

9.2 Streptoccocal cellulitis. Note the well-defined red area and the formation of bullae, one of which has ruptured.

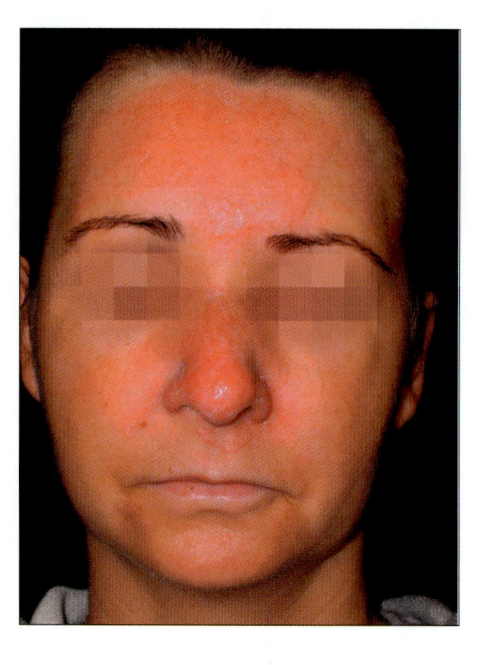

9.3 Erysipelas. Note the sharply demarcated areas of erythema.

Prognosis

Recurrence after antibiotic treatment occurs in about 25% of cases and may be spontaneous or initiated by quite minor trauma. Recurrent cases may require long-term prophylactic treatment with low-dose penicillin or erythromycin.

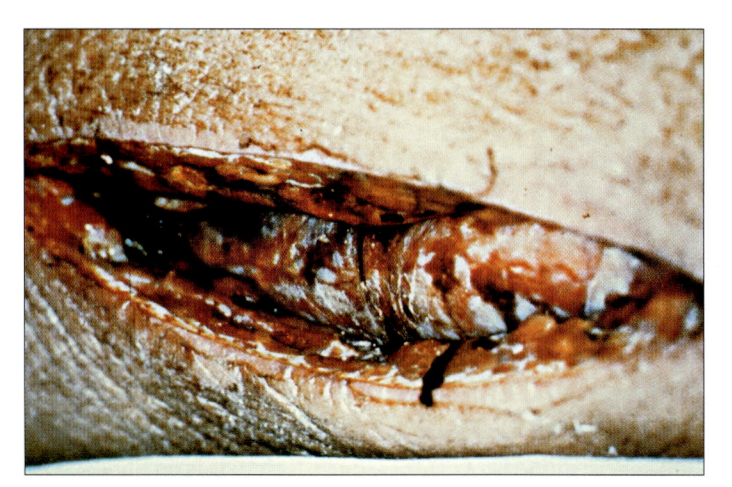

9.4 Necrotizing fasciitis with necrotic muscle.

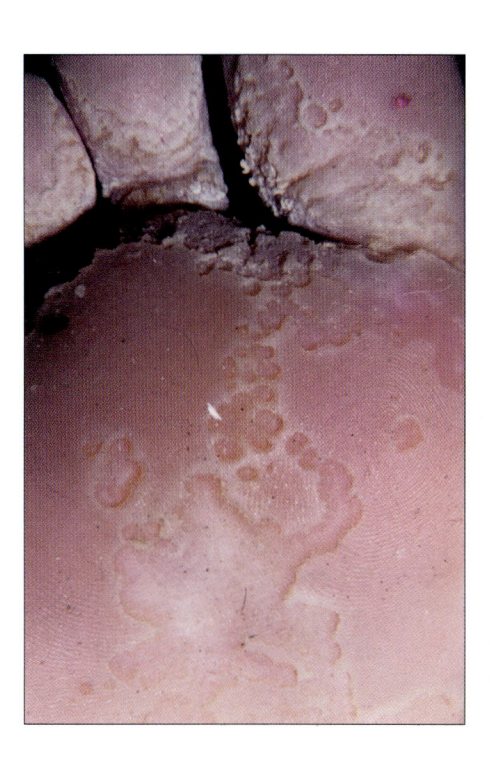

Pitted keratolysis

Introduction

This is a common superficial bacterial infection occurring on the soles of the feet. It usually occurs in those with sweaty feet, or those who wear occlusive footwear, such as work boots or trainers.

Clinical presentation

The skin over the weight-bearing areas appears moist and oedematous with punched out circular pits and furrows, resembling the surface of the moon (9.5). The feet usually have an offensive smell. Several species of bacteria have been implicated including *Corynebacterium*, *Dermatophilus*, and *Micrococcus* spp. These bacteria excrete enzymes that degrade keratin and thereby produce the characteristic pitted surface.

Differential diagnosis

The appearance (and smell) are characteristic; however, it is sometimes mistaken for a fungal infection.

Management

The bacterial infection responds to topical antibiotics such as fusidic acid cream, or acne medications such as clindamycin solution.

Prognosis

It is important to dry the skin of the feet to prevent recurrences. Options include 20% aluminium chloride (Drichlor) or 10% formaldehyde soaks.

9.5 Pitted keratolysis. Note the punched out circular pits and furrows, resembling the surface of the moon, over the weight-bearing areas.

Erythrasma

Introduction
Erythrasma is an indolent skin infection usually of the axillae, groin, or toe webs caused by the bacterium *Corynebacterium minutissimum*. Hot, humid environmental conditions encourage this infection.

Clinical presentation
There are sharply marginated, reddy-brown patches in the axillae or groin (**9.6**), which develop often over many years. Sometimes patients complain of irritation but usually they are asymptomatic.

Differential diagnosis
The coral red fluorescence is typical of erythrasma but pityriasis versicolor and tinea infections can have a similar appearance.

Management
Patients respond well to a range of topical antimicrobials such as fusidic acid, miconazole, or erythromycin (oral or topical).

Prognosis
Without treatment the condition persists indefinitely. If treated, it will relapse if climatic conditions are adverse or personal hygiene is poor.

Atypical mycobacterium infection

Introduction
Fish tank, or swimming pool, granuloma is an infection with *Mycobacterium marinum* – an atypical mycobacterium which grows in culture at 30°C. It is most commonly seen in keepers of tropical fish (the infected fish usually die). It can also be contracted from swimming pools.

Clinical presentation
The lesions usually develop following an abrasion after an incubation period of 2–3 weeks. A nodule develops that may then break down to form an ulcer or remain as a warty plaque (**9.7**). Lesions are frequently multiple and nodules may form along the line of the draining lymphatics, known as sporotrichoid spread (**9.8**).

Histopathology
The pathology varies from nonspecific inflammation to well formed tuberculoid granulomas. Intracellular acid-fast bacilli are only identified in 10% of cases.

Differential diagnosis
The main differential in the UK is bacterial pyoderma. In those returning from the tropics, leishmaniasis and sporotrichosis are alternatives as is a tuberculous chancre (**9.9**).

Management
A skin biopsy should be sent for culture at 30°C but it will take a month for the colonies to grow. Although self-limiting, with spontaneous healing occurring within 6 months, several treatments are advocated, but the optimum treatment has not been established.

Prognosis
Commonly advocated treatment regimens include: minocycline 100–200 mg daily for 6–12 weeks, rifampicin 600 mg and ethambutol 1.2 g daily for 3–6 months, and co-trimoxazole 2–3 tablets twice daily for 6 weeks. Public health authorities should be notified.

Skin infections and infestations   117

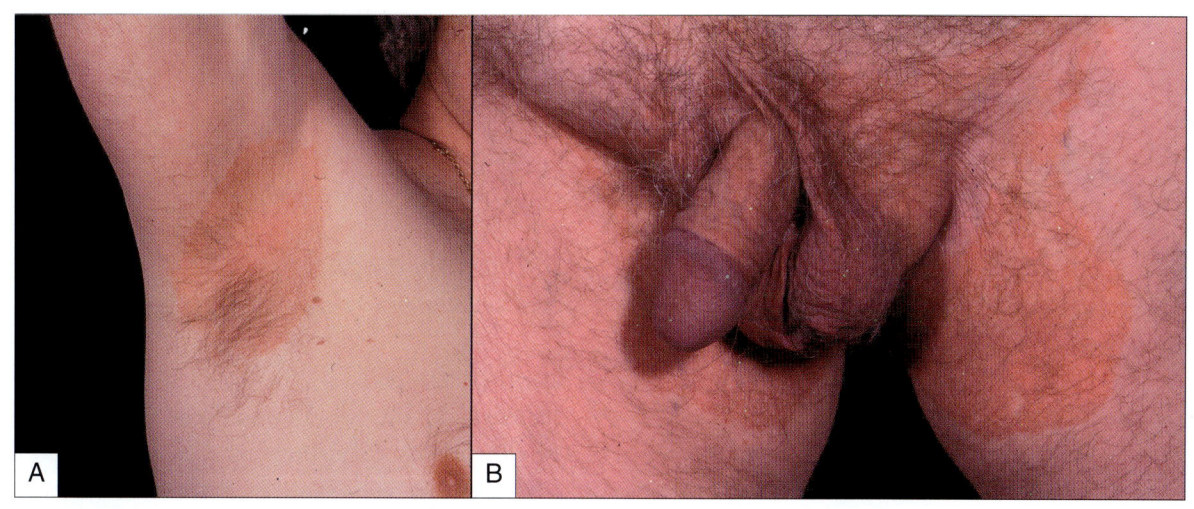

9.6 A, B: Erythrasma. Sharply marginated lesions in the axillae and groin.

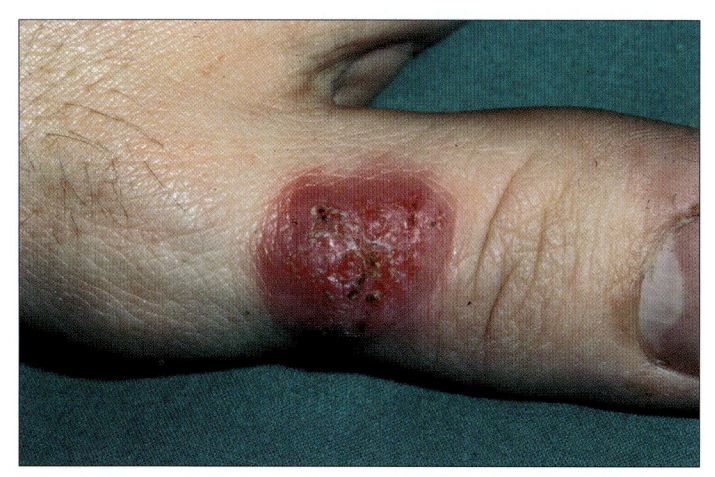

9.7 Atypical mycobacterial infection due to *M. marinum* in a tropical fish keeper, clinically similar to warty tuberculosis.

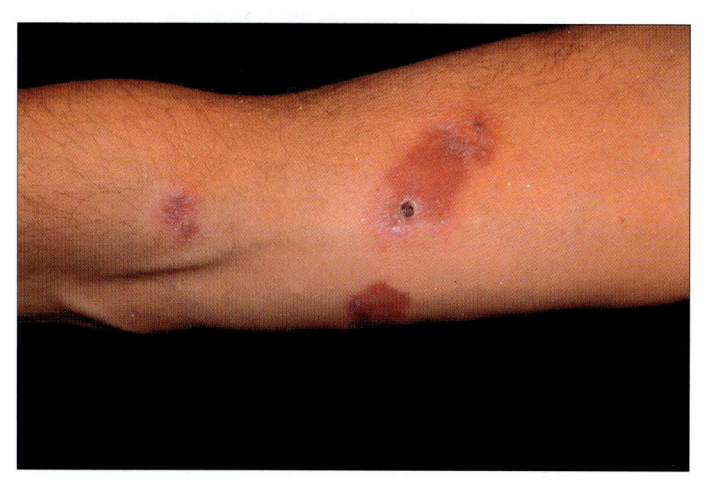

9.8 Sporotrichoid spread in atypical mycobacterial infection.

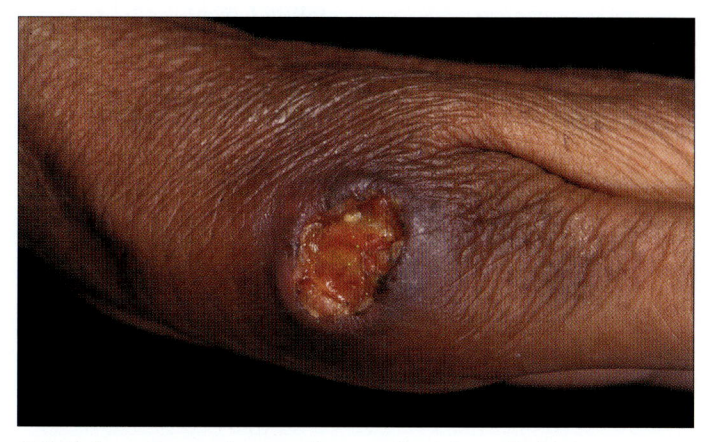

9.9 Tuberculous chancre in a patient from Pakistan.

Anthrax

Introduction
Anthrax is an extremely rare, but often fatal, infection caused by *Bacillus anthracis*. It has recently become important because of its use, by terrorists, as a biological weapon. Natural infection occurs after contact with infected animal hides that have usually been imported from Africa or the Indian subcontinent.

Clinical presentation
Patients present with a vesicle or bulla that enlarges over a week or so, to become haemorrhagic and necrotic, leading to the formation of an adherent back eschar (**9.10**). It is sometimes surrounded by satellite vesicles and is a striking brawny oedema that is surprisingly painless. The lymph glands enlarge and the patient becomes unwell with a low-grade fever.

Histopathology
The bacilli can be seen on Gram staining of the exudate. Culture, polymerase chain reaction (PCR), and serology are helpful.

Differential diagnosis
Acute pyoderma is usually painful and the systemic upset is greater in anthrax. Cowpox is very similar in appearance and clinical course but is benign and self-limiting (**9.11**).

Management
Ciprofloxacin 500 mg bd, initially intravenously, for 14 days.

Prognosis
In 80% of cases the lesion heals over 2–4 weeks and the patient recovers with little scarring. In 20% a bacteraemia occurs followed by a haemorrhagic meningitis and death. Antibiotic treatment does not change the course of the primary lesion and the eschar still forms, but it reduces the bacteraemia and the consequent mortality.

Gonococcal septicaemia

Introduction
Gonorrhoea can on rare occasions present to the dermatologist with one or two pustules with arthritis of one or more joints.

Clinical presentation
The lesions are typical, once recognized, and present as small vesicles with a red halo, which become haemorrhagic pustules (**9.12**). They occur in crops or three to four lesions scattered over the limbs and heal after a few days.

Differential diagnosis
Septicaemia and vasculitis from other causes.

Management
Patients should be referred to a genitourinary medicine department as coexisting sexually transmitted diseases are common; antibiotic-resistant strains are very frequent.

Prognosis
The prognosis is good providing it is treated adequately. Contact tracing is advisable.

Secondary syphilis

Introduction
There is an epidemic of syphilis currently in Europe and probably worldwide. After many decades of syphilis being a rare disease in dermatology clinics, dermatologists in the UK are now beginning to see patients presenting with secondary syphilis.

Clinical presentation
The cutaneous presentations of secondary syphilis are variable, but the commonest to present to the dermatologist is a widespread pityriasis rosea-like rash (roseola) with palmar lesions (**9.13, 9.14**).

Differential diagnosis
These include pityriasis rosea, psoriasis, and urticaria.

Management
Patients should be referred to a genitourinary medicine department as coexisting sexually transmitted diseases are common. Resistance to antibiotics has not occurred. *Treponema pallidum* still responds to penicillin or doxycycline.

Prognosis
The prognosis is good providing it is treated adequately. Contact tracing is advisable.

Skin infections and infestations

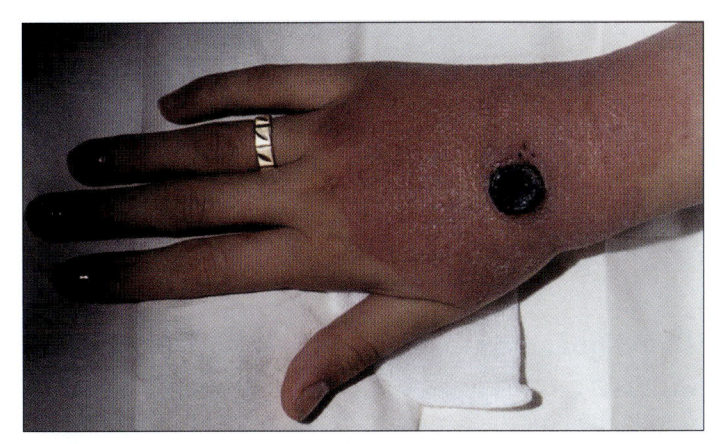

9.10 Cutaneous anthrax. Note black eschar, surrounding erythema and oedema.

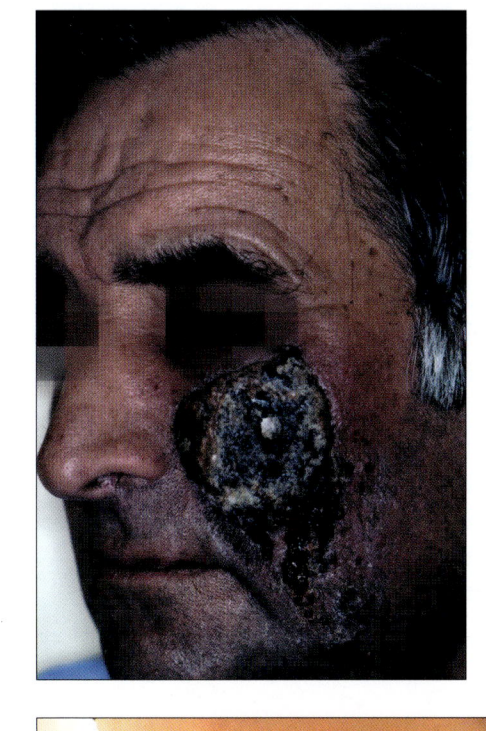

9.11 Cowpox. It is similar to anthrax but self-limiting and benign. Contact with cows or cats should be investigated.

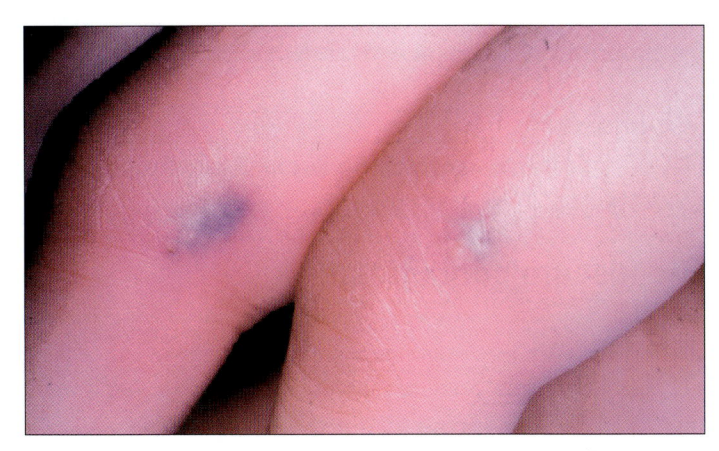

9.12 Haemorrhagic gonococcal pustules on the fingers.

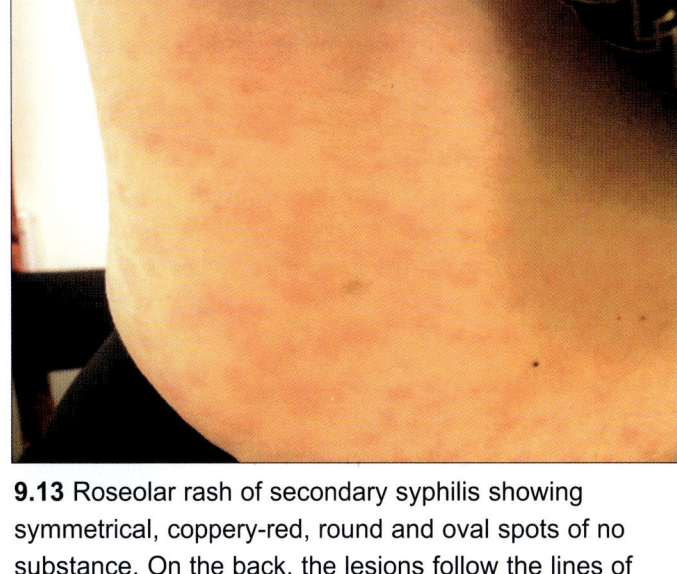

9.13 Roseolar rash of secondary syphilis showing symmetrical, coppery-red, round and oval spots of no substance. On the back, the lesions follow the lines of cleavage resembling pityriasis rosea.

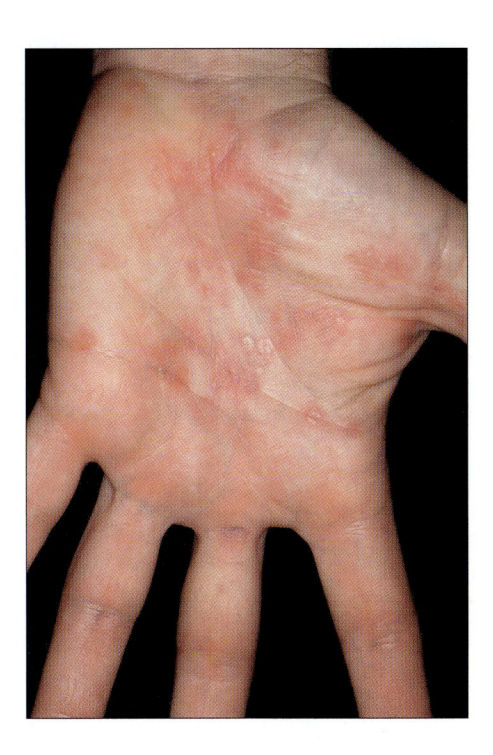

9.14 Psoriasisform papules of the palms or soles help make the diagnosis of secondary syphilis.

Viral infections

Herpes simplex

Introduction
Herpes simplex is a common viral infection with two phases. After the primary infection, the virus lies dormant in the nerve ganglion. The secondary infections occur when the virus comes out from the reservoir in the nerve. Many primary infections are asymptomatic. It is spread by direct contact.

Clinical presentation
Symptoms start about 3–7 days after contact, starting with a prodromal pain followed by the appearance of vesicles on an erythematous base. They are more scattered in the primary infection than in recurrences (**9.15**). The primary lesions heal in about 2–3 weeks.

Histopathology
The diagnosis is established by electron microscopy and viral culture.

Differential diagnosis
These include Stevens–Johnson syndrome. Patients with eczema are predisposed to develop a widespread infection (eczema herpeticum), which requires aggressive antiviral treatment (**9.16**).

Management
Symptomatic treatment with cold compresses of potassium permanganate is helpful. Oral antiviral agents, such as aciclovir, decrease the duration of viral excretion and new lesion formation, and promote more rapid healing, but need to be started early.

Prognosis
Recurrences average 2 or 3 per year, but can be more frequent and require suppressive antivirals.

Herpes zoster

Introduction
Herpes zoster results from reactivation of the varicella virus that has been dormant in the cutaneous nerves following an earlier infection with chickenpox.

Clinical presentation
A prodromal pain, sometimes associated with fever or malaise, occurs 4–5 days before the lesions appear. Red, oedematous plaques appear that spread to cover the dermatome. Then clusters of vesicles appear on the surface becoming pustules that may rupture to form a crust (**9.17, 9.18**). Lesions generally heal in 3 weeks.

Differential diagnosis
It is frequently impossible to make the diagnosis accurately during the prodromal phase.

Management
The aim is to suppress the inflammation with potassium permanganate compresses, to treat the pain with analgesics, and to treat the infection with antivirals such as aciclovir.

Prognosis
7% of patients have severe pain lasting 3 months or longer.

Molluscum contagiosum

Introduction
This is a common poxvirus infection, most commonly seen in children and is spread by direct contact.

Clinical presentation
Patients present with small (2–5 mm) shiny papules with a central pit, often occurring in groups (**9.19, 9.20**). They are frequently inflamed, following scratching.

Differential diagnosis
When the lesions are inflamed, the secondary eczema may disguise the underlying mollusca. Isolated lesions may resemble intradermal naevi or basal cell carcinomas.

Management
Simply squeezing the lesions with forceps is usually followed by an inflammatory reaction and resolution. Vioform-hydrocortisone ointment can be applied to reduce the reaction. Alternatives include cryotherapy or curettage of individual lesions, or the application of salicylic acid or imiquimod cream.

Prognosis
Mollusca are self-limiting, usually clearing in 9 months but occasionally persisting for as long as 4 years. Often the best treatment is to do nothing.

Skin infections and infestations 121

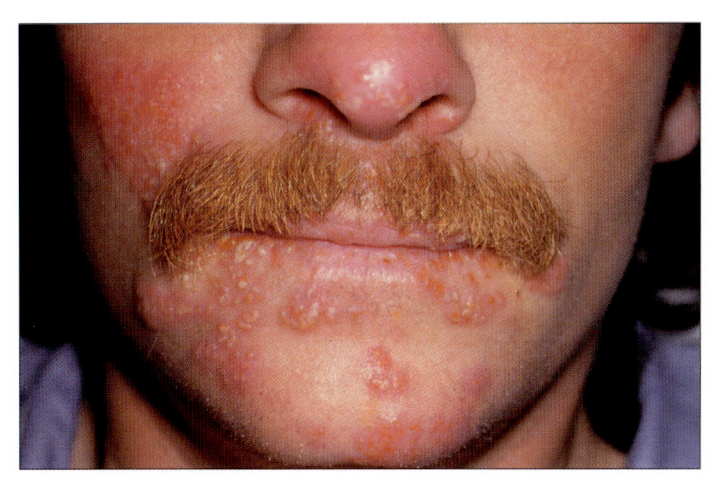

9.15 Herpes simplex. Note scattered lesions of a primary infection with eroded crusted areas arising on an erythematous base.

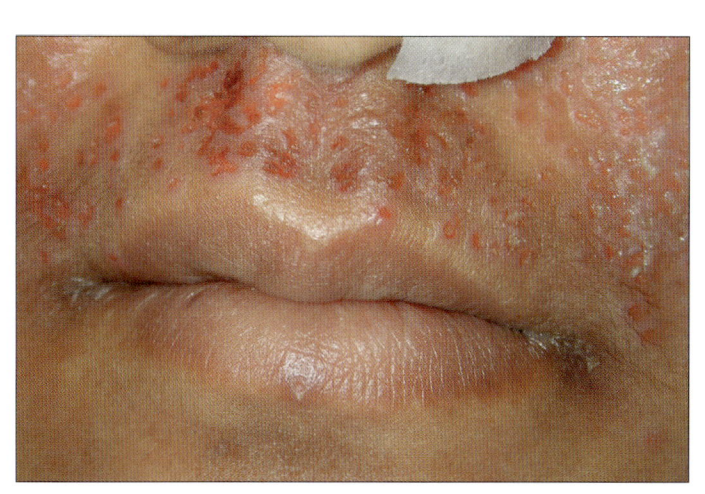

9.16 Eczema herpeticum. Note the large number of lesions.

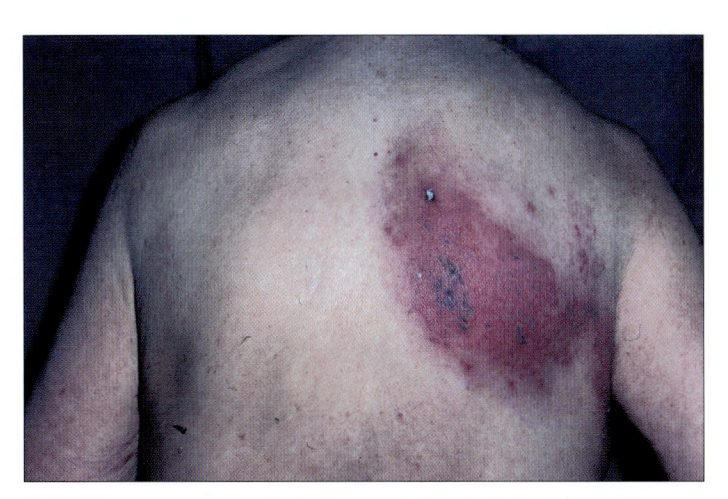

9.17 Herpes zoster. Note the unilateral distribution along the dermatome.

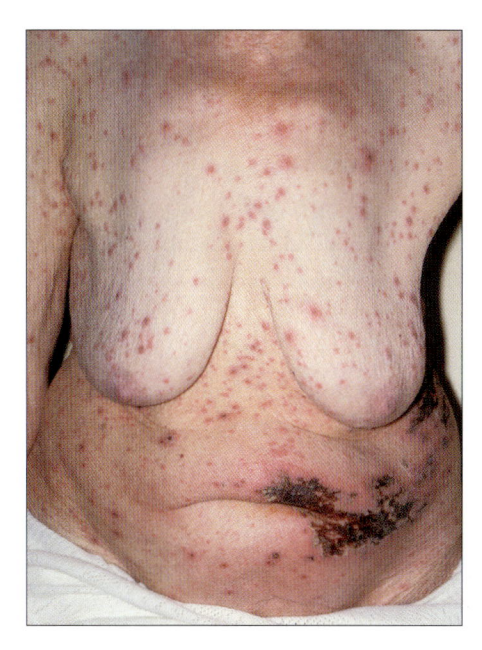

9.18 Herpes zoster. Note the principal lesions along the dermatome but with additional satellite lesions.

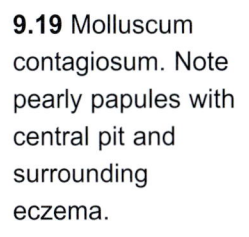

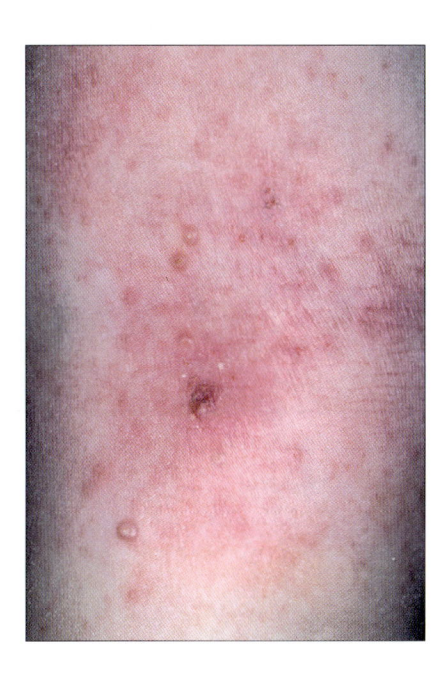

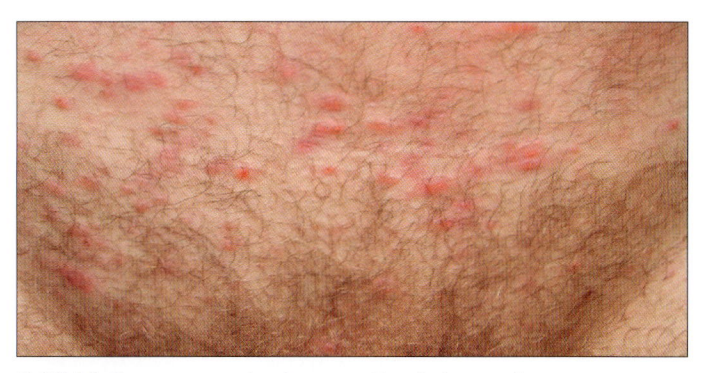

9.19 Molluscum contagiosum. Note pearly papules with central pit and surrounding eczema.

9.20 Molluscum contagiosum. Genital area is a common site in adults.

122 Skin infections and infestations

Viral warts

Introduction
Warts are caused by the human papilloma virus (HPV), of which there are over 100 types. It is transmitted by direct contact with infected skin scales; subclinical infection is common.

Clinical presentation
The appearance varies with the site of the infection. Most commonly a flesh coloured papule appears which then develops a hyperkeratotic surface with back dots, representing thrombosed capillaries which are most easily seen on paring the wart down with a scalpel (**9.21**).

Differential diagnosis
The clinical appearance is usually diagnostic. Periungual warts may mimic periungual fibromas. Verrucas may mimic corns or rare appendageal tumours.

Management
There is no treatment to eradicate HPV. Treatment debulks the wart and stimulates an inflammatory reaction to trigger the immune response required.

Prognosis
Options include simple occlusion with duct tape, salicylic acid wart paints, cryotherapy, and curettage. Warts resolve spontaneously in 40% of cases over 6 months.

9.21 Periungual warts.

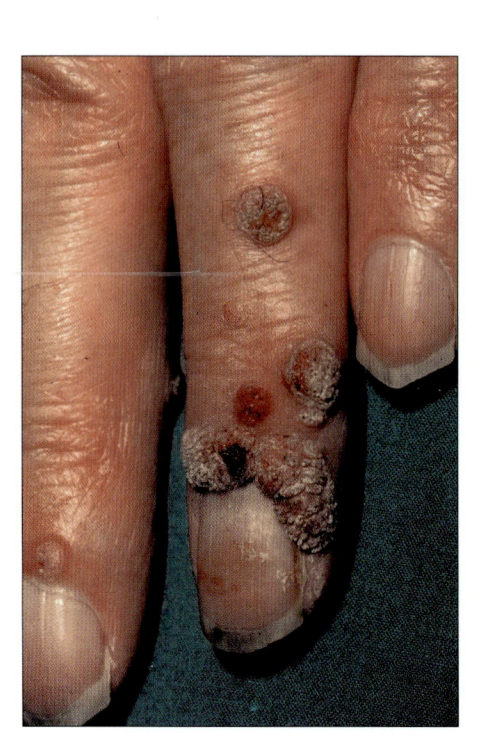

Orf

Introduction
Orf is a poxvirus infection, which is widespread in sheep, mainly affecting young lambs. It is spread by direct inoculation so it is most commonly seen on the fingers of farmers.

Clinical presentation
A firm reddish-blue papule appears after an incubation period of 5–6 days. It enlarges to form a haemorrhagic pustule or bulla 2–3 cm in diameter. It may then form a crust in the centre. It is tender and usually solitary (**9.22**).

Management
Treatment is only needed to prevent or treat a secondary infection.

Prognosis
Spontaneous recovery occurs in 3–6 weeks, but second attacks are quite common.

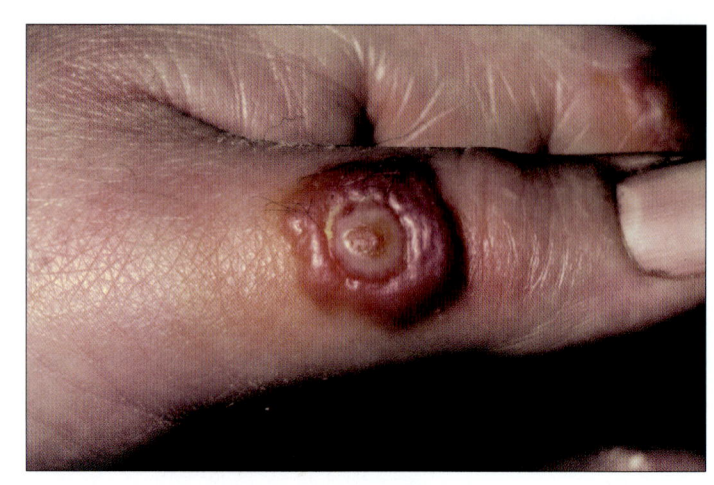

9.22 Orf on the finger of a shepherdess. Note the large bluish pustule.

Fungal and yeast infections

Introduction
Superficial fungal infections (tinea) are common. The fungus only invades the top layer of skin but may stimulate a cell-mediated immune response that varies according to the species of fungus. Common ringworm fungi belong to the groups Trichophyton, Microsporum, and Epidermophyton and may be contacted from another person, either directly or indirectly, or from animals.

Clinical presentation
Clinical presentation is variable, depending on the site and the immune response. There is usually scaling on the surface, and erythema is most marked at the 'active edge' (**9.23**). If the inflammatory reaction is marked there is pustule formation and, if severe, it can transform into a boggy swelling.

Histopathology
Fungus can be seen in the top layer of skin along with neutrophils in a PAS-stained section.

Differential diagnosis
Eczema and psoriasis cause confusion, especially on the hands (beware the one-handed rash! **9.24**). Pyoderma can mimic fungal infection of the scalp.

Management
Scrapings taken from the active edge reveal fungus on microscopy and should be cultured to determine the infecting species. Most superficial infections respond well to terbinafine 1% cream. Deeper infections and those with a marked inflammatory reaction are best treated systemically.

Prognosis
Most infections respond well. It is often necessary to treat the inflammatory reaction with a weak topical steroid. Relapses are common.

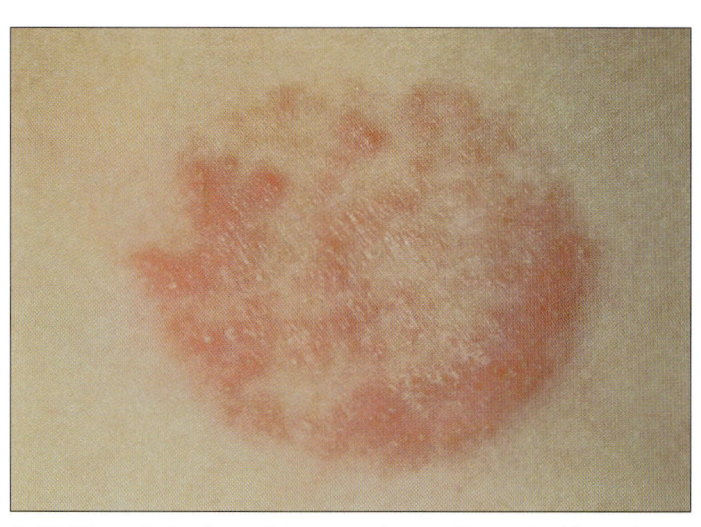

9.23 Tinea infection of the arm due to *T. canis*. Note the ring of active inflammation.

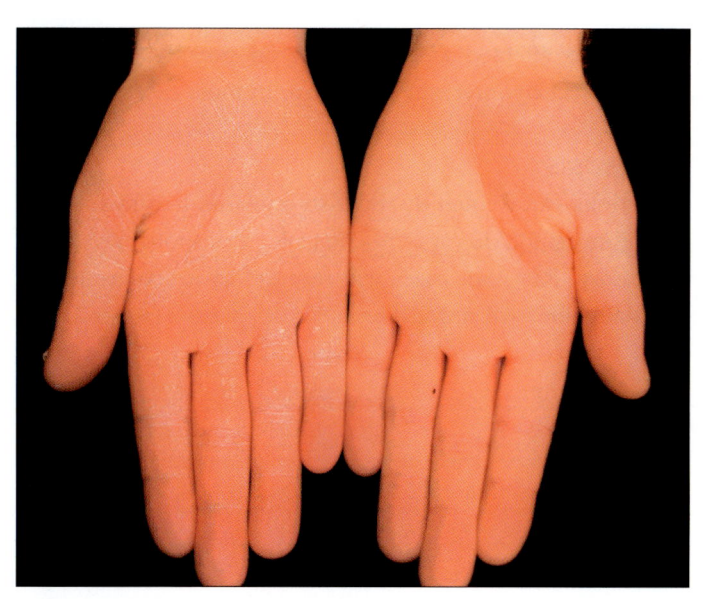

9.24 Tinea infection of the left hand due to *T. rubrum*. Note unilateral distribution.

Pityriasis versicolor

Introduction
Pityriasis versicolor (PV) is a chronic superficial fungal infection of the trunk causing pigmentary changes. It is caused by an overgrowth of the mycelial form of the commensal yeast *Pityrosporum orbiculare* and is particularly common in hot or humid environments. Patients often present following a holiday in a hot climate. It is commonest in young adults and can be spread by physical contact.

Clinical presentation
The condition presents as brown or pinkish, oval or round, slightly scaly lesions on the trunk, upper arms and thighs (9.25). In tanned or dark skin, hypopigmented patches occur due to inhibition of melanogenesis by carboxylic acids released by the organism.

Histopathology
Lesional scrapings treated with potassium hydroxide show the classical 'spaghetti and meatballs' appearance of the spores and hyphae.

Differential diagnosis
The commonest differential diagnosis is that of vitiligo, but in PV a fine scale can be demonstrated if the lesional skin is stretched. Pityriasis rosea, secondary syphilis, and tinea corporis must also be considered.

Management
Topical selenium sulphide or ketoconazole shampoos applied to affected areas and left on overnight, repeated twice at weekly intervals, is effective in most cases.

Prognosis
Infections can frequently recur so repeated treatments with selenium sulphide or ketoconazole shampoos are often necessary. Resistant cases will respond to itraconazole 200 mg daily for 7–14 days.

9.25 Pityriasis versicolor affecting the trunk.

INFESTATIONS

Cutaneous larva migrans

Introduction
Creeping eruption is the most common tropical skin disease seen in returning travellers. Hookworm larvae migrating through the skin cause the tracts. Most commonly it is *Ancylostoma braziliense*, the dog hookworm, which is contracted on tropical beaches from dog faeces.

Clinical presentation
Most patients give a history of tropical travel where they have spent time on beaches. After about 3 weeks an intensely itchy reddish-blue tract appears which grows by about 1 cm daily (9.26, 9.27). The hookworm itself is invisible and lies about 1 cm ahead of the advancing edge of the tract.

Differential diagnosis
There is really nothing quite like it!

Management
Albendazole 400 mg daily for 3–5 days or ivermectin 12 mg single dose is effective.

Prognosis
Untreated the larvae live for about 6 weeks but occasionally for up to 1 year. Travellers should be advised not to walk barefoot on beaches.

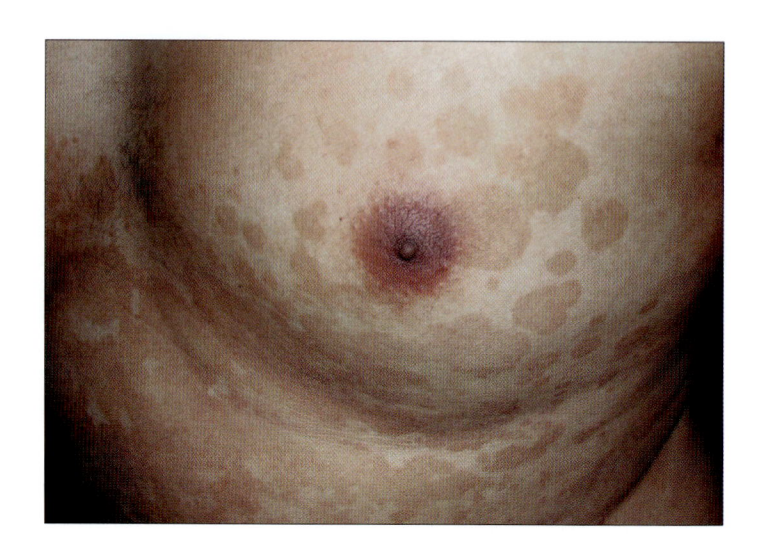

Tungiasis

Introduction
Tungiasis is caused by the jigger, or sand flea found in South America and Africa. Larvae develop in dry sandy soil. The impregnated female burrows into the skin producing a 1 cm nodule, then extrudes its eggs.

Clinical presentation
An intensely itchy nodule, usually on the soles of the feet, appears with a central punctum. Secondary infection is common (**9.28**).

Management
The flea is removed by curettage and cautery of the cavity performed.

Prognosis
Left untreated the flea dies in 2 weeks.

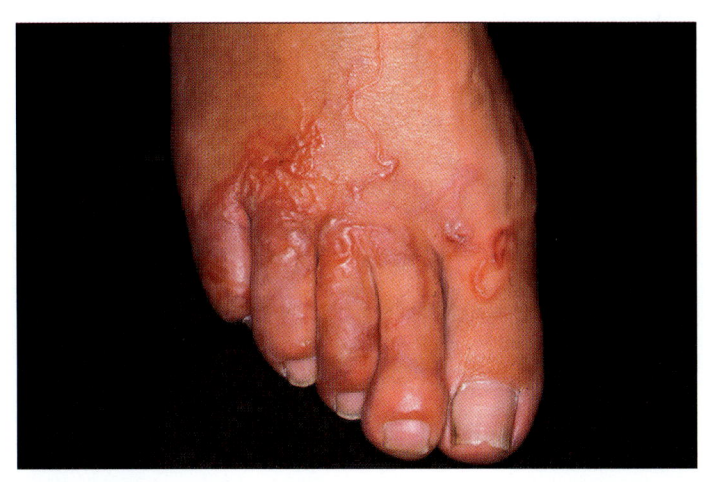

9.26 Cutaneous larva migrans on the foot. Note the advancing tracts.

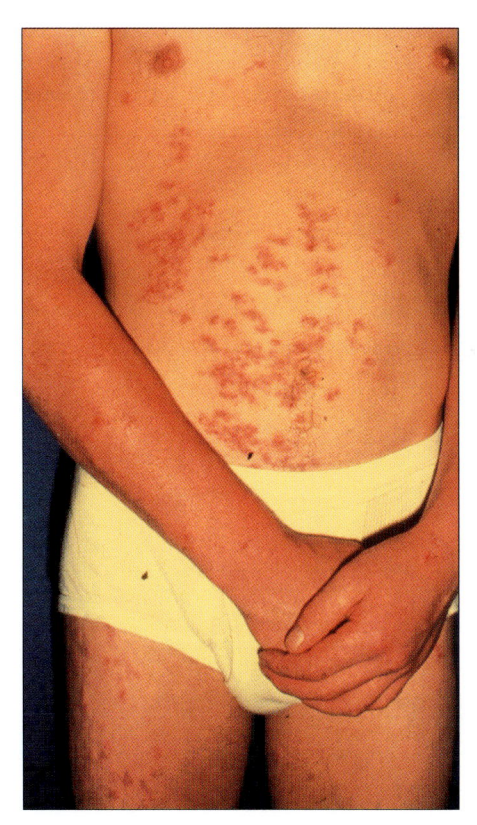

9.27 Cutaneous larva migrans on the abdomen after lying on a tropical beach where locals exercised their dogs.

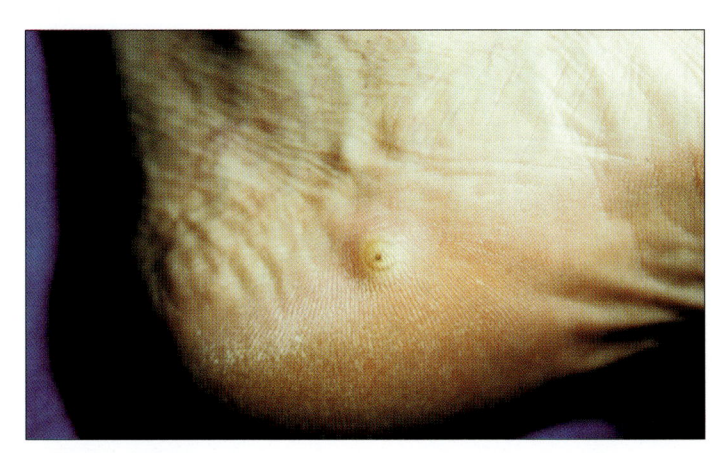

9.28 Tungiasis. Note the white nodule with a central punctum in a typical location on the sole of the foot.

Leishmaniasis

Introduction
Leishmaniasis occurs in South and Central America (the New World), in the Middle East, Asia, Afghanistan, and around the Mediterranean (the Old World). It is caused by a protozoon and transmitted by the bite of an infected sandfly. Depending on the infecting species, it may produce a localized skin lesion or a systemic illness, kala-azar.

Clinical presentation
Patients present with a chronic ulcer, usually on an exposed site, with an infiltrated raised edge and a necrotic base (**9.29, 9.30**).

Histopathology
It is a granulomatous inflammation. In early lesions, intracellular amastigotes may be visible (**9.31**).

Differential diagnosis
Any chronic tropical ulcer may mimic leishmaniasis.

Management
A skin biopsy from the edge of the lesion should be sent for histology and culture. PCR is also useful.

Prognosis
Old World cutaneous leishmaniasis usually heals spontaneously within 1 year. If treatment is needed, simple options such as cryotherapy, itraconazole, or intralesional sodium stibogluconate are best. Those contracted in the New World run a more prolonged course lasting many years and occasionally develop into the mucocutaneous form 'espundia' with destruction of the nasopharynx. These cases require systemic sodium stibogluconate.

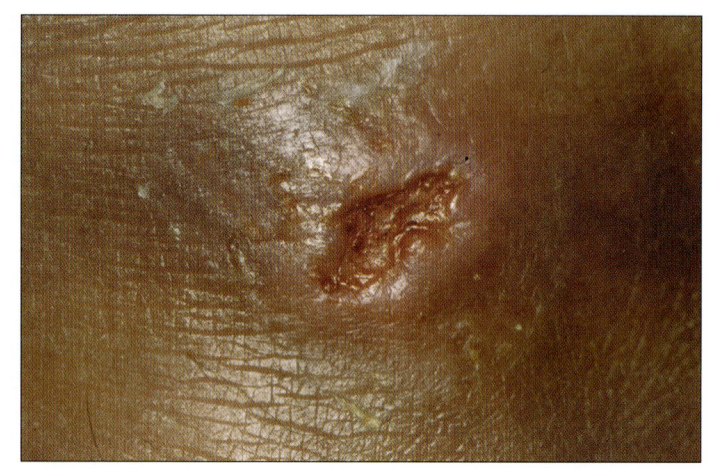

9.29 Leishmaniasis from the Middle East. Note the infiltrated margin and dry base.

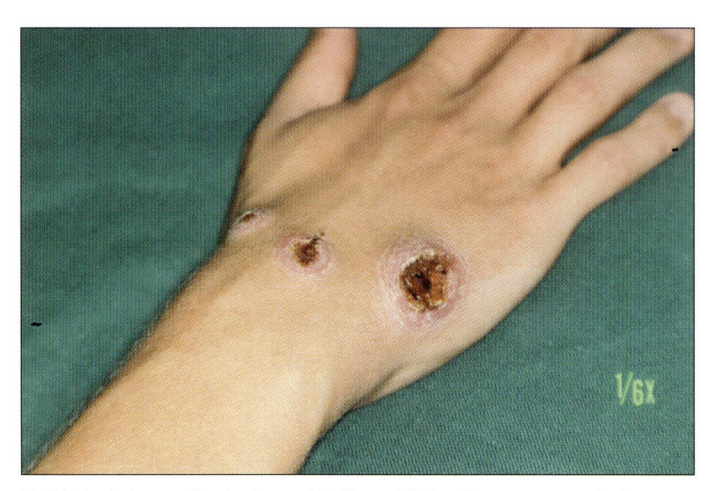

9.30 Leishmaniasis from Belize. Note the exposed site, the multiple lesions, and the raised edge.

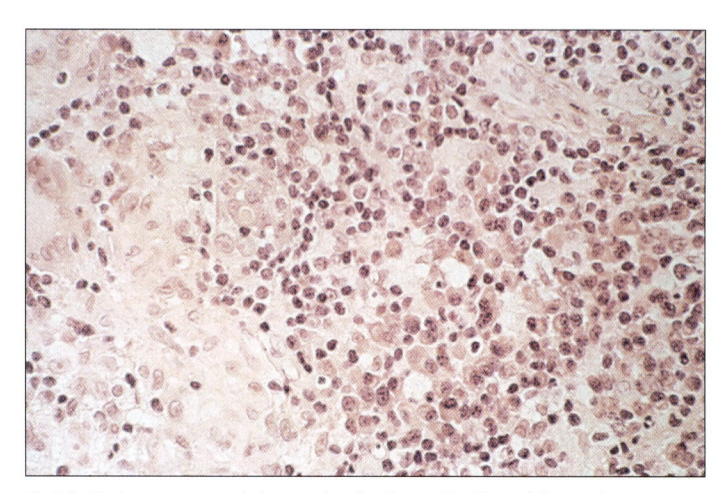

9.31 Cutaneous leishmaniasis from Belize. Note the granuloma formation with giant cells and plasma cells.

Cutaneous myiasis

Introduction
Myiasis is the development of fly larvae in living tissue. It is seen in Africa (tumbu fly) and South and Central America (botfly). The fly captures a flying blood-sucking insect, such as a mosquito, and lays its eggs on the abdomen. The eggs fall off the carrier insect during feeding, and the larvae crawl through the hole into the skin where they develop.

Clinical presentation
A furuncle with a large punctum oozing blood stained fluid (**9.32**) occurs. The spiracle may be seen protruding from the hole from time to time. The patient is aware of the larva wriggling around to enlarge the hole.

Management
The punctum should be covered with petroleum jelly and the larva expressed manually once its spiracle appears (**9.33**). Alternatively, the larva can be excised under local anaesthetic (**9.34**).

Prognosis
If left alone the larva would pupate and extrude itself through the punctum, fall to the ground, then develop into a fly.

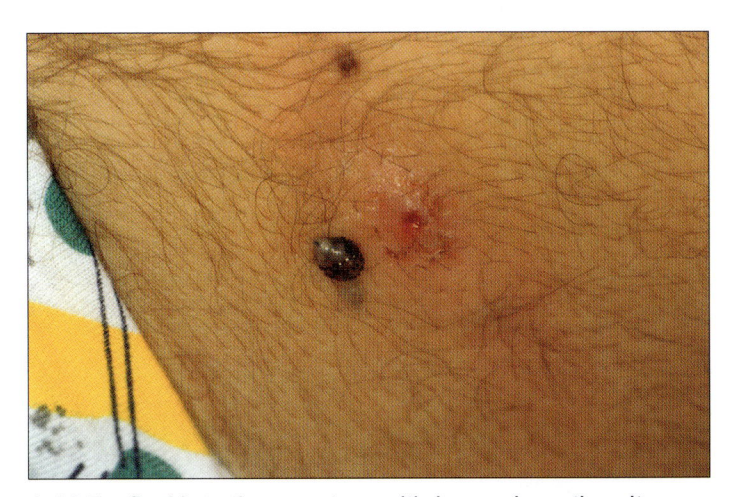

9.32 Botfly. Note the punctum with larva along the site.

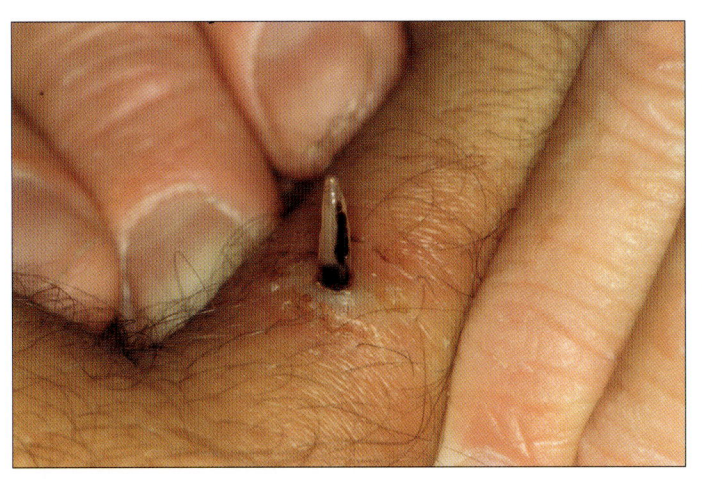

9.33 Botfly larva being expressed manually.

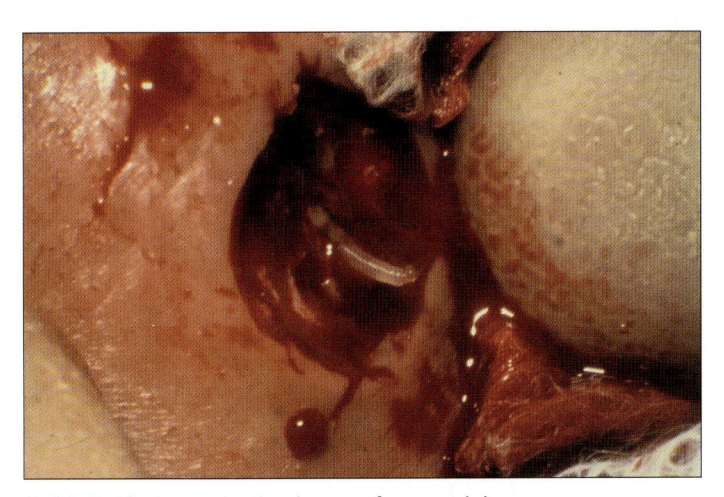

9.34 Botfly larva in the base of an excision.

Further reading

Tyring SK, Lupi O, Hengge UE (2006). *Tropical Dermatology*. Elsevier Churchill Livingstone, Philadelphia.

Habif TP (2004). *Cinical Dermatology*, 4th edn. Mosby, Philadelphia.

Savin JA, Hunter JAA, Hepburn NC (1997). *Skin Signs in Clinical Medicine*. Mosby-Wolfe, London.

Chapter 10

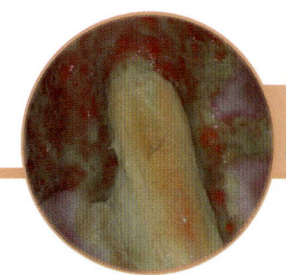

Leg ulcers and wound healing

Anna Rich, RN (Dip BSc Hons) and John SC English, FRCP

Introduction

Leg ulceration is a common and often debilitating problem. A leg ulcer can be defined as a loss of skin below the knee on the leg or foot, which takes more than 6 weeks to heal[1]. They affect 1–2% of the population and are more prevalent in females[2]. Venous leg ulceration is the most common aetiology (70–90%), followed by arterial (5–20%), and mixed venous and arterial ulceration (10–15%)[3]. These ulcers can also be affected by other underlying (e.g. diabetes) and unusual aetiologies (e.g. pyoderma gangrenosum), which may occur simultaneously and may also occur in isolation; they account for 5–10% of ulcers. The key to successful management of leg ulceration relies upon thorough assessment, establishment of a diagnosis, and treating the underlying pathology[4].

This section on leg ulceration discusses the important factors involved in assessment and investigations to be considered. Aetiology of the more common types of leg ulceration will be presented as well as consideration for differing diagnosis. The main principles of leg ulcer and wound management and common therapies will also be discussed.

Clinical presentation

Venous disease

Venous leg ulceration arising from venous disease usually occurs as a result of incompetent valves in the deep and perforating veins. Incompetence of these valves results in a backflow of blood from the deep to the superficial veins, leading to chronic venous hypertension. Predisposing factors such as a previous medical history of deep vein thrombosis (DVT), lower limb fractures, varicose veins, phlebitis, pulmonary embolism, previous venous ulceration or a family history of leg ulceration or thrombosis, as well as standing occupations, limb trauma, or multiple pregnancies may be suggestive of venous disease. Obesity is an increasing cause of venous incompetence.

- Ulcer site: ulcer is most likely to occur around the medial or lateral aspect of the gaiter area of the lower limb (**10.1**, **10.2**).
- Ulcer appearance: venous leg ulcers tend to be shallow in appearance (**10.3**).
- Pain: patients may complain of localized pain or a generalized aching/heaviness in their legs.
- Limb appearance/skin changes:
– Haemosiderin staining: brown/red pigmentation of the skin of the lower limb occurs as a result of the release of haemosiderin (a breakdown product of haemoglobin). It is released owing to distension of vessel walls and leakage of red blood cells into interstitial space (**10.4**).
– Varicose eczema: eczema of the lower limb associated with venous hypertension; can be aggravated by allergic contact dermatitis from the medicaments used (**10.5**).
– Ankle flare: chronic venous hypertension can result in the distension of tiny veins on the medial aspect of the foot/ankle (**10.6**).
– Atrophy blanche: areas of white skin, stippled with red dots of dilated capillary loops (**10.7**).
– Varicose veins: distended veins, a sign of chronic venous hypertension usually due to damaged valves in the leg veins, which become dilated, lengthened, and tortuous (**10.8**).
– Dermatoliposclerosis: 'woody' induration of tissues and fat, replaced by fibrosis (**10.9**).
– Oedema: oedema tends to be generalized and worsens as legs are dependent as the day goes on; reduction in oedema is reported upon elevation of the limb(s) or after spending the night in bed (**10.10**).

130 Leg ulcers and wound healing

10.1 Venous ulceration.

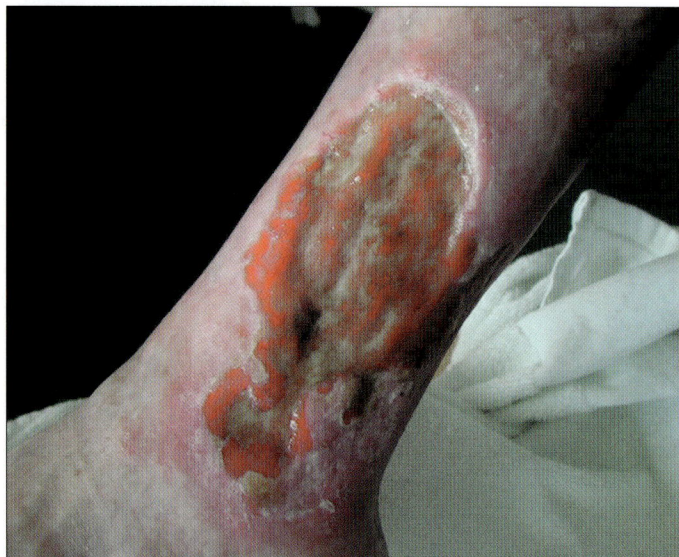

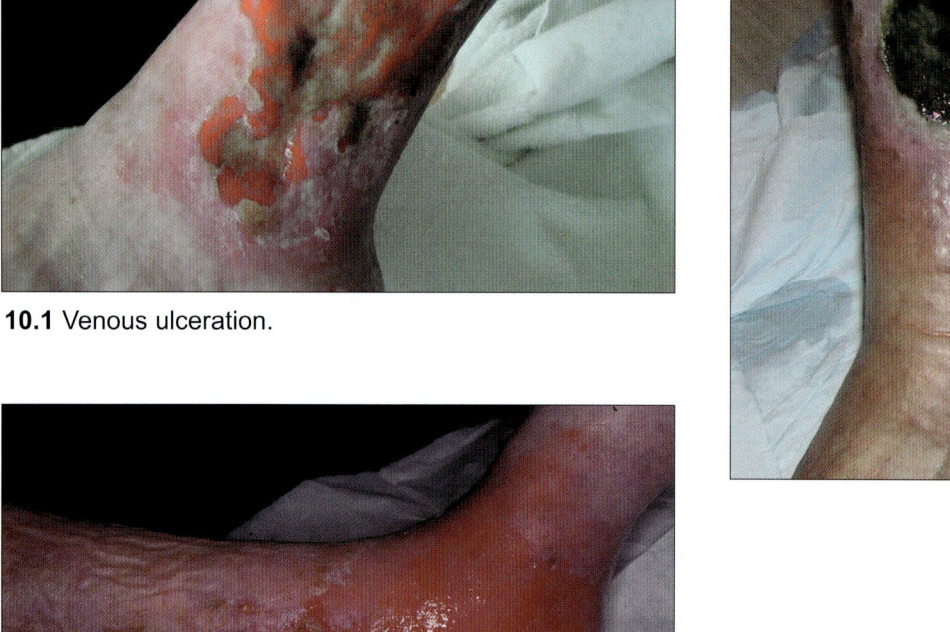

10.2 Venous ulceration with pseudomonas overgrowth. Note the surrounding dermatoliposclerosis.

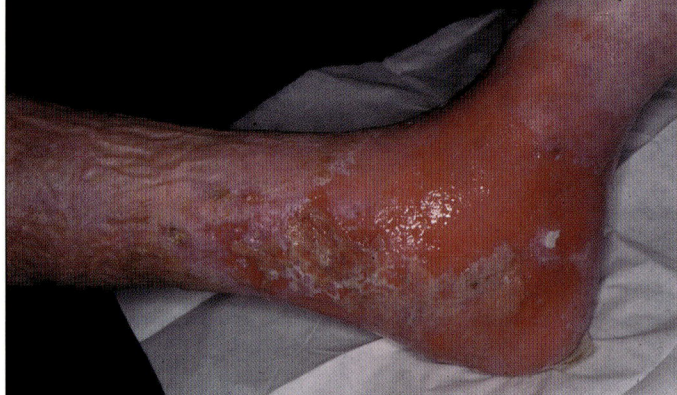

10.3 Venous ulceration and severe maceration from ulcer exudate. A potent topical steroid in addition to the compression will help healing in this situation.

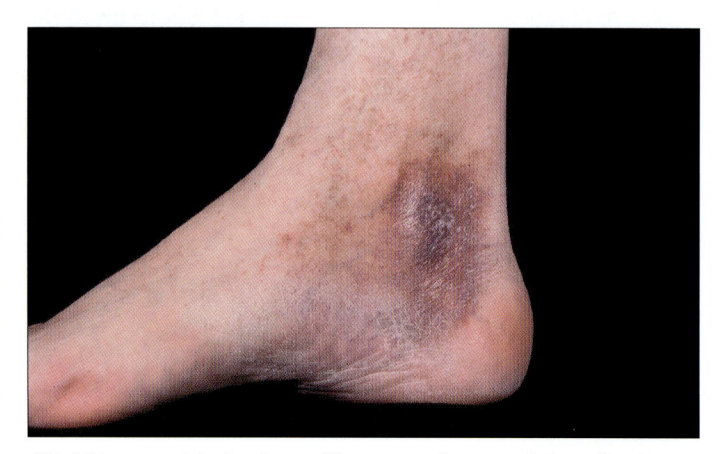

10.4 Haemosiderin deposition over the medial malleolus.

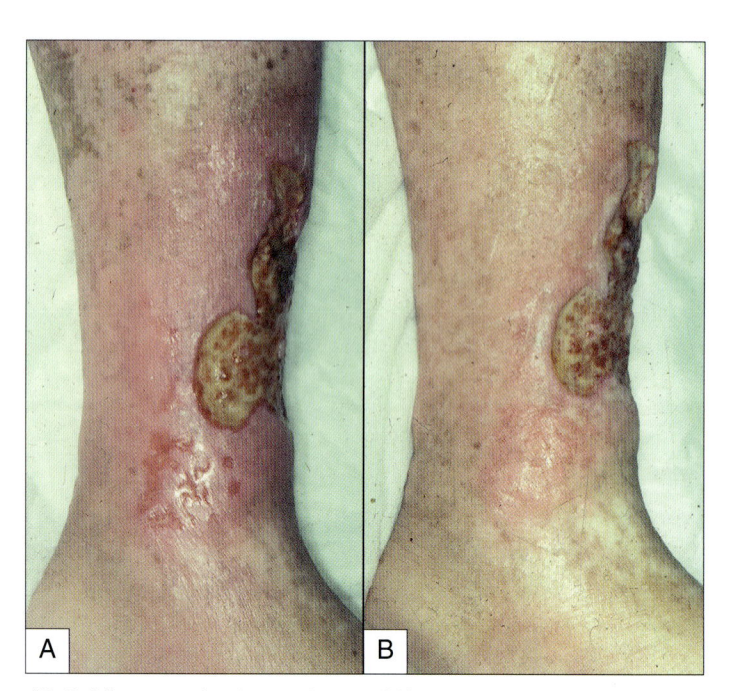

10.5 Allergy to hydrocortisone (**A**) and 2 weeks after stopping the preparation (**B**).

Leg ulcers and wound healing 131

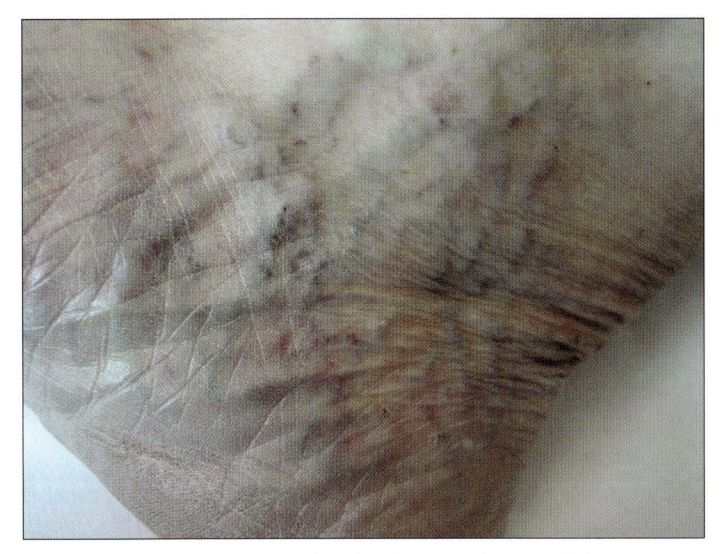

10.6 Distension of superficial veins on the medial aspect of the foot.

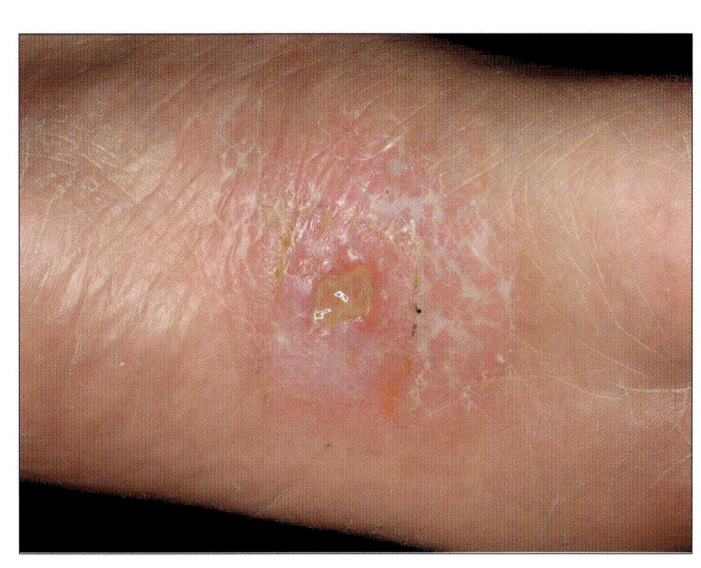

10.7 Atrophy blanche scarring surrounding an ulcer on the sole of the foot.

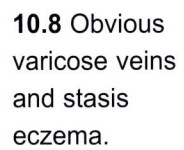

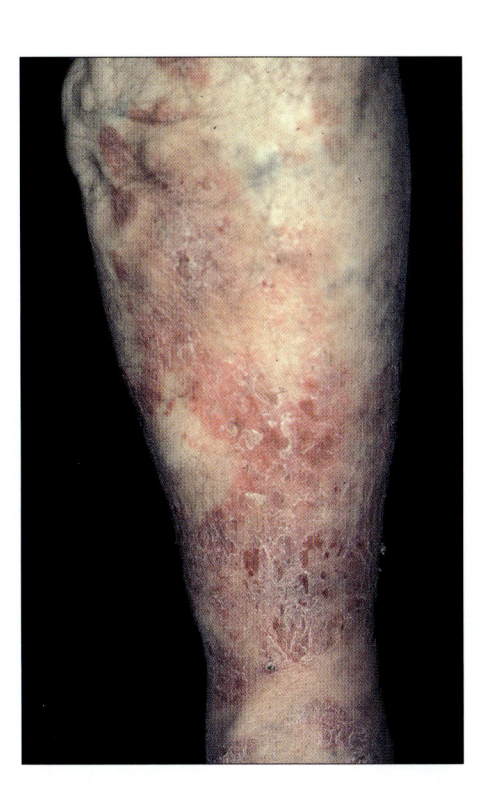

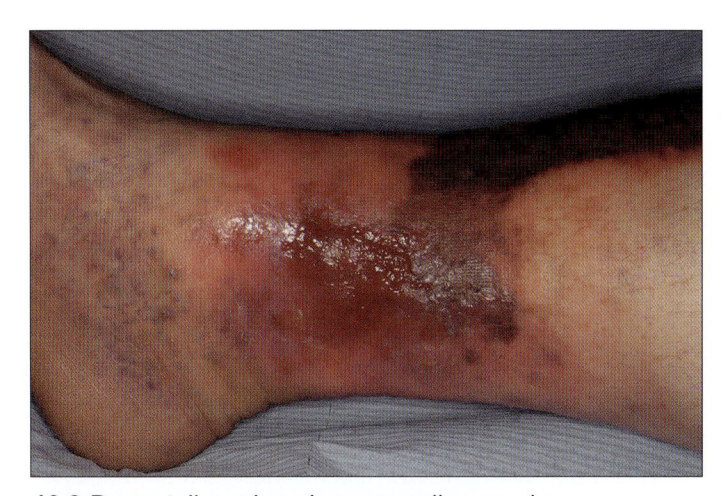

10.8 Obvious varicose veins and stasis eczema.

10.9 Dermatoliposclerosis surrounding an ulcer.

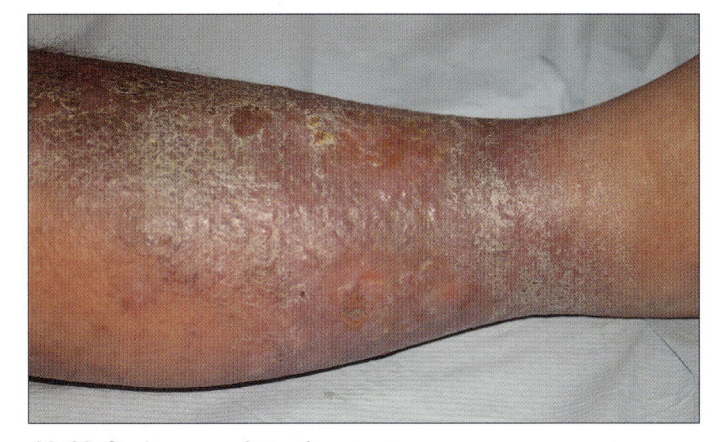

10.10 Oedema and stasis eczema.

132 Leg ulcers and wound healing

Arterial disease
Poor arterial supply as a result of narrowing or occlusion of the vessels may lead to tissue ischaemia and necrosis. Predisposing factors such as a previous medical history of myocardial infarction, transient ischaemic attacks, cerebral vascular attack, hypertension, diabetes, rheumatoid arthritis, peripheral neuropathy or diabetes, or a history of being a smoker may be suggestive of arterial disease.
- Ulcer site: ulcers may be sited anywhere around the lower limb or foot.
- Ulcer appearance: arterial ulcers tend to be deeper and more punched out in appearance (**10.11, 10.12**).
- Pain: patients may complain of severe pain, worse at night or on elevation of the limb. They may also complain of intermittent claudication, cramp-like pain in the calf muscles brought on by walking a certain distance and relieved upon rest.
- Limb appearance/skin changes:
  - Poor tissue perfusion and reduced capillary refill; absent or difficult-to-locate pedal pulses.
  - Loss of hair on the lower leg and the skin may appear atrophic and shiny, with trophic changes in the nails.
  - Muscle wastage in the calf.
  - The limb/foot may be cool to the touch with colour changes evident, pale when raised and dusky pink when dependent (**10.13**).

Mixed vessel
Patients may present with a mixed vessel disease and may be suffering from both venous and arterial disease (**10.14**).

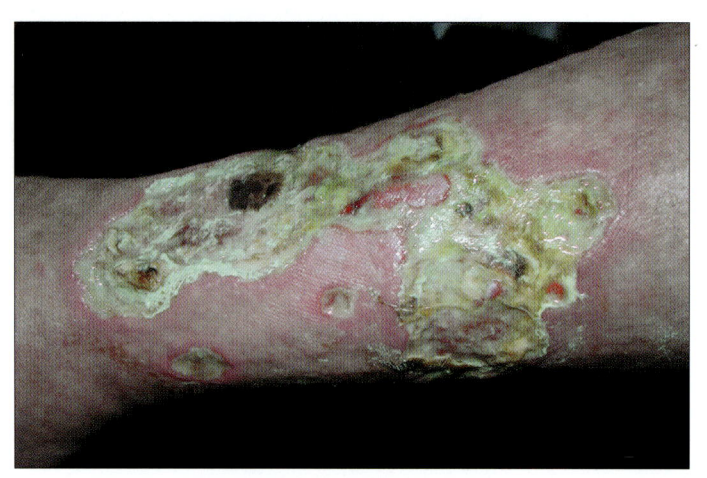

10.11 Arterial ulceration.

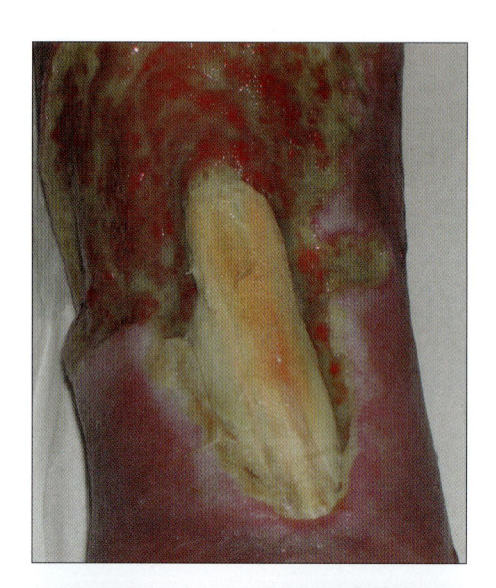

10.12 Arterial ulceration causing the tendon to protrude.

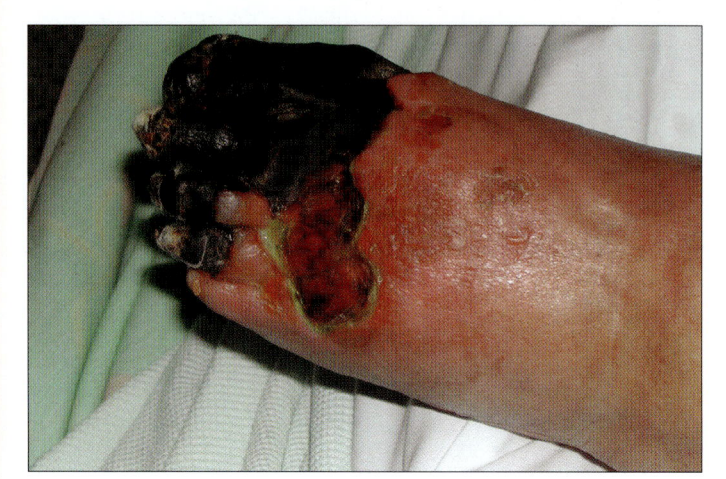

10.13 Gangrene of the toes in severe ischaemia.

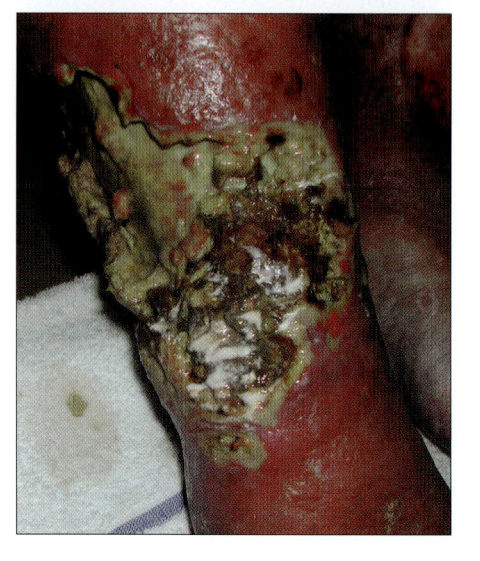

10.14 Severe ulceration in mixed vessel disease. This ulcer responded very well to larva therapy.

Assessment and investigations

The key to successful leg ulcer management relies upon a thorough and accurate assessment. To determine the underlying cause of the ulceration a number of factors should be taken into consideration:

- Cause and history of current ulceration.
- Current treatment and management strategies.
- Any previous history of ulceration.
- Current medication.
- Pain.
- Current and previous medical history.
- Any drug allergies.
- Any known or suspected contact allergies.
- Attention paid to any previous leg problems.
- Site and appearance of the ulcer.
- Levels of wound exudate and any odour.
- Any local problems at the wound site that may complicate or delay healing.
- Appearance of the limb and the skin surrounding the ulcer.
- Social circumstances, paying particular attention to smoking history, diet, mobility, lifestyle, occupation, ability to sleep in bed, and duration of elevation.

Simple investigations such as capillary refill, measurement of the ankle and calf circumferences, wound mapping, and photography of the wound and limb can be performed easily.

Doppler ultrasound

Doppler is a test carried out to establish the blood supply to the lower limb and calculates the ankle brachial pressure index (ABPI). This test should be carried out by a suitably trained and experienced professional and the results should not be considered in isolation but as part of a holistic assessment. This test involves recording a systolic pressure with a hand-held Doppler machine at the foot, usually taken at the dorsalis pedis and posterior tibial pulse, but it may also be recorded at the peroneal and the anterior tibial pulses, and also at the brachial artery. The foot pulse rate is then divided by the brachial pulse rate to obtain a ratio, the ABPI. In a limb with a normal blood supply, an ABPI of around 1.0 can be expected; an ABPI of 0.8–1.0 suggests some arterial involvement, an ABPI <0.79 is likely to indicate significant arterial disease, while an ABPI <0.5 signifies severe arterial disease. Caution should be taken if an ABPI of 1.3 or above is obtained, as it may be a falsely high reading and indicative of arterial calcification.

Foot pulses

The presence of palpable pulses can be checked; however, their presence does not exclude significant arterial disease.

Duplex scan

Colour flow duplex ultrasonography can be used to obtain more detailed anatomical and functional parameters, both on venous and arterial disease.

Differential diagnosis

There are a number of differentials for arterial/venous causes of ulcer. Varicose eczema (gravitational/stasis eczema/dermatitis) is an eczematous eruption as a consequence of venous hypertension. It characteristically originates around the gaiter area of the lower leg; ulceration is not necessary for its development. Its symptoms may include pain, erythema, weeping, maceration, burning, itching, dryness, and scaling (10.8, 10.15). Treatment involves the management of the venous hypertension combined with the application of emollients and topical steroids.

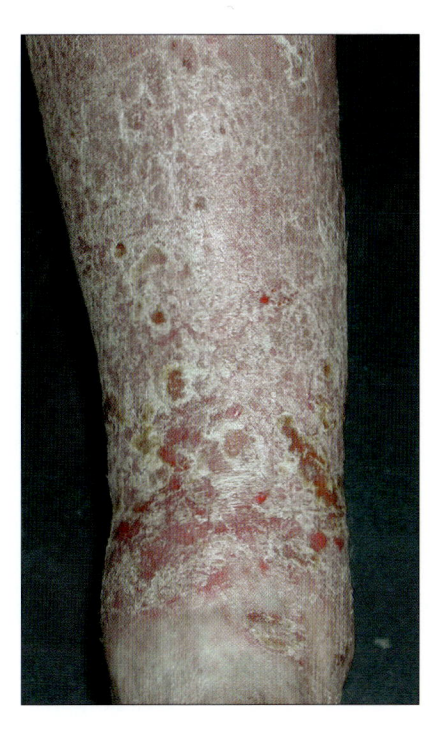

10.15 Severe varicose eczema is often misdiagnosed as cellulitis and does not respond to systemic antibiotics.

134 Leg ulcers and wound healing

Table 10.1 Allergen patch testing in leg ulcer patients

Allergen	% positive	Source
Lanolin	18	In emollients
Fragrances	18	Soaps, body lotions
Neomycin	15	Topical antibiotic
Thiuram	14	Rubber accelerator found in bandages
Colophony	11	Adhesive in hydrocolloid dressings
Formaldehyde	7	Foam baths, some moisturizers
Hydrocortisone	3	Topical steroid

Contact allergy/irritation to components found in topical skin and wound preparations is a common phenomenon in patients with leg ulceration (10.5). Statistics vary, but between 20% and 50% of patients with chronic leg ulceration suffer from contact allergy. The commonest culprits depend upon which products the local healthcare community apply to their patients. In the Nottingham area, thiuram, lanolin, and hydrocortisone are the commonest allergens found on patch testing (*Table 10.1*).

Chronic oedema/lymphoedema is tissue swelling due to failure of lymph drainage, further complicated by limb dependency. Patients may present with primary lymphoedema as a consequence of genetic abnormalities or absent lymphatics. Secondary lymphoedema may occur as a result of cancer or its subsequent treatment, trauma or injury to the lymphatic system, or secondary to venous disease or prolonged dependency of a limb (10.16, 10.17). Management relies upon elevation of the limb, external support, and manual lymph drainage.

Laceration, burns, radiation injuries, and other such trauma can result in ulcers (10.18, 10.19). Where the patient has underlying venous/arterial problems, minor trauma can lead to intractable ulcer.

Iatrogenic causes such as over-tight bandage and ill-fitting plaster cast can cause ulcers. This is a problem particularly when arterial disease has failed to be recognized.

Self-inflicted ulcers can be secondary to IV drug use or caused for psychological reasons in dermatitis artefacta.

Asteatotic eczema occurs in older people with a dry, 'crazy-paving' pattern, particularly on the legs. It is exacerbated by cold weather, central heating, and over washing, and is treated with emollients (10.20).

Pyoderma gangrenosum (10.21–10.23) causes painful ulceration on any area of the skin, the commonest sites being the legs then trunk. When on the lower aspect of the leg, it can be distinguished from venous ulceration by the

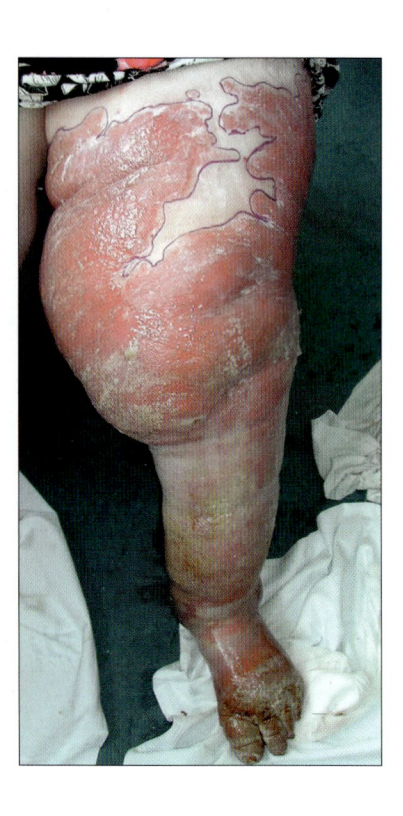

10.16 Weeping stasis eczema and cellulitis.

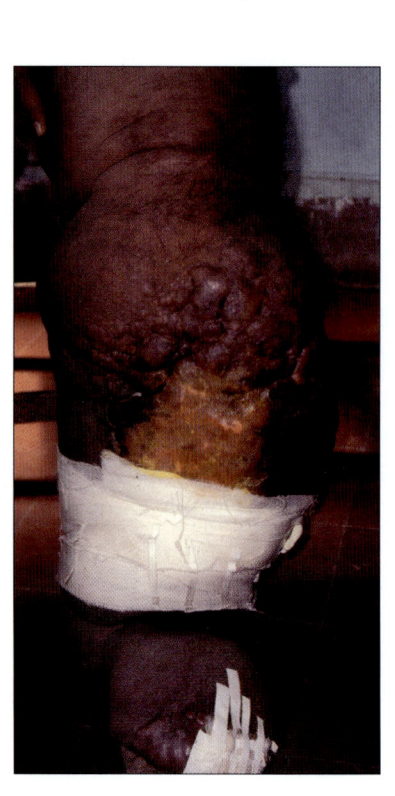

10.17 Chronic lymphoedema due to elephantiasis (worm infestation of the lymphatics).

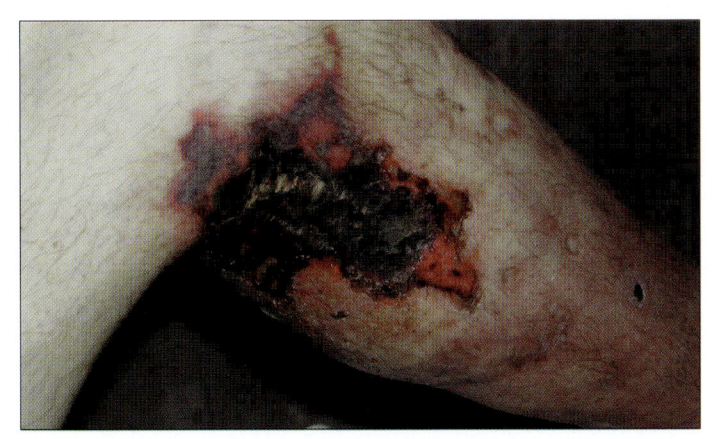

Leg ulcers and wound healing

10.18 Venous ulceration in an IV drug user. The deep and superficial veins are often thrombosed in this group of patients.

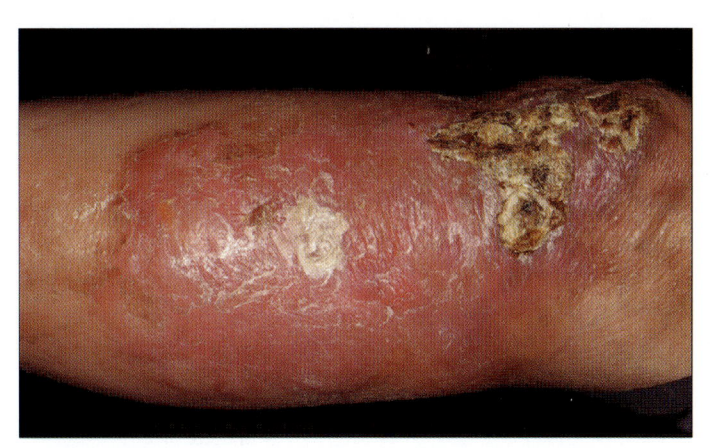

10.19 Chronic thermal burns from sitting too close to the fire. Signs of erythema ab igne are visible around the erythema.

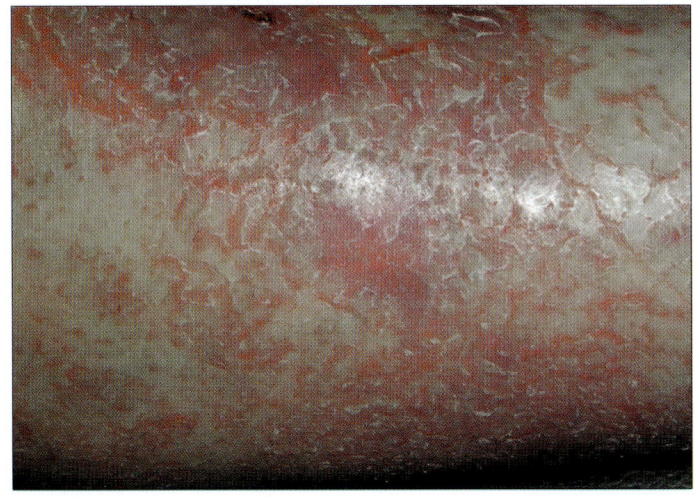

10.20 Asteatotic eczema.

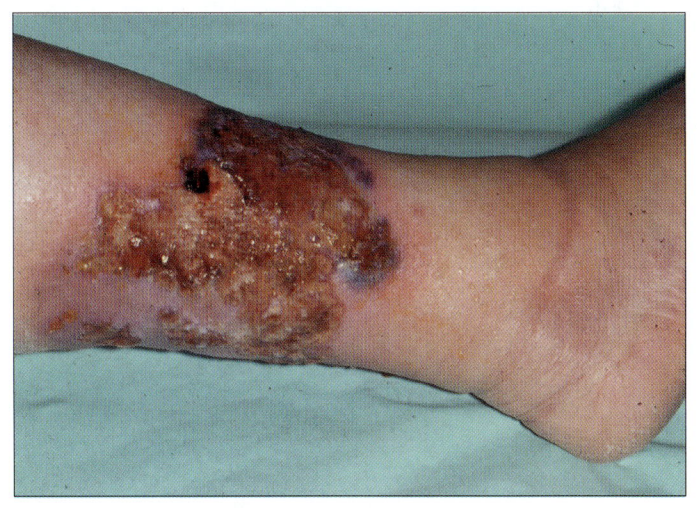

10.21 Pyoderma gangrenosum on the leg.

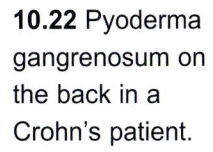

10.22 Pyoderma gangrenosum on the back in a Crohn's patient.

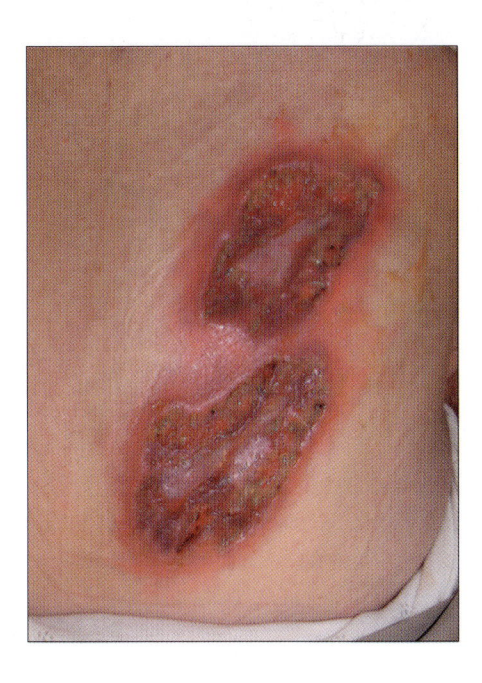

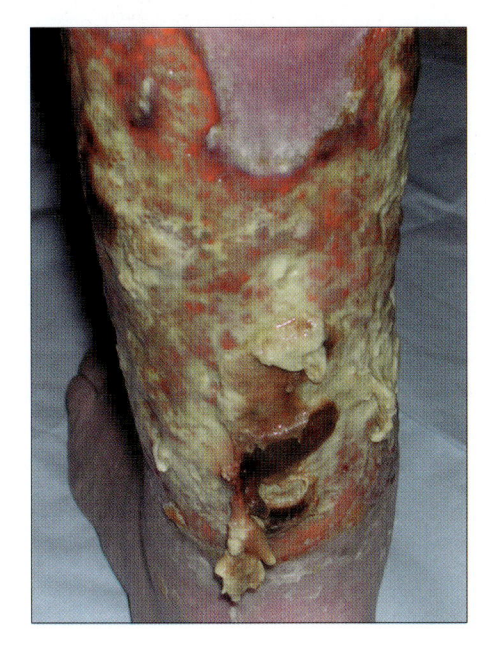

10.23 Low-grade pyoderma gangrenosum, which took 3 years to diagnose.

clinical appearance of a dusky, cyanotic edge to the ulcer, rapid onset, and severe pain. However, sometimes it is a difficult diagnosis to make and low-grade pyoderma gangrenosum is easily missed.

Vasculitis (inflammation of cutaneous blood vessels) will lead to leakage of blood (purpura) and skin necrosis if severe enough (10.24, 10.25). Blood disorders such as polycythaemia, sickle cell, and thalassaemia can cause ulceration. Infections including tuberculosis, leprosy, syphilis, and fungal infections should be considered. However, these are rare causes in the UK, but may be seen in people living in or returning from the tropics (see Chapter 9).

Various malignancies including squamous cell carcinoma (SCC), basal cell carcinoma, malignant melanoma, and Kaposi's sarcoma can cause ulceration. Malignancy is an uncommon cause of ulceration, but the possibility of malignancy should not be overlooked in ulcers failing to respond to treatment. An SCC can develop in a chronic venous leg ulcer (Marjolin's ulcer); it is rare but should be considered if the ulcer has an unusual appearance, particularly overgrowth of tissue at the base or wound margin (10.26–10.28).

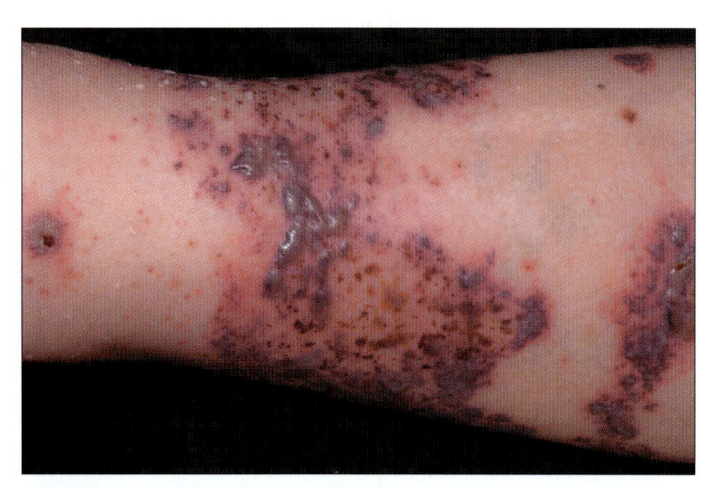

10.24 Haemorrhagic vasculitis.

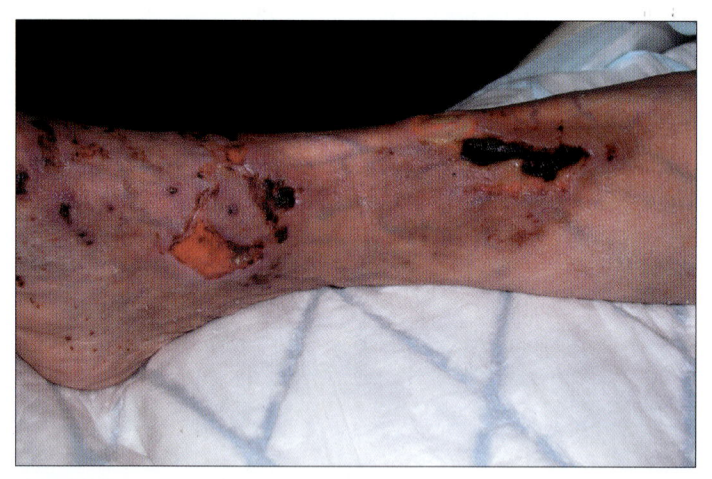

10.25 Vasculitis that has ulcerated.

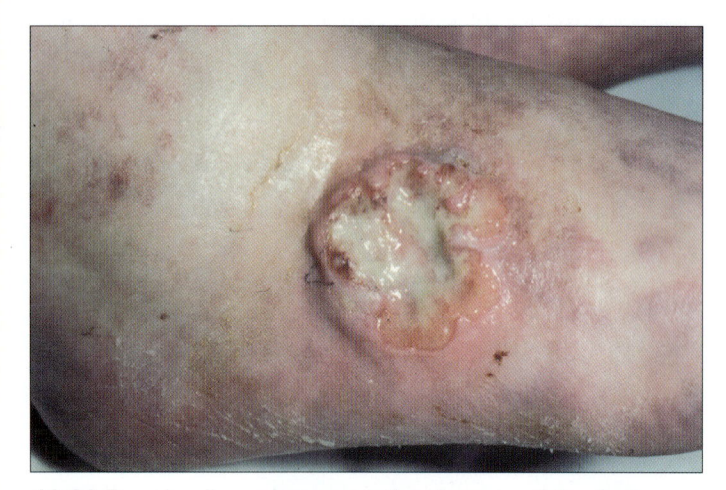

10.26 Basal cell carcinoma on the dorsum of the foot (which looks like SCC).

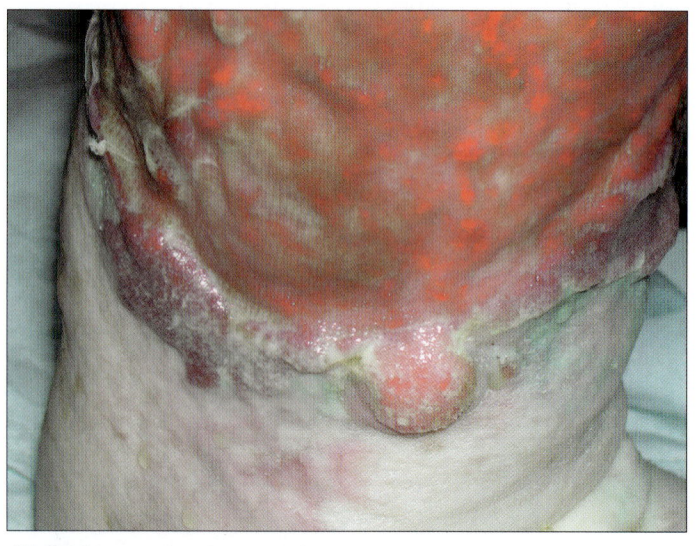

10.27 Hyperplastic granulation tissue mimicking squamous cell carcinomatous change. A biopsy is essential in ruling out malignant change.

Leg ulcers and wound healing 137

In diabetics, ulceration may be due to neuropathy or impaired blood supply. Neuropathic ulcers occur as a result of pressure exerted on the feet that they are unaware of because of loss of sensation due to diabetes. Ischaemic ulcers occur due to damage to arterial circulation as a result of the disease process (10.29). Diabetes also delays wound healing. People with rheumatoid arthritis are thought to develop ulcers due to a combination of local vasculitis, poor venous return due to ankle immobility, and the debilitating effect of prolonged steroid therapy.

Decubitus ulceration occurs at the site of pressure usually associated with immobility (10.30–10.32). An unconscious patient will develop pressure sores within hours on the sacrum or heel if not frequently turned. Prevention is the best treatment. Otherwise, dressings that enhance wound healing and pressure care are the best management.

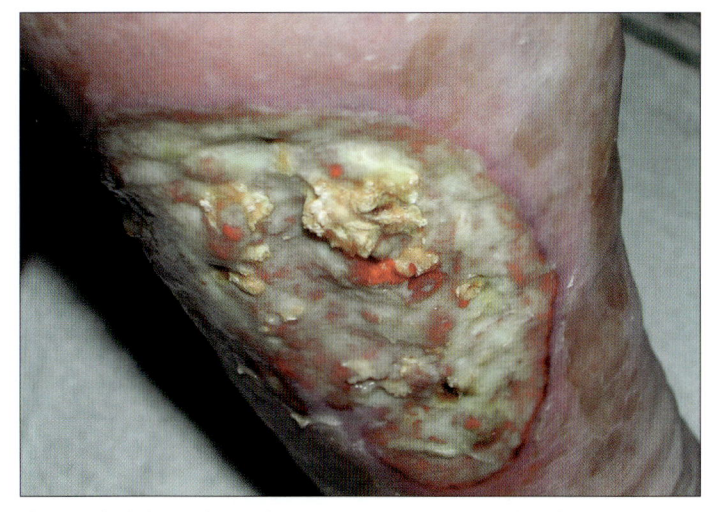

10.28 Calcium deposits can occur in chronic ulcers.

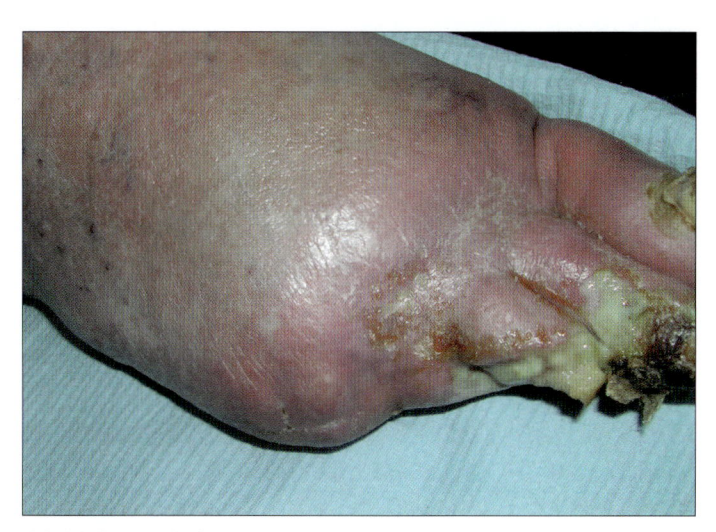

10.29 Diabetic foot.

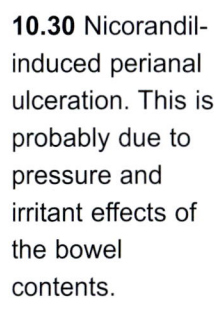

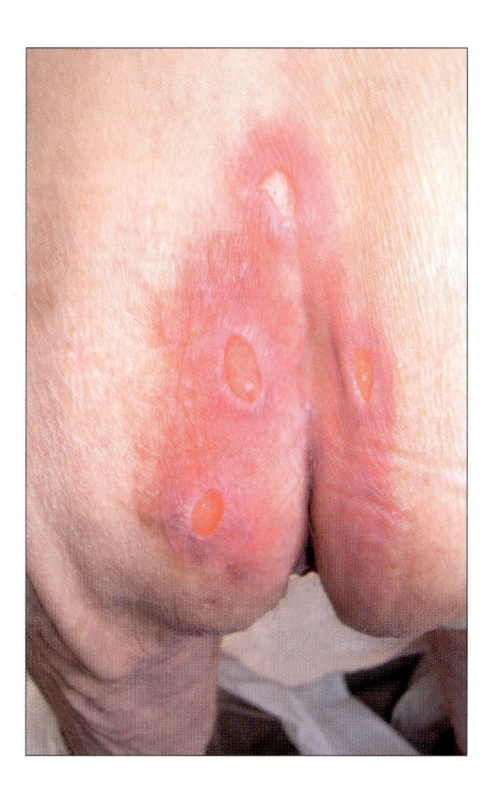

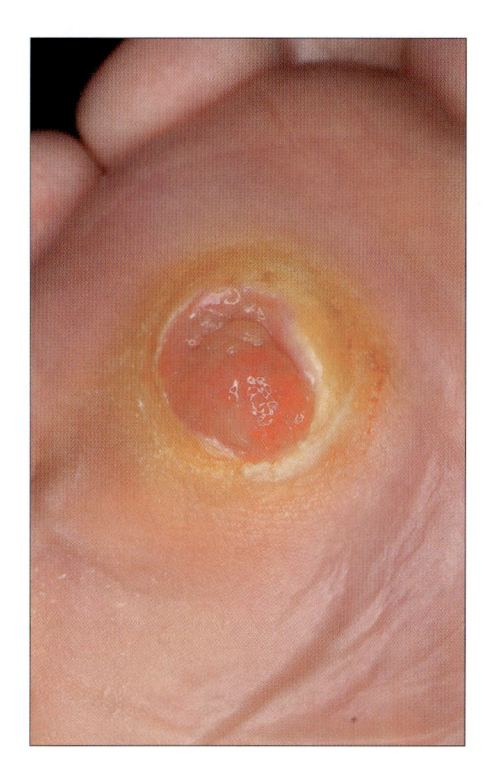

10.30 Nicorandil-induced perianal ulceration. This is probably due to pressure and irritant effects of the bowel contents.

10.31 A pressure sore in a patient with a foot deformity.

138   Leg ulcers and wound healing

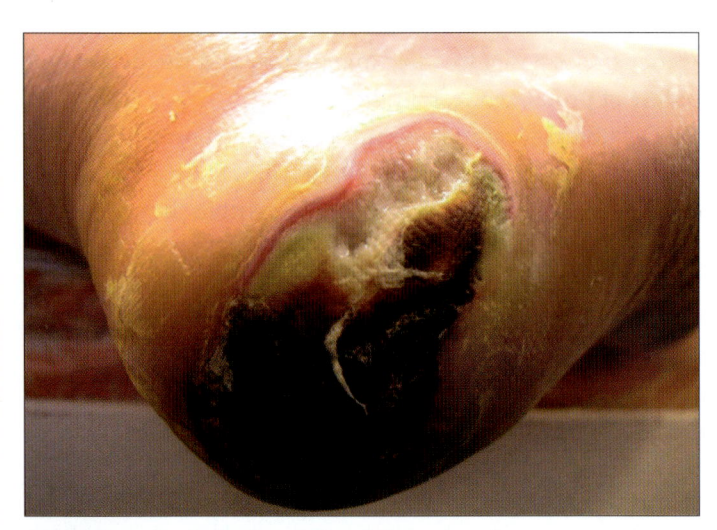

10.32 A typical site for a decubitus ulcer in an immobile patient.

Management

The priority in the treatment of leg ulceration is management of the underlying cause, i.e. improving the venous or arterial circulation, and to create an optimum wound healing environment[4]. It is also essential to address any wider issues that may affect wound healing and work towards preventing complications.

The aim when managing venous disease is to reverse venous hypertension and aid venous return. This can be achieved through the application of graduated external compression (see below) and through elevation and simple exercise of the limb. Management of arterial disease relies upon any feasible surgical intervention and the management of any wound and symptom relief such as pain and exudate control.

Wound healing depends upon the provision of the optimum temperature, moisture, and pH for cells involved in the healing process. It is also essential that any foreign bodies are removed, as is any devitalized tissue, thick slough, or pus. The wound should be protected from any avoidable trauma and the entry of any potentially pathogenic microorganisms, and any clinical infection should be managed. It is important to consider other factors that may delay wound healing such as general health and any illnesses or diseases the patient may have, age, nutrition, certain drug therapies, social environment, infection, the history of the wound occurrence, as well as the identification and management of the underlying cause and the appropriateness of care provision.

Graduated compression therapy can be applied in the form of varying bandaging systems or compression hosiery. Graduated external compression helps to reverse venous hypertension and reduce oedema by forcing fluid from the interstitial space back into the vascular and lymphatic compartments, and by improving venous function. The bandages or hosiery aim to provide graduation of the compression by applying the highest compression (35–40 mmHg) at the ankle and reducing to approximately 17 mmHg just below the knee. By applying the bandages at the same tension all the way up the limb the natural shape of most legs facilitates graduated compression, as the circumference of the limb increases as it gets towards the knee.

There is a vast amount and variety of wound dressings available; however, appropriate dressing selection relies upon the skilled practitioner, with an appropriate dressing leading to the provision of the optimum wound healing environment.

Paste bandages may be applied on their own or can be applied underneath graduated compression bandages and are particularly useful for acute flares of eczema, excoriation, and inflammation. They are also used for softening lichenified skin and act as an occlusive barrier to protect the skin and to help prevent scratching. Zinc paste bandages are often the first paste bandage of choice but may be impregnated with calamine, coal tar, or calamine and clioquinol or ichthammol. Choice will depend upon the desired effect.

The skin on limbs occluded underneath bandages can become dehydrated. Emollients provide a surface lipid film, which prevents water loss from the epidermis, and are most effective when applied after washing when the water content of the skin is at its greatest. Emollients used in the management of leg ulceration should be kept simple and bland to minimize the risk of contact sensitivity.

Topical steroid therapy is the first-line treatment for the management of eczema, and the lower leg is no exception. However, it is important to consider the fact that the potency of the steroid will be increased if applied underneath an occlusive bandage or dressing. It is important also to consider whether the frequency of dressing change may need to be increased to deal with an acute flare of eczema on the lower leg.

Elevation of the limb when at rest is advantageous, provided there is adequate arterial supply to the limb. For patients with venous disease sitting with the legs elevated above the level of the hips helps to reduce oedema by aiding venous return.

Gentle exercise is important for all patients as it aids venous return by activating the calf muscle pump, as well as helping to prevent other complications associated with prolonged immobility.

References

1. Dale J, Callam M, Ruckley C, Harper D, Berrey PN (1983). Chronic ulcers of the leg: a study of prevalence in a Scottish community. *Health Bulletin* **41**:310–314.
2. Gawkrodger D (1997). *Dermatology: An Illustrated Colour Text* (2nd edn). Churchill Livingstone, London.
3. Cullum N (1994). Leg ulcers: a review of research in nursing management in the community. *Bandolier* www.jr2.ox.ac.uk/bandolier/band10/b10-2.html.
4. Falanga V, Phillips TJ, Harding KG, Moy RL, Peerson LJ (eds) (2000). *Text Atlas of Wound Management*. Martin Dunitz, London.

Index

Note: page numbers in *italic* refer to tables in the text

ABCDE criteria 9–10
acne 6, 79–80
  infantile 26, 27
acne excoriée 79, 80
acne keloidalis nuchae 103
acropustulosis of Hallopeau 107
actinic keratosis 48
actinic porokeratosis, disseminated superficial (DSAP) 50
adenoma sebaceum 89
alopecia
  diffuse 105
  scarring 87, 102, 103
  traction 105
alopecia areata 99–100, 110
Ancyclostoma braziliense 124
angio-oedema 33, 34
ankle brachial pressure index (ABPI) 133
anthrax 118, 119
aplasia cutis 18, 19
apocrine glands 3, 4
arsenical keratoses 52
atrophoderma vermiculatum 90
atrophy blanche 129, 131
autoimmune bullous disease 95

bacterial infections 113–19
basal cell carcinoma (BCC) 52–4, 136
biopsies 10
birthmarks 14–19
Bowen's disease (intraepithelial carcinoma) 49
bulla 5
bullous disease
  chronic of childhood 30, 31
  impetigo 44, 45
  pemphigoid 44, 45, 75, 95
burns, thermal 135
'butterfly' rash 87, 88

café au lait macule 16, 17
Candida infection 24
cayenne pepper spots 94, 95
cellulitis 114–15
  dissecting of the scalp 102
cervical intraepithelial neoplasia (CIN) 96
Clark's (dysplastic) naevus 56–8

comedone, senile 60, 62
compression therapy 138
contact dermatitis
  allergic (ACD) 2, 8, 67–8, 70, *70*, 98
  facial 82, 83
  genital area 97
  irritant (ICD) 66, 70, *70*
  wound preparations 134
cowpox 118, 119
Coyrnebacterium spp. 115, 116
crust 7, 8
cutaneous horn 50

Darier's sign 20
DCM mnemonic 8–9
decubitus ulceration 137–8
dermatitis, perioral 80, 81
  see also contact dermatitis; eczema
dermatitis herpetiformis 8, 30, 31
dermatofibroma 47
dermatoliposclerosis 131
dermatomyositis 75, 89
dermatophyte infections 101, 123
  see also tinea
dermis 2
dermographism 33, 36
diabetes mellitus 137
disseminated superficial actinic porokeratosis (DSAP) 50
Doppler ultrasound 133
drug reactions 6, 20, 28, 34, 36, 40, 44
drug use, IV 134, 135
duplex ultrasonography, colour flow 133
dysplasia, genitalia 96

ecchymosis 7
eccrine sweat glands 3, 4
eczema
  asteatotic 134, 135
  atopic 36, 82, 83
  atopic in infancy 24, 25, 26
  discoid 38
  endogenous 69, 70
  genital area 97–8
  hand and foot 65–70, 108
  hyperkeratotic hand (tylotic) 72, *73*
  impetiginized 7, 8

eczema (*continued*)
  nail dystrophy 108
  varicose/stasis 129, 131, 133, 134
eczema herpeticum 120, 121
elephantiasis 134
epidermis 1–2
epidermolysis bullosa 26, 27
epoxy resin allergy 67
erysipelas 114
erythema 7
  toxic 28, 29
erythema ab igne 135
erythema multiforme 44, 45
erythrasma 116, 117
erythroderma 35–6, *41*
erythroplasia of Queyrat 51
'espundia' 126
examination, skin 5–10
excoriated lesions 7

facial rashes
  history and clinical features 77, *78*
  management 78, 79
  see also named conditions
feet
  dermatitis 66–70
  fungal infections 72–3
  plantar pustulosis 74
  scabies 75, 76
  tungiasis 125
  see also nails
fibroma, periungual 111
fish tank granuloma 116, 117
flea bites 34, 35
fly larvae 127
follicular hyperkeratosis 90, 102
follicular plugging 87
folliculitis decalvans 102
fungal infections 123–4
  hands and feet 72–3
  nails 106, 107
  see also tinea

genetic factors
  basal cell carcinoma 52
  melanoma/dysplastic naevi 56
  squamous cell carcinoma 54
genital disease
  diagnosis 91
  see also named conditions
gonococcal septicaemia 118, 119
Gottron's papules 75, 89

granulation tissue, hyperplastic 136
granuloma
  fish tank/swimming pool 116, 117
  pyogenic 20
granuloma annulare 22, 75

haemangioma
  infantile (strawberry naevus) 14, 15
  thrombose 62
Haemophilus influenzae type B 114
haemosiderin deposition 5, 129, 130
hair follicles 2–4
  hyperkeratosis 90, 102
  plugging 87
hair loss
  diffuse 105
  trichotillomania 100
  see also alopecia
hands
  dermatomyositis 75, 89
  eczema 65–70, 72, *73*, 108
  fungal infections 72–3
  palmar pustulosis 74
  psoriasis 71–2, *73*
  see also nails
'heliotrope' rash 89
Henoch–Schönlein purpura 28, 29
herpes simplex 9, 44, 120, 121
herpes zoster 120, 121
herpetiform lesions 8
history taking 4, 77
hookworm, dog 124, 125
human papilloma virus 51, 96
Hutchinson's sign 61
hyperpigmentation 6, 7
hyperplastic granulation tissue 136
hypopigmentation 7, 30

icthyosis 26, 27
immunosuppressive agents 41–2
impetigo 7, 8, 113–14
  bullous 44, 45
insect bites 34, 35
insect infestations 125, 127
intraepithelial carcinoma (IEC/Bowen's disease) 49
investigations 10–11

Jessner's benign lymphocytic infiltrate 88
juvenile plantar dermatosis 32, 66

kala-azar 126
keloid 6
keratin layer 1, 2
keratoacanthoma 55
keratolysis, pitted 115
keratosis
    arsenical 52
    seborrhoeic 62
keratosis pilaris 30, 31, 90
kerion 101
Koebner's phenomenon 40

Langerhans cell histiocytosis 24, 25
Langerhans cells 2, 99
larva migrans, cutaneous 124, 125
leather allergy 67, 68
leg ulcers
    arterial disease 132
    assessment and investigations 133
    differential diagnosis 133–8
    management 138–9
    mixed vessel disease 132
    venous disease 129–31
leishmaniasis 116, 126
lentigo maligna 58–9
lentigo maligna melanoma 60
lichen aureus 5
lichen planopilaris 103
lichen planus 75, 93–4, 109
lichen sclerosus 91–2
lichen simplex 97
lichen striatus 9
lichenification 36, 37, 82, 83
lupus erythematosus 44, 86–8
    discoid 77, 86–7, 104
    subacute cutaneous (SCLE) 86, 88
lymphangioma circumscriptum 16, 17
lymphoedema, chronic 134
lymphoma, cutaneous (mycosis fungoides) 35, 36

macule 5
Marjolin's ulcer 136
mastocytoma 20
medical history 4
melanocytes 2
melanoma, malignant 9–10
    acral lentiginous 60, 61
    desmoplastic 61
    differential diagnosis 62
    early diagnosis 56
    lentigo maligna 60
    management 62
    nodular 47, 60
    precursor lesions 56–9
    superficial spreading 59
    verrucous 61

melasma 86
Merkel cells 2
Microcossus spp. 115
Microsporum canis 101
milaria 23
molluscum contagiosum 120, 121
Mongolian blue spot 18, 19
Mycobacterium marinum 116, 117
Mycoplasma pneumoniae 44
mycosis fungoides 35, 36
myiasis 127
myxoid cyst 111

naevus
    compound melanocytic 58
    congenital melanocytic 16, 17
    dysplastic 56–8
    epidermal 18, 19
    halo 57, 58
    intradermal 6
    junctional 57
    Meyerson's 58
    papillomatous 57
    sebaceous 18, 19
    spider 22
    strawberry 14, 15
naevus depigmentosum 30
naevus flammeus (salmon patch) 15
naevus sebaceus 104
nail folds, telangiectasia 89
nails
    alopecia areata 99, 110
    eczematous dystrophy 108
    lichen planus 109
    median dystrophy 111
    neoplasia 60, 61, 111
    onychogryphosis 110
    onychomycosis 106, 107
    Pincer 110, 111
    psoriasis *41*, 107–8
    yellow nail syndrome 110
nappy area 14, 23, 24, 26, 27
necrotizing fasciitis 114, 115
neonatal rashes 23–7
neurofibromatosis 16
nickel 8
nodules 5, 6

oedema, lower limb 129, 131, 134
onychogryphosis 110
onychomycosis 106, 107
oral disease
    bullous autoimmune 95
    diagnostic difficulties 91
    lichen planus 93
    malignant lesions 96
orf 122

paediatric dermatoses 13
    rashes 14, 23–32
    skin lesions *13*, 14–22
palmo-plantar pustulosis *41*, 74
papular lesions 5, 6

paste bandages 138
patch 5
patch testing 10, *10*, 11, 67, 98
pemphigoid 75
    bullous 44, 45, 95
    cicatricial 95
pemphigus 95
penile intraepithelial neoplasia 96
petechia 7
phospholipid syndrome 76
pigmentation 2, 7
pilomatricoma 20, 21
Pincer nail 110, 111
pityriasis alba 30, 31
pityriasis amiantacea 101
pityriasis rosea 28, 29
pityriasis versicolor 124
Pityrosporum orbiculare 124
Pityrosporum ovale 84
plantar dermatosis, juvenile 32, 66
plaque 5, 6
pompholyx, recurrent of palms/soles 69
port wine stain 16, 17
pressure sores 137–8
'prickle cell' layer 1–2
Propionibacterium acnes 79
pseudopelade of Brocque 104
psoriasis 6, 8, 39–42
    arthropathy 40, 42
    clinical features/differential diagnoses *41*
    erythrodermic 35, *41*
    facial 84, 85
    hands and feet 71–2, *73*
    in infancy 26, 27
    nail involvement 107–8
    palmo-plantar pustular *41*, 74
    with seborrhoeic dermatitis 84, 85
psychological factors 4, 100
punch biopsy 10
purpura 7
pyoderma gangrenosum 134–6
pyogenic granuloma 20, 62

radiation-induced keratoses 51
rheumatoid arthritis 137
rhinophyma 81
ringworm 101, 123
'rodent ulcer' 52, 53
rosacea 80–1
rubber allergy 67, 68

salmon patch (naevus flammeus) 15
sand flea (jigger) infestation 125
scabies 42–3, 75, 76
scalp disorders 99–105
    aplasia cutis 18, 19
    basal cell carcinoma 53
    psoriasis 39, *41*
sebaceous glands 3, 4
sebaceous naevus 18, 19
sebo-psoriasis 84, 85

seborrhoeic dermatitis 84
    infantile 24
seborrhoeic keratosis 62
'shagreen patch' 89
skin anatomy and physiology 1–4
skin prick tests 10, 11
skin scrapings 10
smoking 96
spider naevus 22
sporotrichosis 116, 117
squamous cell carcinoma 54–5, 92, 96, 136
    in situ (intraepithelial carcinoma) 49
staphylococcal scalded skin syndrome 28, 29
Staphylococcus aureus 38, 43, 102, 114
striae 32
syphilis, secondary 118, 119

target lesions 44, 45
telangiectasia, nail-fold 89
telogen effluvium 105
tinea infections 123
tinea capitis 101
tinea corporis 38
tinea facei 87, 88
tinea manum 73, 123
tinea pedis 106
trachyonychia 109
Treponema pallidum 118
Trichophyton tonsurans 101
trichotillomania 100
tuberculous chancre 116, 117
tuberous sclerosis 89, 111
tungiasis 125
'twenty nail dystrophy' 109

ultraviolet (UV) radiation 41, 48, 49, 52, 54
urticaria 2, 33–5
urticaria pigmentosum 20, 21

varicose veins 129, 131
vasculitis 7, 75, 76, 136
vesicle 5
viral infections 9, 44, 120–2
vitiligo 30, 31
vulval eczema 97
vulval intraepithelial neoplasia 96
vulval ulceration 98
vulvo-vaginal-oral syndrome 94

warts, viral 122
wound preparations 134, 138

xanthogranuloma 20, 21

yellow nail syndrome 110

Zoon's balanitis 94
Zoon's vulvitis 95